AF449119

Tympanoplasty

Tympanoplasty

Osteoplastic Epitympanotomy

Horst L. Wullstein
Sabina R. Wullstein

Translated by P. M. Stell
Foreword by John Conley

290 Illustrations

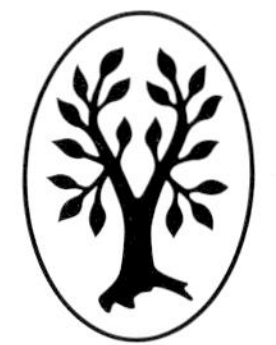

1990

Georg Thieme Verlag Stuttgart · New York
Thieme Medical Publishers, Inc., New York

Horst L. Wullstein †, M.D.
Professor Emeritus
ENT Clinic
Julius Maximilian University
Würzburg
West Germany

Sabina R. Wullstein, M.D.
Professor
ENT Clinic
Julius Maximilian University
Würzburg
West Germany

Wullstein Clinic
Oberer Neubergweg 10 a
8700 Würzburg
West Germany

P.M. Stell, CH.M., F.R.C.S.
Professor
Dept. of Otolaryngology
University of Liverpool
Royal Liverpool Hospital
Prescot St.
P.O. Box 147
Liverpool L69 3BX
England

John Conley, M.D.
Clinical Professor of Otolaryngology, (Emeritus), Columbia University, College of Physicians and Surgeons; Attending Otolaryngologist Columbia Presbyterian Medical Center; Attending Head and Neck Service, St. Vincent's Hospital and Medical Center of New York. N.Y.

Deutsche Bibliothek Cataloguing in Publication Data

Wullstein, Horst L.:
Tympanoplasty : osteoplastic epitympanotomy / Horst L. Wullstein ; Sabina R. Wullstein. Transl. by P.M. Stell. Foreword by John Conley. – Stuttgart ; New York : Thieme ; New York : Thieme Medical Publ., 1990
    Dt. Ausg. u.d.T.: Wullstein, Horst L.: Tympanoplastik
NE: Wullstein, Sabina R.

Important Note: Medicine is an ever-changing science. Research and clinical experience are continually broadening our knowledge, in particular our knowledge of proper treatment and drug therapy. Insofar as this book mentions any dosage or application, readers may rest assured that the authors, editors and publishers have made every effort to ensure that such references are strictly in accordance with the **state of knowledge at the time of production of the book.** Nevertheless, every user is requested to examine carefully the manufacturer's leaflets accompanying each drug to check on his own responsibility whether the dosage schedules recommended therein or the contraindications stated by the manufacturers differ from the statements made in the present book. Such examination is particularly important with drugs that are either rarely used or have been newly released on the market.

This book is an authorized and revised translation from the 1st German edition, published and copyrighted 1986 by Georg Thieme Verlag, Stuttgart, Germany. Title of the German edition: Tympanoplastik. Osteoplastische Epitympanotomie.

Some of the product names, patents and registered designs referred to in this book are in fact registered trademarks or proprietary names even though specific reference to this fact is not always made in the text. Therefore, the appearance of a name without designation as proprietary is not to be construed as a representation by the publisher that it is in the public domain.

This book, including all parts thereof, is legally protected by copyright. Any use, exploitation or commercialization outside the narrow limits set by copyright legislation, without the publisher's consent, is illegal and liable to prosecution. This applies in particular to photostat reproduction, copying, mimeographing or duplication of any kind, translating, preparation of microfilms, and electronic data processing and storage.

© 1990 Georg Thieme Verlag, Rüdigerstrasse 14, D-7000 Stuttgart 30, Germany
Thieme Medical Publishers, Inc., 381 Park Avenue South, New York, N.Y. 10016

Typesetting by R. Hurler, D-7311 Notzingen, typesetted on Linotronic 300
Printed in Germany by K. Grammlich, D-7401 Pliezhausen

ISBN 3-13-745701-7   (GTV, Stuttgart)
ISBN 0-86577-301-7   (TMP, New York)   1 2 3 4 5 6

Dedicated to
GEORGE E. SHAMBAUGH, JR.

Foreword

I write this preface in friendship and respect for the late Professor Horst Wullstein and his wife, Professor Sabina Wullstein, who carries on with his work and tradition.

My introduction to Professor Wullstein came first in the early 1960s through Professor Franz Altman, who had come to the United States from Vienna and who was a distinguished otolaryngologist at the Columbia-Presbyterian Medical Center in New York. Both he and Horst Wullstein were scholars, clinicians, researchers and friends in the vanguard of the remarkable changes that were occurring in the field of otology and otologic surgery. An active interchange of information, ideas and visits developed over the next three decades in all of the developing specialty groups in the field of otolaryngology, but those occuring in otology and head and neck surgery had special emphasis. It was due, in part, to these rich communications that I became familiar with the work and the resources of Professor Horst Wullstein. He instinctively understood the potential, historical development and expansion of otolaryngology into head and neck cancer, facial plastic and reconstructive surgery, and labored with unmatched energy to create the realities of this clairvoyant perception. His perspicacity and success at molding these aspects into the curriculum of otolaryngology helped to establish a new professional era. It took a large volume of his time, his intelligence and his energy. He also initiated a series of annual courses at the "Kopfklinik" of the University of Würzburg, where he was director of the ENT division, dealing with cancer in the head and neck and plastic and reconstructive surgery. With a distinguished faculty, his courses became a hallmark of advanced teaching in these subjects in Europe at the time.

In 1968 he married Sabina, who studied and collaborated with him in every aspect of his work. Her support in his professional and personal life since that time, and particulary during the past twelve years, was both critical and incalculable. This book is a condensation of Professor Wullstein's life's work with the collaboration and support of Sabina Wullstein.

In their book the Wullsteins announced the historical presentation of the microsurgical concept of tympanoplasty in 1950. This concept was enhanced in 1970 by the introduction of osteoplastic epitympanotomy. Their initial work in this field established guidelines for the treatment of chronic infections, cholesteatomas and the rehabilitation of certain types of deafness. These fundamental principles are still applicable today and have also led to new concepts.

The early introduction of a self-made surgical microscope and, later, use of a Leica camera for microphotography (1953), combined with subsequent improvements in optics by Zeiss, made a significant contribution to the research and study possibilities of the concealed and individualistic anatomical portions of the middle ear. The text is richly amplified by microphotographs of silhouettes of the temporal bone, histopathologic preparations of both the middle ear and temporal bone, depicting all conceivable variations in anatomy and pathology. There are slide preparations of specific areas of abnormalities that are highly germane. One of the most attractive features of the book is the art work, which is strongly illustrative and graphic and still retains a high artistic style.

In addition to the detailed presentation of the past and present state of the art on tympanoplasty with all of its biologic, anatomic and surgical ramifications, there is superb information on cholesteatomas, trauma to the temporal bone, facial nerve involvement, hearing problems, eustachian tube function, congenital and autoimmune abnormalities. The authors have established this book, not only as a historical and academic reference text, but one that bears the fruit of years of long and hard work and advanced experience. This makes it a particularly valuable asset to the otolaryngologist, the micro-otolaryngologist, the micro-otologic surgeon and the academician.

John Conley
Emeritus Professor of Otolaryngology
– Head and Neck Surgery
Columbia-Presbyterian Medical Center
New York

Preface

Originally, an English edition of the monograph *Operationen zur Verbesserung des Gehöres: Grundlagen und Methoden* by H.L. Wullstein and his colleagues (Georg Thieme Verlag, 1968) was planned. However, revisions were necessary before this could be undertaken. At that time the intraoperative study of the primary foci of disease and of the histopathology of the soft tissue structures of the middle ear had been so far advanced by the junior author (S.R.W.) that the concept of the etiology of otitis media had been fundamentally changed to take account of the decisive part played by the mucosal folds.

The original publication dealt with all reconstructive procedures, and is still valuable as a reference work and as a guide to the literature today. The revisions resulted, however, instead in the publication of a new German book on tympanoplasty, of which this is the updated translation. Material from the earlier book is repeated in Chapter 3.

Tympanoplasty presents problems of the most varied and unusual kind: in addition to achieving absolute healing of the middle ear infection, a free air-containing space must be created. This type of problem is not faced by any other surgical discipline.

The senior author (H.L.W.) has lived through an era of fundamental change of surgical concepts and technique in the temporal bone. He remembers with gratitude his teachers who taught him the theoretical and clinical basis and gave him responsibility in an area of surgery fraught with lethal complications. He would like to record his debt of gratitude to the pathologist Dr. W. Ceelen, the physiologist Dr. W. Trendelenburg, to Dr. O.F. Ranke for his friendship, to the internists Dr. A. Lichwitz and Dr. F. Parkes Weber. In otorhinolaryngology, he is grateful for his training under the strict discipline and logic of Dr. J. Zange, and also to the precise clinical observations of Dr. Th. Nuehsmann. Finally, he is especially grateful to his own father, Ludwig Wullstein, for his early operative surgical training.

The junior author had the good fortune to study under the anatomists Dr. D. Perovic, Dr. J. Krmpotić-Nemanic, Dr. A. Šercer and, later, Dr. B. Gušić. Dr. G. Kelemen was her teacher in the histopathology of the temporal bone, and guided her in the reordering of the collection of about 500 temporal bone sections in the Würzburg Clinic, built up over many decades since the time of Dr. A. von Tröltsch, especially by Dr. P. Manasse. During the war all the sections had become completely mixed up and their records burned.

The authors intend this monograph to be based on their own conclusions rather than to be a review. They ask the authors of many very important contributions to this subject to understand and forgive them.

The authors are also very grateful to several colleagues who have taken great trouble with the translation of the previous book: for the Japanese working group assembled by Dr. Kamio; for the Spanish edition, to Dr. J. Bartual-Pastor; and for the Russian translation, to Dr. N.A. Preobrashensky. The authors also wish to record their great gratitude to Dr. and Mrs. Buckingham for the English edition which unfortunately did not appear, for reasons explained above.

The senior author has good reason to feel grateful to Georg Thieme Verlag for their support over many decades. He was introduced to the publishers, particularly Dr. h.c. Bruno Hauff, by his teacher Dr. J. Zange, and received a sympathetic reception for his manuscript "Die Labyrinthitis and Paralabyrinthitis im Roentgenbilde", which contained many photogravure prints. At that time, the publishers themselves were in the first phases of postwar recovery. The book was printed immediately after the currency reform of 1948. The subject of the work was the explanation of an all too often lethal otogenic disease, osteitis of the bony labyrinth, and its progressive pathological and clinical course over many months, in contrast to that of membranous labyrinthitis. Its natural history can no longer be learnt because of the prompt use of antibiotic therapy, although many inflammatory otological complications still occur. The author is fully aware that he would not have made the step to one-stage tympanoplasty without a detailed knowledge of osteitis lying in the center of the temporal bone, where it has direct contact with the two cranial fossae and the internal meatus.

At this point we wish to express our great personal thanks to Dr. h.c. Hauff for the confidence that he has displayed in us both, and his encouragement to strive for the highest standards. However, these high standards were also the cause for the long delay: the continuous flow of new ideas demanded clinical confirmation before they were recorded. These new concepts made it possible to expose the pneumatic spaces of the temporal bone in all directions, beginning at the site of origin of the disease, and yet to restore a middle ear normal in depth and shape.

The genesis, clinical appearances and surgery of cholesteatoma form a central theme of otology and otological surgery. Congenital cholesteatomas of the petrous temporal bone tend to invade the middle and posterior cranial fossae. The authors are very grateful to Dr. W.T. Koos, Director of the Neurosurgical Unit at the University Clinic of Vienna, for permission to reproduce three operative pictures (Figs. **278a**, **b**; **279**) from his *Color Atlas of Microneurosurgery.*

We are very grateful to Mr. Storz for his selfless support in providing the endoscopic observations and illustrations.

The authors have learnt through working for many months with Georg Thieme Verlag how difficult it is to prepare a manuscript with many high-quality illustrations. Georg Thieme's staff have been tireless and very kind in their cooperation and explanation of the publishing process. For this we thank Dr. Volkert, Mr. Datz and Mr. Zeller.

The authors are most grateful to their colleagues in the Clinic for their unflinching support during the last ten years. We wish to record our recognition and hearty thanks to Ms. Marion Ittensohn and Ms. Antje Schlagmüller for their masterful revision of the incomplete text and illustrations, which they carried out in addition to their other duties.

Horst L. Wullstein and Sabina R. Wullstein
Würzburg, Spring 1986

The morning of his last calling the final agreement for the English translation of this book arrived. Horst Ludwig Wullstein was no longer able to experience the joy of this news. The task of completing the English edition helped give me the strength needed to heal my loneliness. I found in Georg Thieme Verlag the warmth, understanding and great support I was searching for. I extend my sincerest thanks and gratitude to Dr. h.c. G. Hauff, and also to Mr. Achim Menge, for this. Our long-time friend Dr. John Conley, has written the foreword. For this I would like to express my warmest thanks. I am also very grateful to Dr. Jacqueline Vignaud and Dr. Hasso for permission to reproduce the MRI picture (Fig. 216b).

Through the English edition, I became acquainted with new co-workers of the medical publishers, Mrs. Hadler and Dr. Robertson, who worked with me on this book with great care and effort. I also thank Mr. Zeller for the high quality of the layout that forms an essential part of this book.

My very special thanks, however, go to Dr. P.M. Stell for his unending contribution and subtle sensitivity in translating this book.

My husband wished to present this English edition especially to his American friends and colleagues, and dedicate it to Dr. George E. Shambaugh, Jr.

Sabina R. Wullstein   *Würzburg, Summer 1990*

Contents

Operative Methods for Individual Osteoplastic Exposure of all Middle Ear Cavities 58

Endoscopy and Endoscopic Operations 78

Tympanoplasty in Chronic Inflammation of the Middle Ear 82

Cholesteatoma 101

Conductive Deafness of Inflammatory Origin 137

The Eustachian Tube 152

Tympanoplasty in Trauma of the Temporal Bone 157

Congenital Cholesteatoma, Aneurysms of the Internal Carotid Artery, Congenital Anomalies, Facial Nerve, Dysplasias 164

Healing and Hearing 173

Summary 189

References 191

Index 199

Introduction

Tympanoplasty was an entirely new concept in otological surgery when it was introduced in the early 1950s, at the time when the microscope first began to be used regularly in surgery. Osteoplastic epitympanotomy developed from the concept of tympanoplasty; its basis and method date from 1970–1972. It is suitable for every anatomical and pathological situation, and for the complete orthotopic reconstruction of normal contours.

The accent on embryology in this operative manual might be thought to be unusual. However, it should be remembered that scarcely any other anatomical region of the body has such difficult access. The upright posture, the demands of the neurocranium for space, and the position of the two main sensory organs are the main factors in the development of the complex aeration of the temporal bone which allow concealed infections and their complications to develop. This phylogenetic situation is complicated by the exceedingly rich variation in embryological development.

The pathology of the very narrow area separating the air-containing environment within the temporal bone from the delicate, permeable membrane leading to the inner ear, the cerebrospinal fluid (CSF) spaces of the base of the skull, and the two cranial fossae with their thin bony walls should urge every otologist to master the basic principles of this monograph. Treatment of this region remains the central task of otology: the disease may be either acute or chronic and concealed for years, but it can lead suddenly to a lethal situation, despite advances in diagnosis and treatment.

Microsurgery was first used on the temporal bone and owes its development to tympanoplasty. Initially, its use spread only slowly into other branches of surgery; firstly, into ophthalmology and then laryngology. The microscope has been used since 1966 in neurosurgery, which nowadays would be unthinkable without it, and vascular surgeons now use it regularly.

The present book covers an span of more than 50 years of clinical otology. Since 1933, the senior author (H.L.W.) had extensive experience of oto-genic complications, including circumscribed external and internal pachymeningitis, phlebitis of the sinus wall, thrombosis of the various sinuses, and cerebral abscess, but in particular, the many forms of labyrinthitis and osteitis and the resulting labyrinthogenic meningitis. For more than ten years, from 1936 to 1948, with an interruption by the war, H. L. Wullstein investigated the differential diagnosis of osteitis of the inner ear capsule, the critical interface between the upper airway and the sensorineural system of hearing. The result was the first synopsis of the interplay among otitis media, membranous labyrinthitis, osteitis of the inner ear capsule and paralabyrinthine and labyrinthine cholesteatoma. Based on this pathological and clinical foundation, he established in 1951 one-stage reconstruction of the destroyed and infected middle ear, using free tympanic membrane grafts. He introduced the term tympanoplasty for this operation. His publications attracted immediate interest from 1952 onward.

It is tympanoplasty and not antibiotics which has reduced the danger of chronic otitis media. Drugs can neither heal chronic inflammation nor halt its unseen progress. Once complications have set in, the only hope of preventing a lethal outcome is radical surgery. Tympanoplasty is reconstructive rather than destructive, and it can be a prophylactic operation. Even if surgical improvement of hearing was slight or even illusory, the principle of tympanoplasty justified surgeons in embarking on prophylactic surgery. Furthermore, it made the early pathological stages the keypoint of planning of surgery in an attempt to recreate a completely healthy, newly enclosed airspace in the temporal bone. This explains why the previously common lethal complications of chronic otitis media have now become rare.

The senior author claims credit for the development of *one-stage tympanoplasty* from its very inception; he was the first to carry out a tympanoplasty at a time when the activity of antibiotics in this area was unknown. From the beginning he insisted, on pathophysiological grounds, that tympanoplasty must be a one-stage operation, even in an infected middle ear.

One-stage tympanoplasty represents a break with every otosurgical tradition. Yet it is the only method of immediately achieving the aeration of the middle ear necessary for the satisfactory anatomical and functional healing of severe mucosal inflammations of the epitympanum, large defects due to cholesteatoma and adhesive processes, and tubotympanic inflammation.

Osteoplastic epitympanotomy has replaced the radical operation, which was only rarely carried out, and then only for impending complications, because of the permanent irksome cavity. Dissection begins directly at the site of origin of the disease and extends only as far as the nondiseased pneumatic spaces of the temporal bone. It is a "tailored", nondestructive procedure, which can be used even in early childhood. Before the successes of otosurgery achieved gradually during the last hundred years, purulent complications were the most highly feared causes of death; they were far more numerous than malignancy of the head and neck. Thus, when the senior author began training in 1933, only the departments of surgery and medicine produced more postmortem examinations; a state of affairs which is now scarcely believeable. George Shambaugh Jr. states that this was also true at the Massachusetts Eye and Ear Infirmary at that time.

This extensive danger to the base of the skull from infections in the widely ramifying aerodynamic system prevented the immediate cooperation of the neurosurgeon and the otologist; it only became possible when the otologist eliminated the danger. At the same time, the otologist gave neurosurgery a fresh impetus with the newly developed microsurgery. The age of the "neurosensory centers" based on neurology, neurosurgery, otorhinolaryngology and opthalmology then began, at the same time as a period of frightening increase in severe skull trauma.

Etymology of the Nomenclature used in this Monograph

Tympanum, Epitympanum and Attic

The otological term "attic" may have two etymological origins:
1. *Attica* is derived from the Greek word attikos, a half-story suprastructure over the main cornice of a building, particularly used to carry sculptures and inscriptions, for example, on Roman triumphal arches.
2. *Atticus* is a latinized form first used in the baroque period. It describes a gable room in a sloping roof without an "attica."

These terms from early comparative anatomy were chosen purely on descriptive grounds and had no anatomical significance. The tympanum is the eardrum. The attic is a common medical short form indicating a gable room. Behind that is the *aditus* (an entrance) leading into the *antrum* (a grotto in the hollow system). Both have the same roof, the *tegmen*.

Because of the high degree of functional and anatomical interdependence, logically we should divide the three levels of the middle ear cavity into the mesotympanum, the hypotympanum (with the orifice of the eustachian tube and the sinus tympani) and the epitympanum (with the lever system of the ossicles).

The term "attic" will doubtless remain in everyday use. However in training centers, the succeeding generation should be taught to think clearly and logically about this complex situation in a vital area. Therefore *the term "attic" will not be used in this monograph.*

The protympanic recess, which is so clinically essential, is formed by the anteromedial part of the epitympanum (Hammar 1902, Pernkopf 1960). The aditus and antrum, which are also of anatomical and functional importance, lie posteriorly. In the medial wall of the protympanic recess lies the "anterior point of danger," i.e., the antelabyrinthine trigone.

The photographs of the anatomical preparations and those of the operations were mainly taken by the junior author (S.R.W.); the few that were taken in earlier years by the senior author are so indicated. Photography was not possible with the microscope which he constructed himself in 1948–1949. As soon as the first microscope arrived from Zeiss in 1953, a Leitz movie camera was mounted on one eyepiece, and monocular photographs were taken. The camera was mounted on one eyepiece for the first three operative films taken through an operative microscope for the 6th International ENT Conference in 1957. Surgery and filming were monocular because at that time neither photadaptors nor co-observation tubes were available.

Functional Anatomy of the Middle Ear

Anatomical details have gained in importance as middle ear surgery has developed from a destructive procedure whose sole purpose was to heal, to reconstructive surgery, which has both a healing and a reconstructive intent. The many anatomical variations of the temporal bone are particularly significant in one-stage osteoplastic exposure and orthotopic reconstruction of the ear. If knowledge of these variations is combined with the ability to expose the disease from its site of origin to the limit of its extent, the following questions can be answered about a particular patient:

- Why has the pathological and functional disorder developed in this and in no other way?
- Wherein lies the problem with respect to exposure?
- What surgical difficulties should be anticipated in the individual case?

Before explaining why a chosen operative procedure is preferred, it is essential to discuss the developmental processes which have given rise to anatomical variations and which contribute to the various clinical pictures.

Unlike the rigid definition of the term "congenital", the concept of a genetically determined process defines only the outer limits and the preferred direction of development. The model of this concept of an epigenetic landscape, described by the British developmental physiologist Conrad Waddington (1975), demonstrates this clearly (Fig. 1).

How a pathological lesion arises and how it regresses depend solely on the construction of the middle ear spaces at a given moment, the vitality of the mucosa, and on the intensity and duration of the insult. It is wrong to speak of a genetically determined hypertrophic, atrophic or dystrophic phase of inflammation or of pneumatization. Any prolonged chronic insult which exceeds the ability of the mucosa to adapt causes irreversible damage.

The potential of the mucosa to resist damage is enhanced by a mucociliary transport system, which forms part of the resistance complex of the middle ear. It lies not only in the bony walls, the constitu-

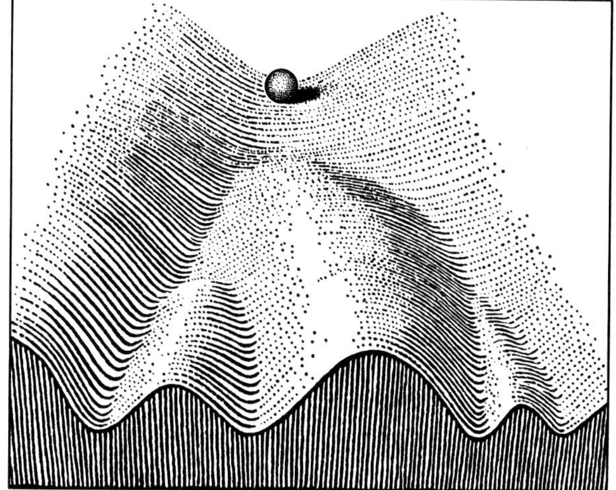

Fig. **1** In this **model of an epigenetic landscape,** a ball rolls down a sloping surface toward the observer. The hill and dale structure of this surface forms the genetically programmed spatial conditions under which any animal or man — symbolized by the ball rolling down the surface — can develop during his lifetime. Environmental influences acting in a lateral direction allow the ball to roll temporarily up one or other side as it continues its path in the prescribed valley (Waddington 1975)

ent parts of the middle ear cavity and the internal surface of the tympanic membrane, but also in the system of mucosal folds. One of the most interesting facets of the folds is their varying character in different areas, determined by their function.

Knowledge of the varying anatomy and function at different times is of great importance in understanding the course of the disease, as well as the individual developmental processes of the ear and their variations. The following subjects are included in this chapter to demonstrate these developmental processes:

- the temporal bone and the base of the skull;
- the growth centers of the skull and the growth phases of the temporal bone;
- the development of the air spaces in their bony

casing and of the structures which are of a decisive significance in aeration and drainage;
– the origin of the mucosal folds;
– the arrangement of the mucosal folds; Koerner's septum;
– the middle ear: its niches, prominences and recesses, especially the tympanic sinus, the facial recess, the pretympanic and supratubal recesses,
– the aeration and drainage system of the middle ear;
– the first and second constrictions in the aeration system of the middle ear;
– the anterior and posterior sector in the aeration system of the middle ear;
– the tympanic diaphragm; the anterior and posterior tympanic isthmi;

– the relation of the sigmoid sinus and the jugular bulb to the tympanum and the retrotympanic spaces;
– the lateral epitympanic air cushions acting as a vibration damper.

Diseases of the eustachian tube will not be dealt with here (see p. 152), but it must be pointed out that the function of the eustachian tube directly correlates with the shape of the skull; meso- and brachycephalic persons have good tubal function, whereas dolicocephalic subjects often have poor tubal function.

The Temporal Bone and the Base of the Skull

The human skull is a complex of two functional units: the neurocranium and the viscerocranium, the latter being subdivided into the masticatory and respiratory cranium. The various organs and their functions vary widely in the intensity and timing of their growth, and this effect is most clearly seen at the base of the skull. In the early developmental phase, the growth centers of the sphenoid bone without doubt play a crucial role. No other part of the skeleton demonstrates so many controversial, general and specific points of skeletal and skull morphology. For surgery, however, the temporal bone is certainly the most important part of the base of the skull.

The origin of the shape of the base of the skull and of its congenital anomalies lies in the region between the basisphenoid, basiclinoid, intrasphenoid and spheno-occipital synchondroses and the anlage of the petrous temporal and the occipital bones. This area is bounded by the superior sphenopetrosal ligament, running from the posterior clinoid process to the superior sphenoidal apex on one side, and on the other side, by the inferior sphenopetrosal ligament, lying close to the foramen lacerum and the lingula of the sphenoid and the sphenoidal process of the petrous apex above the fibrocartilage which forms the sphenopetrosal synchrondosis. It thus lies on the posterior edge of the carotid groove (see also p. 164 in regard to the anlage of congenital epidermoid and congenital epidermoid cysts arising in the embryonal phase).

The number of bone centers in the fetal sphenoid bone varies; there may be up to 19 ossification centers in the sphenoid anlage. There are also differences between right and left sides, as well as in the development of the synchondroses. The presphenoid begins with the ossification of the sphenoethmoidal cartilage on the medial side of the optic canal, extending as far as the anterior clinoid process; it fuses with the orbitosphenoid, which later forms the lesser wing of the sphenoid bone. Asymmetries vary in severity up to a complete unilateral defect of the orbitosphenoid, including the sphenoid arch, with prolapse of the frontal lobe and displacement of the eyeball anteriorly and inferiorly, in the presence of a completely normal opposite side. The presphenoid is followed by ossification of the basisphenoid, which fuses with the basiclinoid to form the clivus. The two alisphenoids, which later become the greater wings of the sphenoid, develop on the basisphenoid (Fig. 2).

Ossification of the cartilaginous phase lasts from the prenatal period to the end of the first year of life (Fig. 3). The variations of shape of the neurocranium arise from the base of the skull, and are due to the the ossification of the synchondroses between parts of the sphenoid, temporal and occipital bones. These fuse at various times and in various forms, which may be symmetrical or asymmetrical. These variations of shape are influenced by the growth of the mass of the brain itself. The shape of the neurocranium changes slowly throughout life.

The aerated cells surround the sound transport system of the middle ear and the sensorineural hearing organ, permeate the entire base of the skull and extend from the ethmoid bone, along the eustachian tube, inferior to the tegmen tympani as far as the attachment of the tentorium to the occipital bone.

The cause of congenital lesions can be understood from the disorders of two early developmental phases:

1. incomplete closure of the neural groove;
2. the development of the bony centers (especially those of the sphenoid bone), including the bony eustachian tube and its anomalies.

In the first case the defects range from simple anomalies to the most serious defects in the closure of the neural groove, and include complete or partial dysraphias extending from the nasion through the basion to the vertebra, as well as the more serious forms of facial cleft, cyclopia and proboscis, etc. (Bosma 1976). More important in everyday clinical practice are the mild forms, including occult dysraphias of the soft palate affecting the musculature of the nasopharynx and the cartilaginous eustachian tube.

The length of the presphenoid compared with the basisphenoid and the basiclinoid affects the angulation of the base of the skull: a short presphenoid is associated with a flat clivus; a broad floor of the posterior cranial fossa, with platybasia and slight angulation of the temporal bone. The brain is then said to undergo *occipitopetal development*, in contrast to *frontipetal brain development,* in which a long presphenoid is associated with a steep clivus, a deep posterior cranial fossa and marked angulation of the petrous pyramid from front to back.

This relation of the presphenoid to the basisphenoid together with the alisphenoid determines the length, angulation and diameter of the bony eusta-

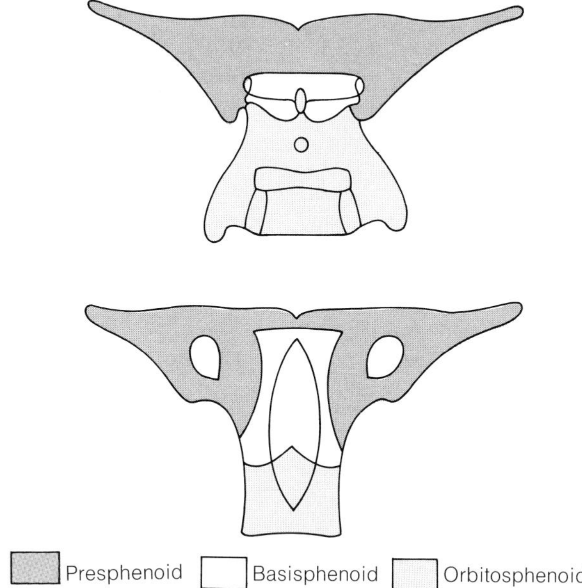

Fig. **2 Developmental anlages of the sphenoid.** The upper figure shows a view from above, and the lower the view from in front (Bosma 1976)

chian tube. An abnormal position of the condyles of the occipital bone, or a short or aplastic clivus can cause a basal impression. The base of the skull changes not only during childhood but throughout life, and has lasting effects on the eighth cranial nerve, the shortest cranial nerve, lying in the subarachnoid space between fixed points.

The ear develops within the temporal bone, a mixed bone composed of membrane bone (the tympanic and squamous parts) and enchondral bone (petrosal and mastoid parts) (Strack 1975). The

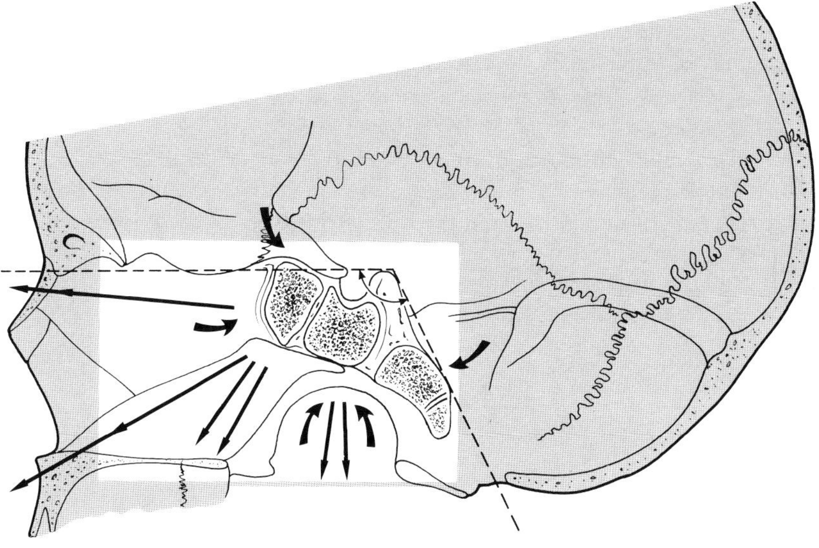

Fig. 3 **Postnatal development of the sphenoid-clivus angle.** The arrows show the effective force on the angulation of the base of the skull due to frontipetal or occipitopetal development of the brain (Roche and Lewis 1976)

evolution of the ear's function as a sensory organ determined this position, where it is exposed to all the biomechanical effects, resistances and pressure on the base of the skull; these define its external and internal shape.

The inner ear capsule is a completely independent bony organ embedded in the temporal bone. It is surrounded by the loose spongiosa of the petrous pyramid, which is fixed between the rigid cortical bone of the two surfaces of the petrous pyramid. The inferior surface is under the influence of the caroticobulbar vascular angle. Isolated tears of the capsule following slight shock illustrate the sensitivity of the enchondral and endosteal layers of the inner ear to distortion transmitted via the spongiosa. Progessive remodelling of bone of the inner ear capsule over many years as a result of distortion due to shifting, tilting and torsion of the petrous pyramid is conceivable.

The biodynamic processes and the pressure of the maturing cell structure within the intercellular tissues demonstrate, and require, increased metabolism during the growth phase. These processes determine the degree of change of position of the temporal bone within the base of the skull, so long as this is being molded anteriorly or posteriorly by the development of the brain. The site and timing of this adjustment of the temporal bone around the vertical and horizontal axes and around its own axis is influenced by numerous genetic and epigenetic factors (see Fig. 1).

Two groups of variations of shape of the temporal bone and their mutual interaction should be determined as far as possible before an operation:

a) The Position of the Petrous Temporal Bone Within the Base of the Skull. The variations of shape and the change of position of the petrous pyramid in the base of the skull are very numerous and have been fully investigated by Šercer 1959, Krmpotic 1960 and others. Both authors regarded these anomalies of position as a cause of otosclerosis, a unique and frequent form of chronic bony remodelling. The credibility of this concept is supported by the gradual changes which arise from the central region of the base of the skull (the sphenoid with its greater wings) which act as mechanical factors on the neurocranial part of the temporal bone. the kyphosis of the base of the skull alters with the upright posture, leading in turn to a change of the sphenoid-clivus angle. Normally the angulation of the base of the skull decreases due to the growth process from 135° at birth to about 110° in adulthood.

The rotation and torsion of the pyramid (Šercer 1959) depend not only on the frontipetal or occipitopetal cerebral development but also on the degree of angulation of the base of the skull around the two petrous pyramids. The orientation of the posterior surface of the petrous pyramid relative to its upper surface changes synchronously with cerebral development. The two surfaces form an angle, termed the "roof angle."

The torsion of the petrous pyramid and the reduction of the roof angle influence the angle between the bulb of the jugular vein and the internal carotid artery where they enter or leave the petrous pyramid inferior to the inner ear capsule. The base of the petrous pyramid becomes smaller with a narrow *caroticobulbar angle*, as does the paralabyrinthine region and thus the space for the two inferior cell tracts. This affects the surfaces of the cortical bone of the petrous pyramid and the bony cochlea.

The course of the endolymphatic duct and the extent of the endolymphatic sac are strongly correlated with the caroticobulbar angle. In our investigations it was very small in almost all patients suspected of having Ménière's syndrome.

b) The Development of the Tympanic Plate. The following parameters of the squamous bone, the zygomatic process and the mastoid bone influence the development of the tympanic bone: the height of the tegmen tympani and antri; the development of the recesses; the position of the lateral wall of the epitympanum; the depth of the middle ear cavity; the height of the bulb of the internal jugular vein; the curvature of the external auditory meatus; the anterior displacement of the posterior meatal wall and simultaneous anterior displacement of a very steep sigmoid sinus with a narrow mastoid process; and, possibly, the presence of a Koerner's septum in the aditus (see p. 16).

If the acute angle between the posterior surface of the petrous bone and its superior surface is reduced, the tympanic bone will lie at a higher level. This produces a narrow zygomatic arch, a very curved external auditory meatus and a low-lying middle cranial fossa dura, mainly at the junction with the temporal squama where the posterior ramifications of the impression of the inferior temporal gyrus extend. The combination of this anatomical variation and anterior displacement of the sigmoid sinus with a high jugular bulb reduces the air-containing volume of the middle ear cavity. The smaller the air-containing volume of the middle ear cavity, the greater the danger of temporarily reduced pressure due to air resorption in the epitympanum and the mesohypotympanum until the next physiological refill, and the greater the danger of retraction of the tympanic membrane.

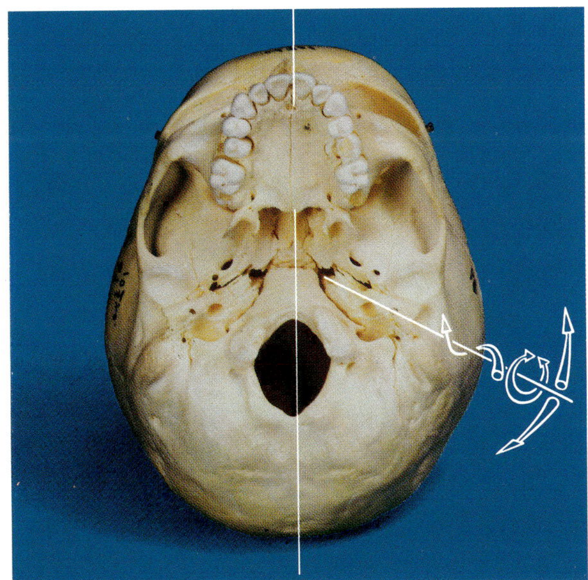

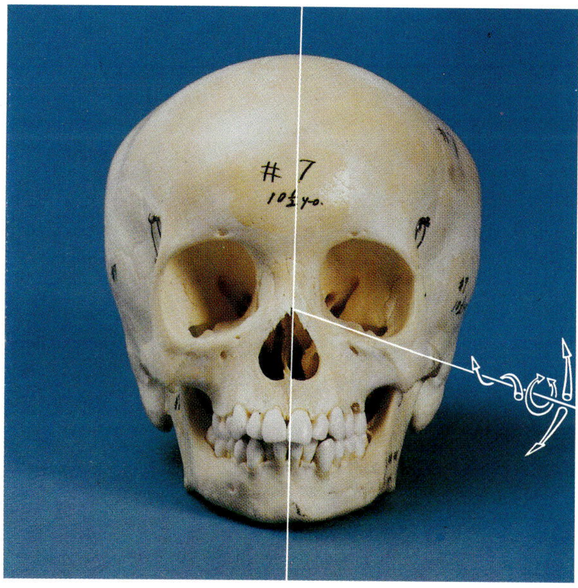

Fig. **4** **Declination of the pyramid.** The lateral angle of the petrous bone becomes larger during frontipetal development of the brain. This is the obtuse angle anteriorly formed by the upper surface of the pyramid and the median sagittal plane

Fig. **5** **Inclination of the pyramid** moves superiorly in frontipetal brain development, and the vertical angle becomes less. This angle is obtuse superiorly between the superior margin of the pyramid and the median sagittal line of the skull. The pyramidal base sinks vice versa in occipitopetal brain development, and the vertical angle increases

The smaller the angle between the sphenoidal plane and the plane of the clivus, the more marked is the curvature of the base of the skull. Thus, not only is the meatus more curved, but its long axis is more vertical. If the sphenoid-clivus angle is greater, the skull base is flatter and the long axis of the external meatus becomes more horizontal.

The position of the tympanic bone is determined by this development. In the frontipetal type, i.e., with more marked inclination and less declination of the temporal bone, the tympanic bone lies more inferior and anterior. This position is reversed in the occipitopetal type (Figs. **4**, **5**). In the case of a simultaneous anterior displacement of the sigmoid sinus with a high jugular fossa, the positional changes usually experienced by the tympanic bone are hindered; this affects the ossification centers and leads to subsequent deformity.

Growth Centers of the Skull and the Growth Phases of the Temporal Bone (Figs. 6, 7)

Understanding of the enormous richness in variation of shape of the middle ear and inner ear can be considered under three headings when describing the pathology, physiology and surgery of this area:

1. the origin of the petrous bone, particularly the biokinetics of bone growth, and its ossification;
2. the development of the air spaces of the ear in the petrous bone, and the origin and function of the fine mucosal structures, including the mucosal folds;
3. the volume of the air-containing space of the middle ear and the strength of its internal pressure.

These three interrelated factors affect the formation and shaping of the temporal bone. They can only be correctly understood on the basis of the kinetics of growth of the entire skull.

The creation of the spatial arrangement by genetic and epigenetic orientation patterns during the *growth phase* can be summarized under three headings as follows:

a) The synchondroses of the skull base (intrasphenoidal, sphenopetrosal, spheno-occipital, petro-occipital and intraoccipital) and the sutures (sphenoethmoidal and sphenosquamous) are responsible for the *first growth phase* of the temporal bone from birth to the second year of life.

In man, the brain is the most active structure to mold the skull, the skull base and the organs embedded in it. In the second embryonal month, the development of the brain is extremely eccentric. The expansion of the mass of the brain is evident from the extensive growth of the superolateral face of the hemisphere, where the mesenchymal capsule is weak. The growth of the surface of the basal part of the brain is slow; it is therefore denser. The mesenchymal tissue lying below this part of the brain which forms the precartilaginous base of the skull cartilage begins to develop within it, and this process begins where the mesenchyme is densest.

The neurocranium undergoes accelerated development during the prenatal period so that it has already reached 25% of its ultimate volume by birth, at which time the viscerocranium begins to develop. According to Pankow (1949/50), an increasing deceleration in the curvature of the base of the skull occurs between the second and third year of life, because 90% of the development of the brain is then complete. After the sixth year of life there follows a

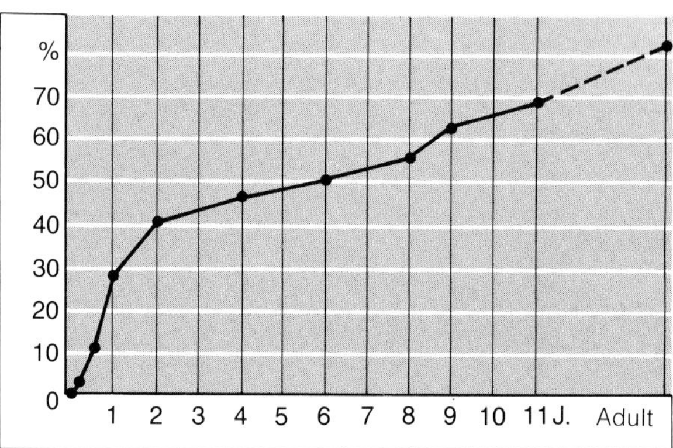

Fig. **6** **Average growth curve of the temporal bone** (Dahm 1970)

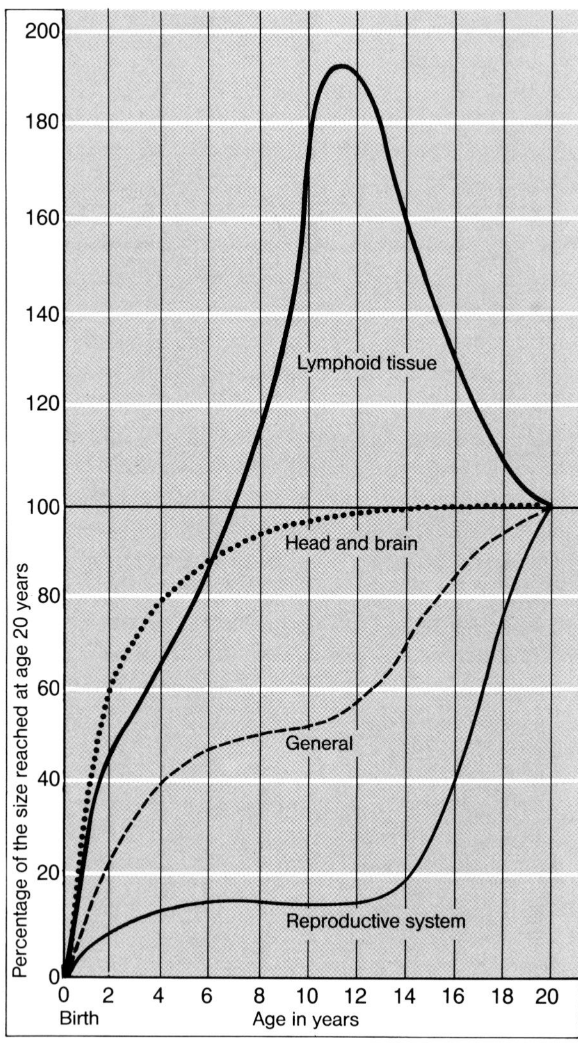

Fig. **7** **Postnatal growth curve of various tissues expressed as a percentage of total gain from birth to maturity** (Scammon 1930)

further growth spurt lasting until puberty. Whereas the growth of the neurocranium persists until the end of the second year of life and then continues evenly until adulthood, the viscerocranium demonstrates several phases of varying speed of growth. The volume of this part of the skull triples in the first year of life. At the beginning of the second year of life, it has reached only one quarter of the adult size and in the eighth year, only half the size of the fully developed adult face reached at 23 years of age.

Premature ossification of individual synchondroses of the skull base and change of the curvature of the skull base in the angle between the sphenoidal plane and the clivus is associated with inhibition of growth of the temporal bone and the central part of the face.

b) The hyaline cartilage of the temporomandibular joint is responsible for the *second growth phase* of the skull between the second and seventh years of life.

It is also responsible for the development of the mandible. Its activity as a *growth center* is strongly correlated with the development of the central part of the face, i.e., the zygomatic bone, the zygomatic arch and hence, the tympanic bone. A broad zygomatic root, a broad zygomatic arch, and a broad, flat lateral epitympanic wall sloping inferiorly indicate a high epitympanum, a high tegmen tympani, and a high middle cranial fossa dura. If the lateral epitympanic wall is almost vertical, which can be deduced from the height and breadth of the epitympanum, the protympanic recess will be found to be deep. The tensor fold divides the protympanic recess from the supratubal recess. Its position determines whether the protympanic recess is wide and the supratubal recess shallow, or vice versa.

If the zygomatic arch is narrow and the lateral epitympanic wall is almost horizontal, the epitympanum will be small and the dura low. Furthermore, the position of the dura mater and thus the profile of the petrous bone can be deduced from the temporal line. The closer the temporal line runs to the suprameatal spine, and the narrower the zygomatic arch and its root, the lower the dura and the smaller the epitympanum.

After freeing the skin of the external auditory meatus at the start of an osteoplastic procedure, inspection of the root of the zygoma, the temporal line, the curvature of the bony meatus and the lateral epitympanic wall often suffice to estimate the size and extent of the epitympanum.

The greater the curvature of the external meatus, the more obliquely the lateral epitympanic wall lies, and the deeper the dura. A very curved meatus is also narrow because the zygomatic arch is similarly narrow, and the anterior meatal wall formed by the temporomandibular joint then bulges more markedly. The tympanomeatal angle is difficult to view clearly. The narrower the meatus, the smaller the tympanic (Rivini's) notch; but the anterior tympanic spine and the bony projection on the tympanosquamous fissure are more prominent. In this case the hypotympanum is often shallow, the lateral sinus displaced anteriorly and the bulb of the interior jugular vein high.

The zygomatic process increases in length by approximately 50% from birth to the end of the second year of life. The second growth spurt is completed between the eleventh year of life and adulthood.

The first anlage of the tympanic bone is visible from about the ninth week of embryonic life. The tympanic ring has reached its final size at the end of pregnancy. It fuses with the squamous bone; this point is marked by a groove, the tympanic notch. The aperture of the opening of the external meatus was originally bigger. The conversion of this opening to form the fundus of the external acoustic meatus (the porus) is achieved by outgrowth of two bony struts from the anterosuperior and posteroinferior wall of the tympanic ring. These struts fuse during the first year of life. Above this bony bridge lies the external acoustic porus. The underlying bridge closes by ossification before the fifth year of life.

c) The suture system of the central part of the face (frontomaxillary, zygomaticomaxillary, zygomaticotemporal, pterygopalatine and sphenozygomatic sutures) is responsible for the *third growth phase* from the seventh year to adulthood.

During this phase, the entire skull grows by extensive apposition of bone on the surface, with simultaneous resorption within.

The cartilaginous growth of the nasal septum is important in the sagittal and vertical growth of the central part of the face. In addition to general constitutional factors, the many functional demands of the viscerocranium have an extensive formative influence. The pneumatization of the viscerocranium develops indirectly and directly, including the mastoid process during this phase of growth of the upper jaw when the nose, the nasal septum, the nasopharynx and the eustachian tube are being developed.

The postnatal development of the individual bony parts to form one temporal bone does not proceed evenly, either in time or space. A hollow space forms at the point where the petrous, squamous and tympanic bones unite. This space is the middle ear, joined by two sutures, the petrosquamous and the tympanosquamous. These sutures later ossify. The points at which they are still partially open are the fissures: these are often wide defects through which the dura mater is related directly to the mucosa of the middle ear. The fissures form the pathway of least resistance for the spread of infection within the skull or to the external surface. Their position determines the course of the blood vessels supplying the middle ear; for example, the entrance of the anterior tympanic artery and the exit of the chorda tympani nerve from the petrotympanic fissure. Finally, they indirectly determine the arrangement of the mucosal folds which develop around the viscera of the middle ear. For example, the position of the tensor fold determines the size of the protympanic and supratubal recesses.

The external petrosquamous suture arises at the point where the squamous and petrosal bones unite. The internal petrosquamous suture runs through the roof of the antrum and the tympanum, i.e., it is intra-antral and intratympanic, but extratubal. It does not take part in the growth of the eustachian tube. Its intra-antral part may persist as a bony plate (Koerner's septum) which divides the antrum into medial and lateral segments.

The suture between the petrous and occipital bones is occasionally of clinical significance, since an aberrant island of epidermal cells may persist on the posterior surface of the petrous pyramid when the neural groove closes, and from these cells a congenital epidermoid later arises.

After birth, the squamous and mastoid bones change from a vertical to an oblique position, and then become more upright again within the first year of life, synchronous with the formation of the mastoid process.

The progress of the displacement of the growth centers can be defined by phases of cell proliferation, cell determination and cell differentiation of varying length. The sequence of these phases is programmed, and the biodynamics of their progress are important for each succeeding phase. The first short phase extends over the first two years of life, the second from then until the sixth or seventh year, followed by the third long growth phase encompassing the two marked bony growth spurts and lasting until adulthood.

The second growth phase of the temporal bone is often included with the third phase. It is characterized by slow ossification, but by *marked development and maturation of the lymphatic tissue and the local mucosa and submucosa.* The middle ear mucosa therefore reacts more rapidly and more briskly to external stimuli. Gelatinous tissue masses are found everywhere in the recesses and niches of the middle ear, which is still undergoing growth, so that the relative extent of the active surface of the middle ear mucosa is reduced. A small swelling of this highly vascularized lining or of the mucosal folds decreases the air volume, leading to a marked variation of the internal pressure. Feedback reinforces the response of the still immature mucosa because immunological stability has not yet been achieved. The two constrictions in the aeration system of the middle ear, the first being the eustachian tube and the second the tympanic diaphragm, are obstructed, interrupting aeration and drainage. The entire mucociliary resistance system is thus paralyzed. Seromucinous middle ear infections, and their sequelae, including primary inflammatory cholesteatoma, are frequent at this time of life; their origin lies in this feedback system.

Differentiation of the individual parts follows the displacement of the growth centers. Its kinetics are controlled by simultaneously modelling of bone, formation of the air-containing space and the strength of the intrinsic internal pressure. The change of position and shape of the temporal bone, especially of its pneumatized part, is coordinated with ossification. An increase in the air-containing space induces ossification. So long as the internal pressure within the middle ear remains the same, the increase of volume continuously adapts to it. The interaction of the following three factors ultimately determines the size of the air-containing middle ear space:

1. biokinetics of bone growth and its ossification;
2. development of the air spaces of the middle ear in their bony housing;
3. the internal pressure.

Development of the Air Spaces of the Middle Ear (Fig. 8)

Origin of the Mucosal Folds

In the newborn almost the entire middle ear space is full of gelatinous tissue, and the soft tissues of the medial and lateral walls are in apposition. The air-containing middle ear space develops due to the growth of the tympanic plate and the adaptation of a vertical position by the tympanic membrane.

Air enters the middle ear cavity soon after birth. It is almost certain that amniotic fluid is present in the cleft of the middle ear cavity during pregnancy — it is known that the fetus begins to swallow before birth. The surface covered with mucosa enlarges during the fetal period, due to a decrease in the gelatinous tissue. At the same time, four projections push forward from the primary tubotympanic tube. These are the *saccus anterior, medius, superior and posterior* (Hammar, 1902).

The further development and modification of these projections, especially of the posterior saccus which forms the hypotympanum, coincides with the increase in breadth and size of the middle ear due to the growth of the tympanic plate. The tympanic membrane, the malleus and the eustachian tube change from a horizontal to an oblique position. At the same time three eminences (pyramidal, chordal and styloid) appear. All these factors determine the depth of the tympanic sinus and the facial recess.

If the sacs form normally and uniformly according to the principle of the "pneu," then an octahedron can be recognized at the point of contact between the saccus posterior, medius and superior. The membranous tension of the sacs is uniform at all points. They meet at an angle of 120° at constant internal pressure.

As there are so many variants of form, it was not easy to find appropriate material, but after a long search we found a specimen from the fifth foetal month in Bollobas's collection in Budapest, which allowed us to verify this construction of the "pneus" (Fig. 9).

The first evidence of the middle ear cavity can be clearly recognized in the 125-mm foetus. The first pouch forms on the medial wall between the tensor tendon and the long process of the incus. This is the saccus medius, which aerates the greater part of the antrum. In the 160-mm fetus the epitympanic and tympanic segments of the middle ear cavity can be

---

* A "pneu" is a system in which a tensile (stretchable) cover separates a pliable mass within under pressure from another pliable mass without.

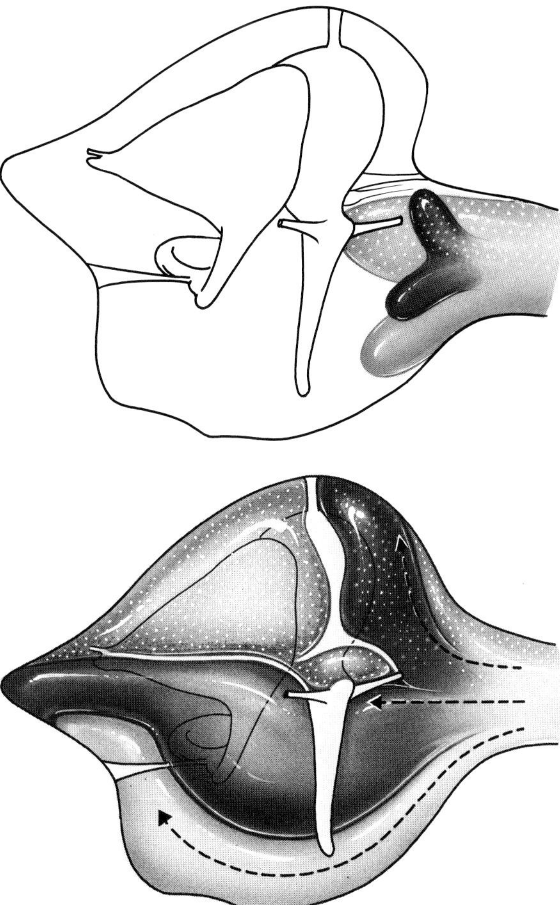

Fig. **8 Development of the sacci and the air-containing spaces of the middle ear** (Proctor 1964)

distinguished from each other. The further development of the middle ear cavity in a fetus of 222 mm is completed with the formation of the anterior, superior and posterior sacs, which develop last. Mucosal folds arise at the points where the sacs meet each other, and they incorporate the structures on which the saccus impinged during its development: the tensor and stapes tendons, the ossicles, the ligaments, the blood vessels and the chorda tympani. Such folds include:
- the tensor fold between the saccus medius and anterior;
- the folds of von Tröltsch, and the mallear and incudal folds between the saccus medius and superior:
- the stapedial folds between the saccus superior and posterior.

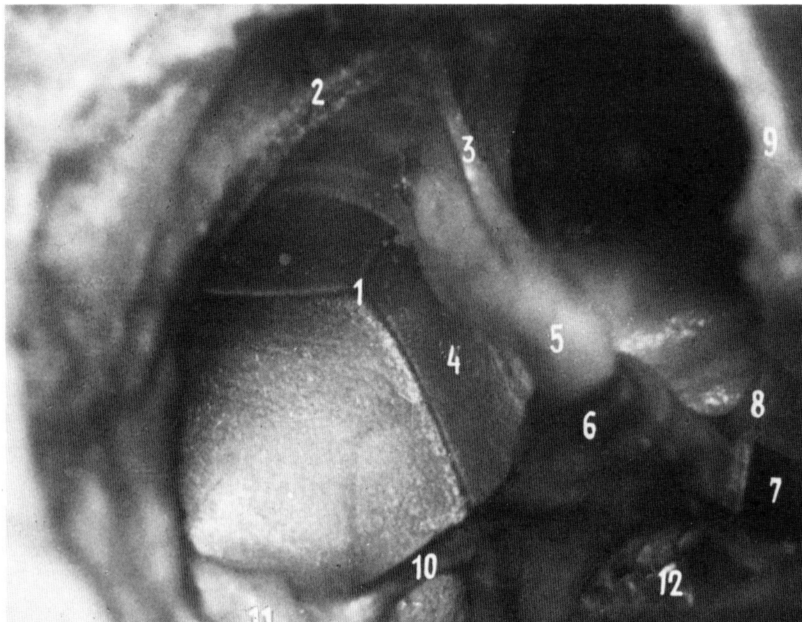

Fig. **9 Air spaces of the middle ear determined by the "pneu" constriction system.** The membrane tension is uniform at all points, with three interrelated vesicles, the saccus posterior, medius and superior, and the walls are uniform angle of 120° to each other (1).

1. Tympanic sulcus
2. Chorda tympani
3. Long process of the incus
4. Incudostapedial joint
5. Pyramidal eminence
6. Stapedial tendon
7. Posterior crus of the stapes
8. Facial canal
9. Anterior crus of the stapes
10. Octagon formed by the posterior, medial and superior saccus (Bollobas 1972)

In addition to these obligate, typical localized folds there are other obligate but irregular folds: the various mallear and incudal folds, the folds of the chorda tympani and, also, the accessory irregular folds (see p. 16).

A narrow point, the tympanic isthmus, can be recognized in the 285-mm human fetus. At this point the chorda tympani and its fold extend from the lateral side into the lumen of the middle ear cavity, and the facial nerve and canal as well as the tensor canal and the tensor fold extend from the medial side. The saccus medius and superior appear to be constricted at the site of the isthmus. The ligaments are clearly recognizable as connective tissue cords which form a barrier leading to the development of further sacs and many small mucosal folds.

The styloid eminence appears in the 33-mm fetus in the zone of the saccus posterior. The pars flaccida and Prussak's space are created by extension of the saccus medius medially around the mass of the malleus and incus above the tympanic isthmus to contact the saccus anterior. The latter develops more slowly. The position of the tensor and superior malleoincudal folds depends on the extent of the saccus anterior and medius and on the passive resistance of the ligaments.

At this stage the anterior and posterior folds of von Tröltsch as well as the lateral mallear and incudal folds have developed from the saccus medius and superior. Small stapedial folds develop from the saccus posterior and these later fuse, to form the obturator membrane of the stapes at the time when the dura begins to develop.

After birth the number of mucosal folds is reduced as the gelatinous tissue is resorbed. Those folds which have developed around the viscera of the middle ear cavity and its blood vessels are retained and have some functional significance. Their aggregation and arrangement is inversely proportional to the size of the air-containing volume of the middle ear cavity, which may be expanded even further by epitympanic cell recesses. The greater the volume, and thus the mucosal surface of the walls, the smaller the number of persisting mucosal folds.

The Mucosal Folds (Figs. **10–16**)

The delicate mucosal folds of the middle ear cavity are arranged in cords around the ligaments and tendons attached to the ossicles. The collagenous and infrequent elastic fibers between their layers are dense and lie almost parallel. Their surface is exposed to air on both sides; it is covered by a single layer of flat or cubical epithelium and by one or two layers of cuboidal and columnar epithelium along the aeration pathway. The population density of the ciliary and secreting cells is concentrated around the aeration and drainage pathways as follows:

- in the incudal fossa, i.e., on the stapedial folds and on the lateral and medial incudal folds;
- in the anterior epitympanum, i.e., on the tensor fold and on the anterior and medial mallear folds;
- in Prussak's space, i.e., around the small lateral mallear folds, around the anterior and posterior folds of von Troeltsch and around the accessory folds.

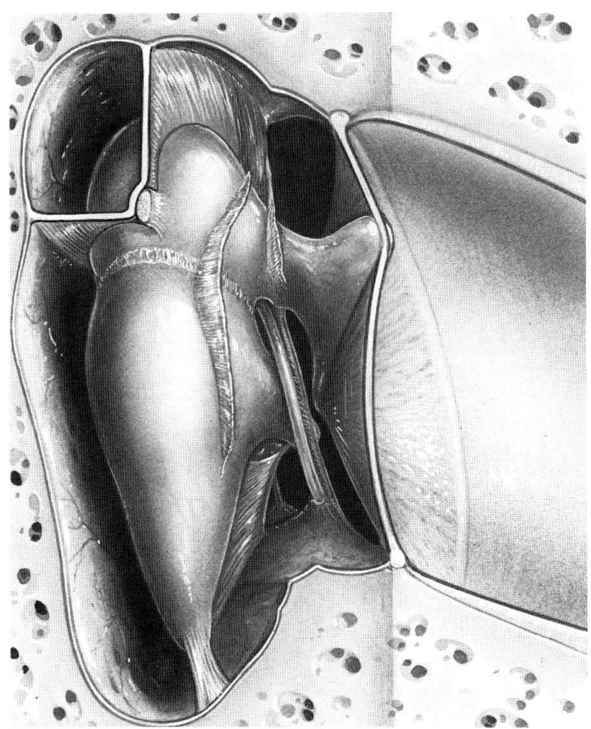

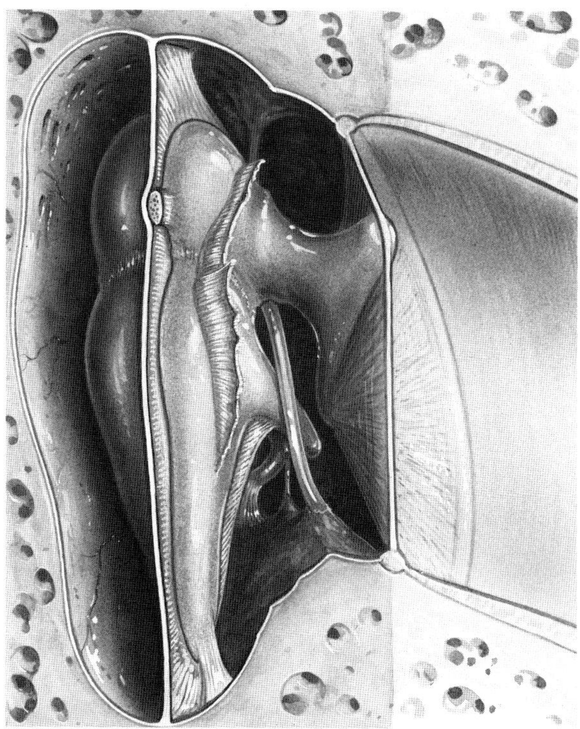

Fig. **10   Diagram of the irregular folds:** the lateral incudal fold is merging with the chordal fold. The medial mallear fold divides the medial segment of the epitympanum into an anterior and a posterior segment. The anterior fold of the malleus adheres to the anterior tympanic wall at the petrotympanic fissure

Fig. **11   Superior sagittal malleoincudal fold.** The lateral incudal fold stretches between the long process and the body of the incus

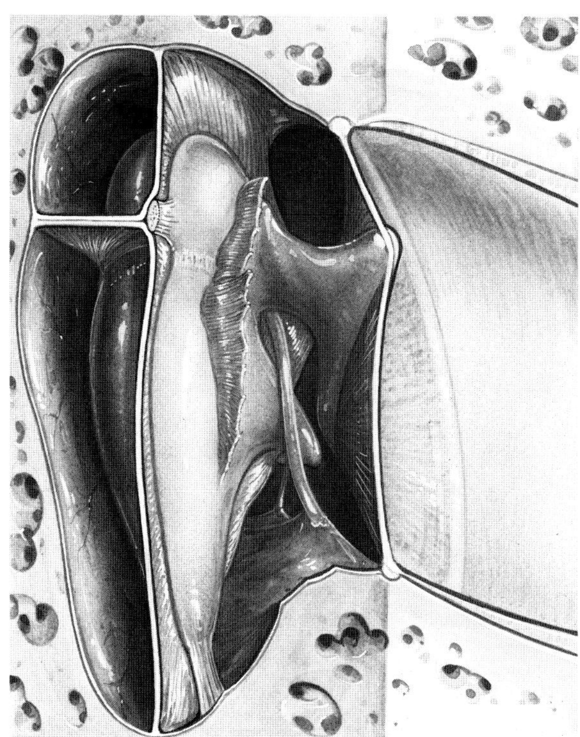

Fig. **12   The anterior mallear fold merging into the superior sagittal malleoincudal fold.** The medial mallear fold divides the medial segment of the epitympanum into an anterior area (also called the protympanic recess) and a posterior part. One of the interossicular folds stretches between the neck of the malleus and the long process of the incus. The lateral incudal fold is also shown.

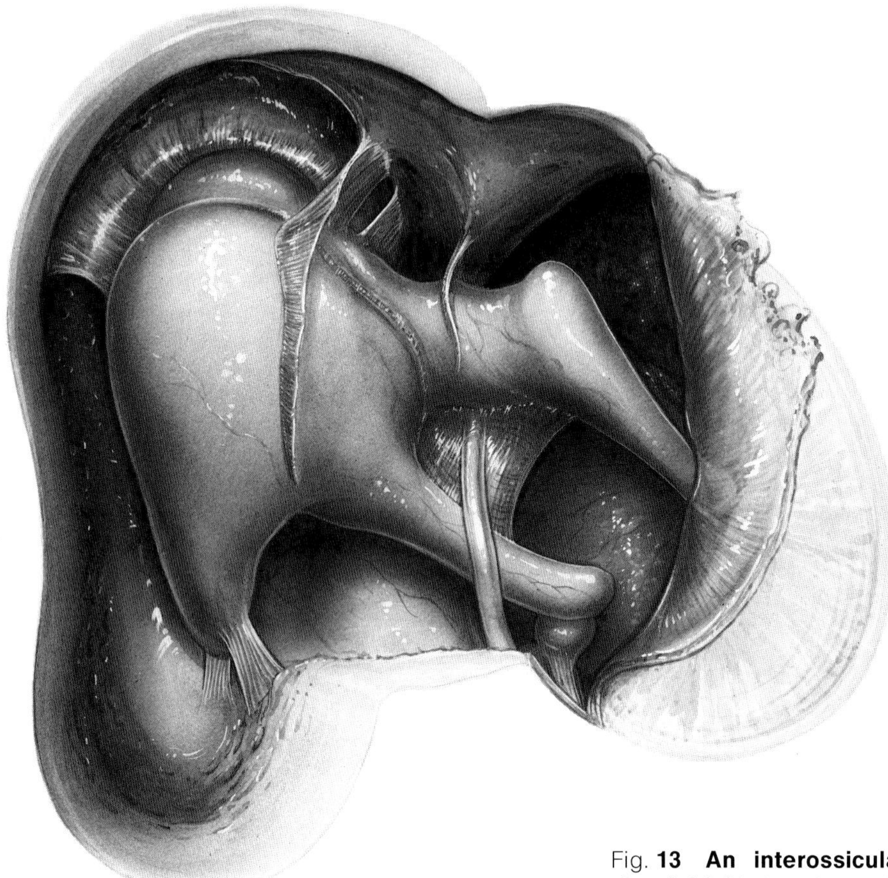

Fig. **13 An interossicular fold merging into the chordal fold.** Anterior mallear fold

There are few ciliary cells, but the epithelium has the potential to modify very rapidly to produce this type of very active transport cell.

The loose and very thin stroma is rich in small blood vessels and lymphoid capillaries, but contains few nerve fibers. Some Pacinian corpuscles can be found in the stroma and are supposed to be responsible, as in the skin, for deep pressure and for fine regulations of the movements of the ossicular chain and tympanic membrane. It is also possible that variations of pressure in the middle ear can be perceived and adjusted via these neural structures. The air cushions formed by the mucosal folds in the epitympanum and filled with residual air, are ideal for transporting this information to the neural structures.

The slightest dilatation of the vessels or transudation of fluid lead to marked swelling and increased density of the stroma of the mucosal folds. Simultaneous resorption of air and increased production of secretions lead rapidly to adherence of the folds. It is then easy to deduce from the morphology and topography what changes and sequelae are to be expected and their site. For example, the obstruction may lie at the second constriction (p. 19) if a lesion in the epitympanum does not resolve even after the mucosa of the tube and of the hypomesotympanum has largely recovered and regenerated.

The resorption of the embryonic mesenchymal tissue depends on the manner in which the air-containing space of the middle ear cavity is shaped by ossification and a constant internal pressure. This determines how the mucosal folds develop relative to each other, how they are placed and how they regress.

The folds extend from the middle ear viscera to the walls of the middle ear and follow the blood vessels which supply it. The vessels enter the middle ear through the fissures and foramina, which thus determine the position of the folds.

Fig. **14   Serial 2 mm section of a decalcified temporal bone illuminated by a 30° endoscope introduced through the eustachian tube into the middle ear.** Photographs were taken with the Zeiss microscope from above, downward (Opmi 6 zoom automatic Contax camera). View from the tegmen tympani into the epitympanum toward the ossicles to assess their spatial arrangement and the mucosal folds more accurately

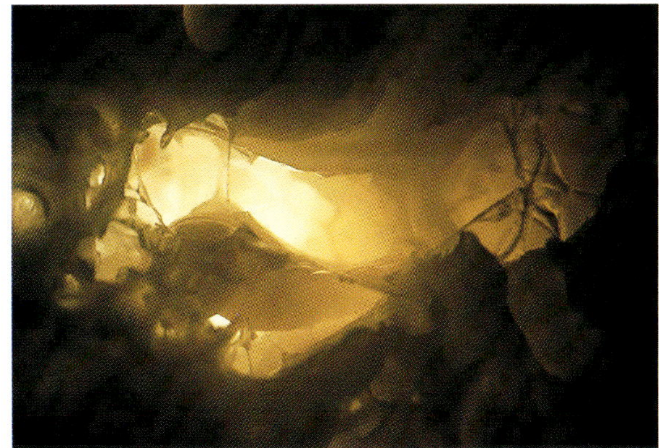

Fig. **15   Serial section of the same decalcified temporal bone shown in Fig. 14, but in this view, 2 mm more inferiorly.** The lateral wall of the epitympanum forms the upper border of the photograph, the medial wall with the divided semicircular canal below. The anterior wall of the epitympanum with the anterior crest is also cut. The protympanic recess is anterior to the head of the malleus, and the supratubal recess lies left and below it in the depth

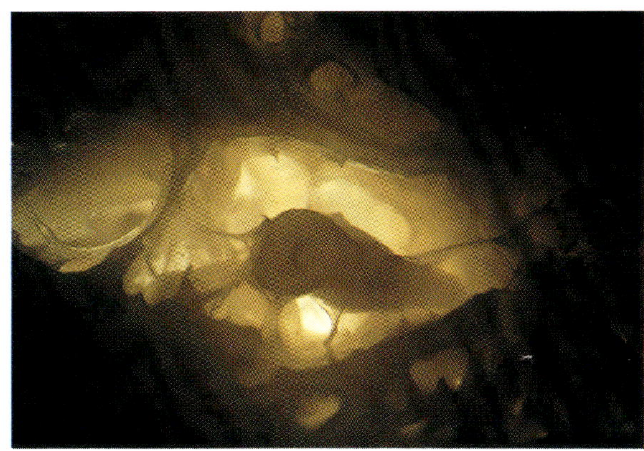

Fig. **16   Serial section of the same temporal bone shown in Fig. 14, but 4 mm inferiorly.** The divided neck of the malleus is shown above the middle, and the junction of the body and long process of the incus is shown below. There are numerous irregular mucosal folds between them and the walls of the epitympanum. This is the region of the tympanic diaphragm, here constricted by the folds

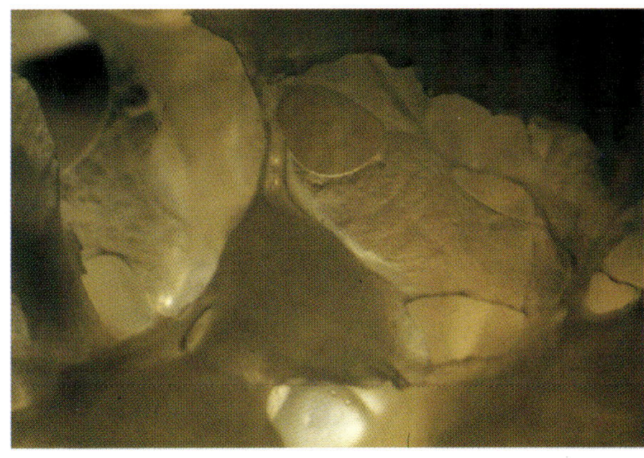

Obligate, Typically Localized Main Folds

The *tensor tympani fold* stretches between the tensor tympani tendon and its canal and the anterior mallear ligament. It encompasses the anterior process of the malleus as far as the transverse crest or the petrotympanic fissure. It divides the anterior segment of the tympanum into a supratubal and a protympanic recess. If the fold were not normally present, there would be a direct connection from the eustachian tube to the epitympanum, and its aeration would be provided not by a superior aeration pathway which branches at that point, but via an independent pathway bypassing the anterior tympanic isthmus. In fact the air flows inferior to the tensor tympani canal and around the cochleariform process via the anterior and posterior tympanic isthmus. According to Hammar (1902) the tensor tympani fold is only seldom absent; Siebenmann (1902) considers it to be often incompletely developed, whereas Aimi (1971) could not find it (possibly for pathological reasons) in 10% of specimens.

The following two folds are always present:

The *anterior fold of von Tröltsch* envelops the anterior mallear ligament, the anterior process and the neck of the malleus, and extends to the anterior tympanic stria as the anterior fold of the mallear ligament.

The *posterior fold of von Tröltsch* surrounds the chorda tympani and then unites with the *chorda tympani fold*. The chorda tympani can, however, run freely within the middle ear cavity from its eminence over the long process of the incus and possess its own independent fold.

The *lateral folds of the malleus and incus* extend between the head of the malleus and the body of the incus and the lateral epitympanic wall in two layers, one above the other. The mucosal folds of the lower layer can fuse with the anterior fold of the mallear ligament in the anterior segment. The folds of the upper layer can divide the epitympanum into a medial and a lateral segment, if the superior saccus has budded anteriorly, frontally and laterally during development.

These inferolateral mallear folds cover *Prussak's space* and form the floor of the *second tier*, i.e., the lateral epitympanic air cushion, which is limited superiorly by the superior mallear-incudal fold (Fig. **41**). Prussak's space forms the *inferior tier.*

The lateral incudal fold can be limited to its posterior part, which includes fibers of the posterior incudal ligament; it can then be regarded as the *posterior incudal fold.*

Obligate but Atypically Localized Folds

These subdivide the epitympanic space anteriorly, superiorly, medially and laterally, but not always in the same manner.

The *superior* and *inferior* malleosquamous folds are determined by connective tissue bundles containing blood vessels. Like the *lateral* mallear fold they belong to the system of membranous compartments lying above Prussak's space (Fig. **37**). They vary in number and size, and were first described by Politzer (1878).

The *medial incudal* and *mallear folds* run from the medial side of the ossicles to the medial wall of the epitympanum, dividing it into an anterior and posterior segment. These folds are responsible for the concealed growth of an anteromedial cholesteatoma isolated in the depths of the petrous bone, or of (p. 108) a posteromedial cholesteatoma in the antrum (p. 110).

Inconstant Folds

These are small folds that mainly lie around the long process of the incus as well as in front of and behind the oval niche, and extend to the pyramidal process and the facial canal.

There may be a *posterior,* a *superior,* and an *anterior stapedial fold* and an *obturator membrane* around the stapes, depending on the process of the budding of the three sacs (medius, posterior and superior). The *superior stapedial fold* can be a prolongation of the incudal fold; the others largely atrophy.

The *interossicular fold* bridges the space from the tensor tendon to the malleoincudal joint and the long process of the incus. The chorda tympani runs partially between its layers (von Tröltsch 1858; Hammar 1902). The interossicular fold is often absent in adults, but microsurgery has shown how frequent it is.

Koerner's Septum

During the development of the mastoid process, a thin bony partition can persist, lying in an almost sagittal plane at the site of the petrosquamous suture. However, the suture almost always fuses in such a manner that the communal antrum arises from a temporary petrosal and squamosal antrum; it is open to the epitympanum through the aditus. Persistence of this thin bony dividing wall to form a *petrosquamosal (Koerner's) septum* has great significance for the pathology of the middle ear. If this septum is present (Fig. **17**), the squamosal antrum is small. Drilling in this area is particularly difficult, due to increased hardness of the bone, and may also result in breakage of the, bony lid. The septum should therefore be borne in mind during antrotomy by the postaural or transmeatal route. The lid lies in this case rather superficial and gives the false impression that the inner cortex has already been reached. If the operation is carried out from the epitympanum and the Koerner's septum is not removed, the antrum remains unopened, whereas at an operation carried out from the mastoid, the epitympanum remains unopened.

If the bony lid breaks, the lateral part which belongs to the temporal squama is removed with it. The medial part belonging to the petrous temporal bone can then be drilled off and the cell system cleared. This loss of bone substance does not need to be replaced; on the contrary: removal of the septum produces a large air-containing antrum and can be beneficial to drainage.

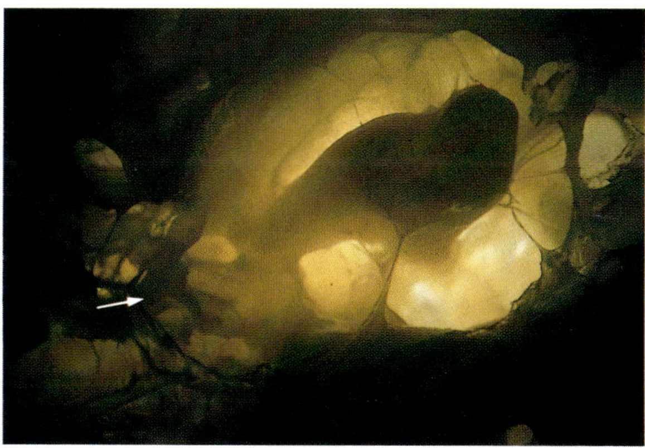

Fig. **17 Serial section of a decalcified temporal bone illuminated by a 30° endoscope introduced through the external meatus and observed from above through the Zeiss microscope.** A dividing wall lying horizontally, the Koerner's septum, can be seen at the entrance of the antrum indicated by an arrow

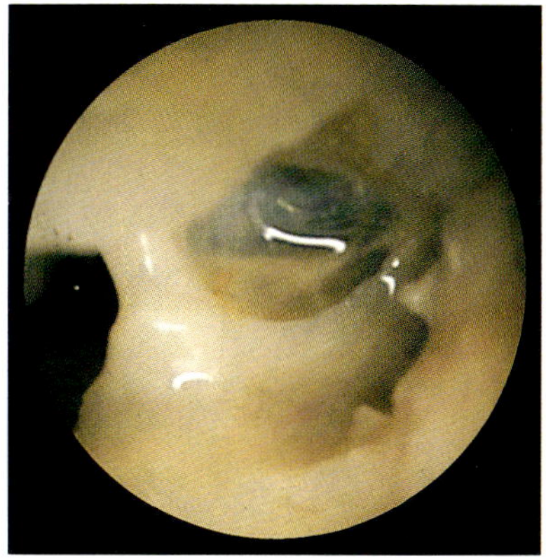

Fig. **18 Protympanic recess demonstrated endoscopically from the medial side of the ossicles.** In the depth, the tensor fold is shown, which in this preparation assumes a more frontal position. The same specimen as in Fig. **46**

Niches, Eminences and Recesses of the Middle Ear

The most anterior segment of the epitympanum acquires its final depth and breadth only after the growth of the zygomatic, tympanic and petrosal bones is complete. A cranial part can be distinguished at this point:
— the *protympanic recess* (Fig. **18**), which is divided by the tensor fold from the underlying.
— *supratubal recess* (Figs. **21, 25**), which is often interpreted as a widening of the tubal ostium.

During the study of the developmental history of the middle ear, particularly the spatial arrangement of the epitympanum, anatomists beginning with Hammar in 1902 have commented on the interdependence of the protympanic and supratubal recesses, which are both very underdeveloped in the infant. They only achieve their final size and depth in the second phase of growth of the temporal bone. They arise as a result of the formation of an air-containing space in the zone of the saccus medius and anterior. The tensor fold is formed at the point where the sacs meet. Their position is sometimes vertical and sometimes more oblique, depending on the development of the sacs. The saccus medius is the fastest to develop. If it extends far anteriorly, the tensor fold lies horizontally, and the protympanic recess, the space above it, is well formed. The saccus anterior, being the smallest, lags behind in its development. It extends only as far as the tensor canal and influences the formation of the anterior fold of von Tröltsch. However, if the saccus anterior

reaches the tegmen because the saccus medius is less well developed at this point, a large supratubal recess forms, often termed a tubal cell. Otherwise, it appears only as a further recess of the tympanic ostium of the tube. The position of the tensor fold in this case is more vertical; or it may remain rudimentary, in which case an anterior mallear fold forms between the anterior process of the malleus and the tegmen.

The space anterior to the head of the malleus is of great clinical significance. Its medial wall forms the sides of a triangle above the geniculate ganglion: anterior to the anterior crus of the anterior semicircular canal, superior to the tensor canal, and inferior to the cortex of the middle cranial fossa. If the bone is well pneumatized, the anterosuperior cell tract leads from here to the pyramidal apex. At this point (the anterior point of danger), a relatively uninfected choleastoma can invade the soft spongiosa deeply without causing symptoms, leading to very serious complications (H. L. Wullstein 1971).

The anatomy of the sinus tympani and the facial recess has become more familiar to surgeons because access is gained via a posterior tympanotomy in the closed techniques of tympanoplasty. Here the surgeon does not have a view of the protympanic and supratubal recesses, although they are of great importance in pathogenesis. Only the anatomy of the two areas considered together allows the surgeon to deduce the cause of the pathology in every case of otitis media.

The formation of the posterior and inferior segments of the middle ear cavity is mainly completed in the first rapid growth phase of the temporal bone between birth and the second year of life. During this phase the child learns to stand upright and to walk; the neck becomes stronger and develops more quickly than the skull. The tympanic membrane turns from its original, more horizontal, position to an oblique position; the tympanic ring rotates externally, due to the growth of the tympanic bone; the mastoid process develops; the antrum lies more deeply; the sternocleidomastoid muscle becomes more strongly developed; the *sinus tympani* (Figs. **19, 20**) is molded from the ossification centers of Reichert's cartilage; and the eustachian tube assumes its final position.

Proctor (1969) and Anson (1973) distinguish a more lateral part of the sinus tympani from a more posterior part which is very variable in size, depth and position. It is very important in operative surgery because it is one point of origin of recurrent or residual cholesteatoma. The *facial recess* lies between the chordal eminence and the second genu of the facial canal; the sinus tympani extends from this point inferiorly beyond the styloid eminence. In addition, these niches are divided from each other by small bridges with overhanging ledges. The ponticulus runs from the chordal eminence to the pyramidal eminence, an important anatomical landmark in facial decompression with preservation of the middle ear structures (H. L. Wullstein 1957); the intervening depression is termed Grivot's fossula.

The subiculum, the bony overhang which forms the round window niche, conducts the air stream through the inferior aeration pathway directly to the round window membrane. During dissection of the round window it may be necessary to drill this down, but drilling should be kept to a minimum to avoid disturbance of function. Such a situation is particularly difficult when removing cholesteatoma matrix from this recess, or very thin epidermis in an atelectatic ear or in an adhesive process. If the facial recess is connected to Poganny's cell, (a very large periantral pneumatized cell), then it is probable that the matrix cannot be removed without an undercut.

The relationship between the position of the two window niches and the declination or inclination of the petrous bone, and hence the size of the sphenoidal angle, is also of interest. Šercer and Krmpotić (1960) confirmed this correlation with the angulation of the skull base by measurements on anatomical preparations of the skull and temporal bone. For this reason Padovan (1961) recommends a preoperative mediosagittal radiograph of the skull to determine the position of the windows (and thus the depth of the sinus tympani) based on measurements of the sphenoid-clivus angle. Saito et al. (1971) measured the depth of the sinus tympani using serial histological preparations and found it to be very deep in the black races. It is well known that the sphenoid-clivus angle in these races is larger, as is the piriform aperture of the nose.

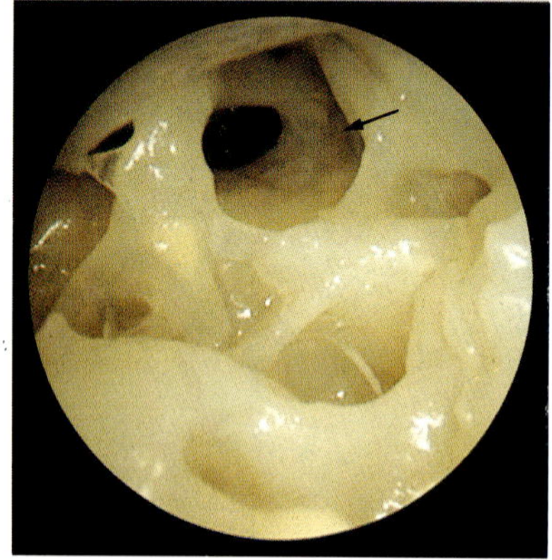

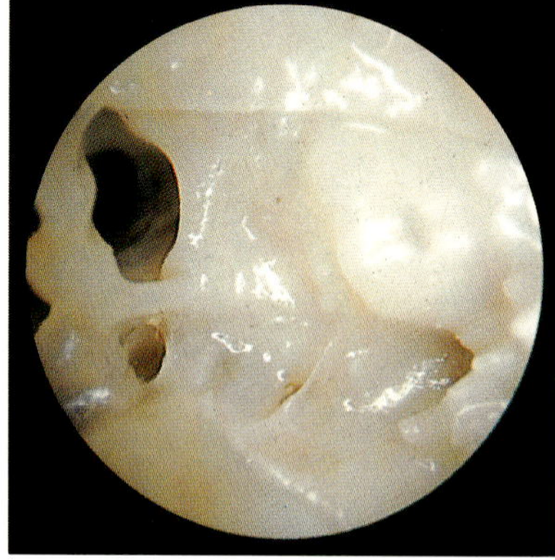

19   **20**

Fig. **19** **Sinus tympani with many deep niches, overhanging ledges and small bridges.** The posterior tympanic isthmus is marked by an arrow, and is wide open

Fig. **20** In contrast to Fig. **19**, the sinus tympani here is shallower. A niche extends inferior to the vertical course of the facial nerve

Aeration and Drainage System of the Middle Ear (Figs. 21–22)

First and Second Narrowing in the Aeration System of the Middle Ear

Osteoplastic epitympanotomy showed clearly that aeration of the middle ear system is regulated by two narrowings:
- the eustachian tube forms the *first narrowing;*
- the *second narrowing* is formed by the tympanic diaphragm between the anterior and posterior segments of the middle ear, one of the boundaries between the first and second branchial arches.

The second narrowing is a bottleneck at the junction of the mesotympanum and the epitympanum. It lies at the level of the tympanic segment of the facial nerve running between the cochleariform process and the incudal fossa. This second narrowing is determined by the stapes, the stapedial tendon, the pyramidal process and the long process of the incus. It is divided by a series of variable mucosal folds into an anterior and a posterior tympanic isthmus: this bottleneck is termed the tympanic diaphragm. The function of this second narrowing is to collect and consolidate the air of both aeration pathways before it is conducted further into the epitympanum and the retrotympanic spaces. Also, it protects against sudden evacuation, against suction from the posterior segment and from a fall of pressure until the next physiological refill with the requisite air mixture. In this way it helps to maintain a constant air pressure in the middle ear. Whereas the *exchange of fresh air* is limited to the anterior segment of the middle ear, only reserve air is to be found in the posterior segment. The latter is connected with all the mastoid spaces and can be very extensive. Air which has already been humidified and warmed anteriorly in the hypomesotympanum gradually fills the posterior segment only so far as is necessary to replace air lost by absorption. For this reason, healthy mucosa at this point requires almost no glands. Excretion from these inaccessible spaces is thus hardly necessary.

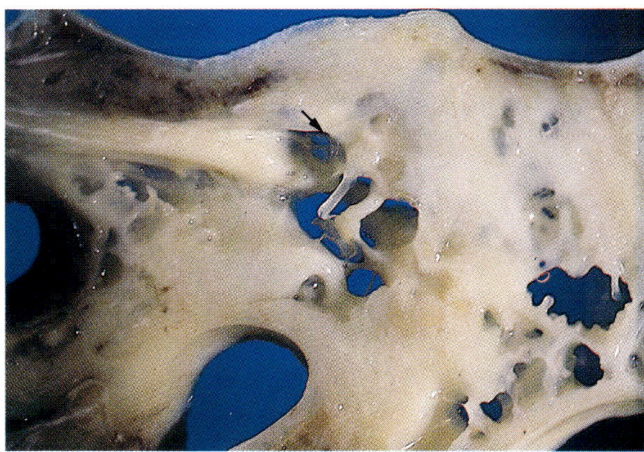

Fig. **21   Coronal serial section of a decalcified temporal bone (2 mm)** to demonstrate the relative position of the supratubal recess (as shown by an arrow) to the middle ear outline with the aeration pathways

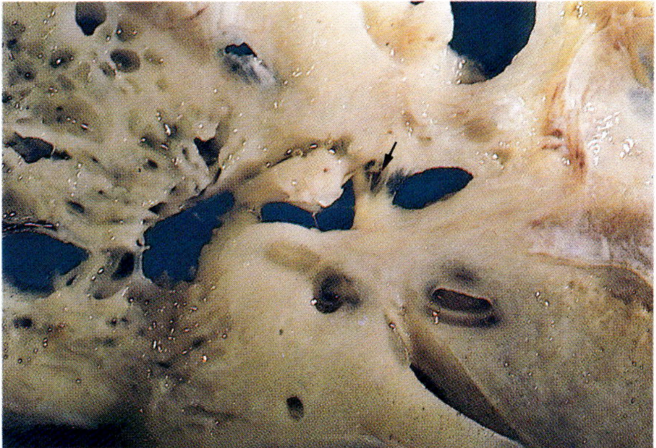

Fig. **22   Horizontal serial section of the temporal bone.** The superior part of the head of the malleus and body of the incus are divided and removed, as is a part of the tensor fold (marked with an arrow). Below and in front of them lie the supratubal recess and the tympanic ostium of the tube. The protympanic recess lies above the tensor fold

Anterior and Posterior Segments in the Aeration System of the Middle Ear

The pathological appearances found during operation can be correlated with the anatomy of the middle ear and its variations. For this purpose the entire pneumatic system of the temporal bone can be divided into two segments:
– the *anterior segment*, formed by the eustachian tube and the hypomesotympanum;
– the *posterior segment*, consisting of the epitympanum and the retrotympanic spaces.

The dividing line between these two segments is formed by the tympanic diaphragm and the tympanic isthmi. Subdivision into two segments is useful on both anatomical and functional grounds. In the anterior segment the air is channelled intermittently through the first narrowing into the middle ear, and then conducted through the middle ear along the aeration pathways to the functionally important sites. Before the air leaves the anterior sector it accumulates in front of the second narrowing and is then conducted to *Prussak's space*, the epitympanum, and the retrotympanic spaces. Here the air surrounds the ossicles, fills the air cushions and then permeates the air-cell system. Conditions in the posterior segment are much more static than in the anterior part. This area is separated from the permanent tubal opening, and the air exchange is much less. The air thus becomes adapted to its environment and is at a constant temperature und humidity. The demands upon the mucosa are much fewer in the posterior segment and the number of ciliated and goblet cells is correspondingly smaller. The air is only slowly absorbed here and requires only to be refilled. It may be called "reserve air", in the sense in which this term is used in the physiology of the respiratory tract. The aditus and antrum also have audiological significance in the presence of standing waves in the mesohypotympanum.

Tympanic Diaphragm, Anterior and Posterior Tympanic Isthmus

(Figs. **23–31**)
As a rule, air cannot reach the epitympanum directly from the eustachian tube. First of all, it encounters the supratubal recess and the tensor fold, and is deflected inferiorly via the inferior aeration pathway to pass through the tympanic diaphragm and thereafter to refill the posterior sector of the middle ear (Fig. **23**).

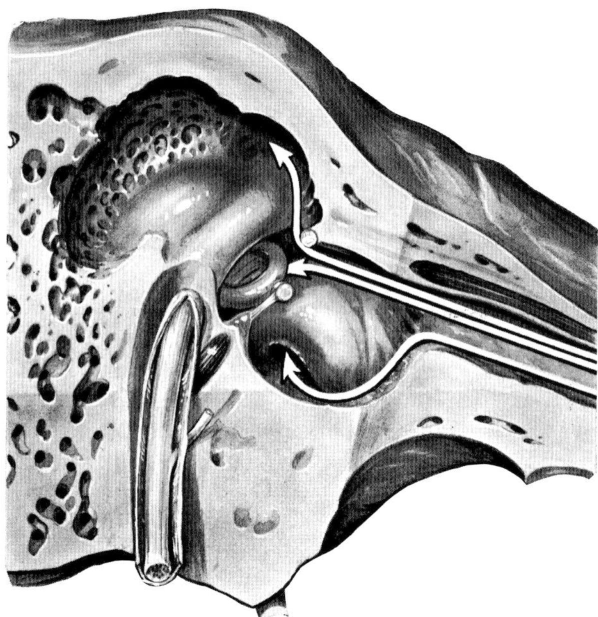

Fig. **23**　**Aeration pathways** (H. L. Wullstein 1952)

The air is warmed and humidified along this short pathway from the nasopharynx via the eustachian tube to the diaphragm by the goblet cells and the mucus-producing glands. The density of ciliary and goblet cells is determined by the physiological demands of warming and humidifying the air and regulation of the internal pressure. The population of these cells falls progressively toward the posterior segment (Fig. **24**).

The aeration and secretory pathways are identical so that mucociliary clearance is via the same route. Breakdown products accumulate at the functionally most important areas of the middle ear which the air stream actively reaches. These are: 1. the oval window reached via the upper aeration pathway; and 2. the round window, lying deeply and presenting a funnel shape toward the lower aeration pathway. Therefore a higher concentration of ciliated and mucus-producing elements is necessary to aid clearance in the anterior sector and particularly along the aeration and secretory pathways. After the incoming air has been warmed, humidified, filtered, etc., in the anterior segment, it accumulates in front of the tympanic diaphragm. The reserve air in the air cushions of the epitympanum and the antrum is passively refilled as necessary at this point. If the air flow continued actively into the posterior segment, the entire mucociliary clearance system of the segment would be overloaded and would cease to function, as happens in an effusion, because the mucosa of the posterior segment possesses almost no morphological prerequisites for self-cleansing.

At the point where the air leaves the tube at the tympanic tubal ostium, it is directed along the canal of the tensor tympani muscle in two directions. One leads directly to the tensor canal, to the anterior tympanic isthmus and to the beginning of the oval niche in the deep groove inferior to the tensor canal (the upper aeration pathway) (Fig. 25). The other is directed toward the tensor fold, where it is intercepted in the supratubal recess and diverted into the lower aeration pathway. This pathway leads through the anterior mesohypotympanic tunnel (Fig. 23) around the promontory to the deepest part of the hypotympanum and beyond it into the round window niche.

Because the umbo of the tympanic membrane lies very close to the bulge of the medial wall of the middle ear (Fig. 26), the air is forced to flow around the promontory along the hypotympanum and further posteriorly and superiorly directly into the round window niche and the sinus tympani. The postulate that the promontory has arisen solely to accomodate the basal turn of the cochlea is thus incorrect. More importantly, it serves to direct the main mass of air to the round window. This explains the position of the round window membrane relative to the oval window, and the presence of the subiculum (Fig. 27).

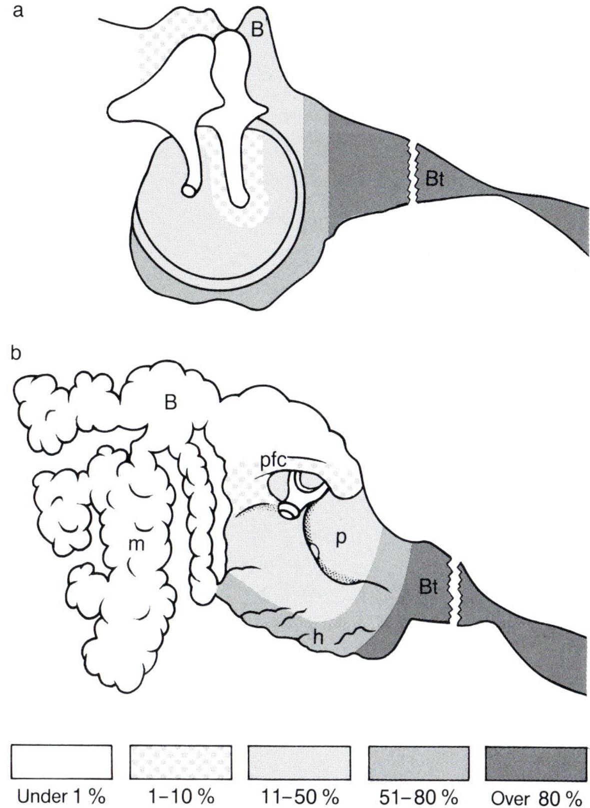

Fig. **24** **The drainage pathways of the middle ear.** The distribution of ciliated cells is shown as described by Lim (1972)

pfc tympanic diaphragm;
Bt eustachian tube;
B antrum;
h hypotympanum;
m mastoid
p promontory;

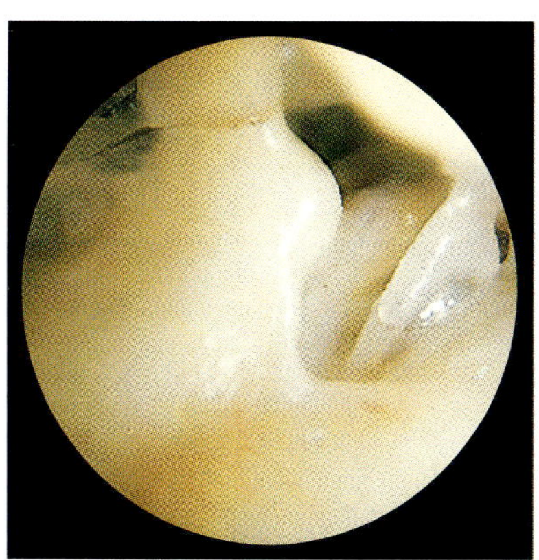

Fig. **25** The upper aeration pathway leads directly beneath the tensor canal around it to the anterior tympanic isthmus and to the oval niche with the stapes. At that point the tegmen tympani can be recognized lying deeply. The obturator membrane extends between the stapedial crura

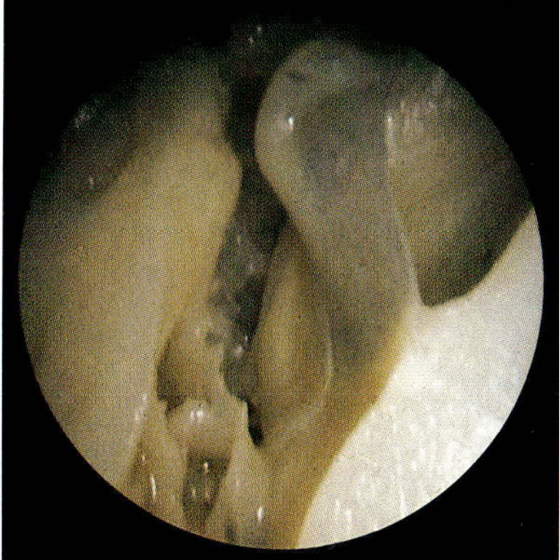

Fig. **26** **The anterior segment of the mesohypotympanic tunnel.** The following points should be observed:
1. the proximity of the umbo to the wall of the promontory of the middle ear; 2. the depth of the hypotympanum with the hypotympanic cells, compared to the depth of the anterior tympanomeatal angle lateral to the tympanic membrane

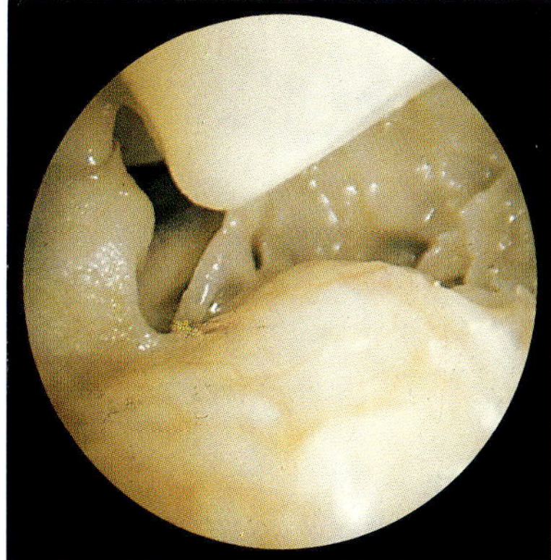

Fig. **27** **View of the tympanic diaphragm from the anterior hypotympanum.** It should be noticed how close the conus of the tympanic membrane lies to the promontory. The deep niche in the tympanic sinus lies to the right of the projection of the promontory

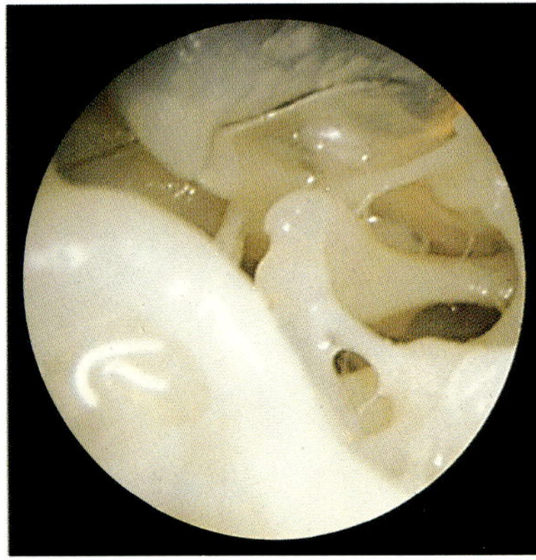

Fig. **28**   **View of the posterior tympanic isthmus and the round window niche with the subiculum.** The entry port to the lateral epitympanic air cushions lies between the pyramidal process, the long process of the incus and the chorda tympani with its fold

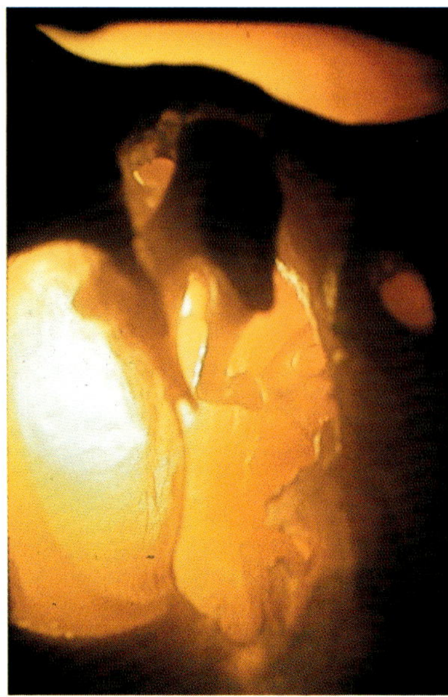

Fig. **29**   **Vertical serial section through the middle ear.** The deep hypotympanum is of greater significance for the perfect function of the middle ear than the depth of the meatal fundus. Any obstruction of the lower aeration pathway, for example, in a high jugular bulb, accordingly severely affects the capacity of the aeration system of the middle ear (see text, p. 24)

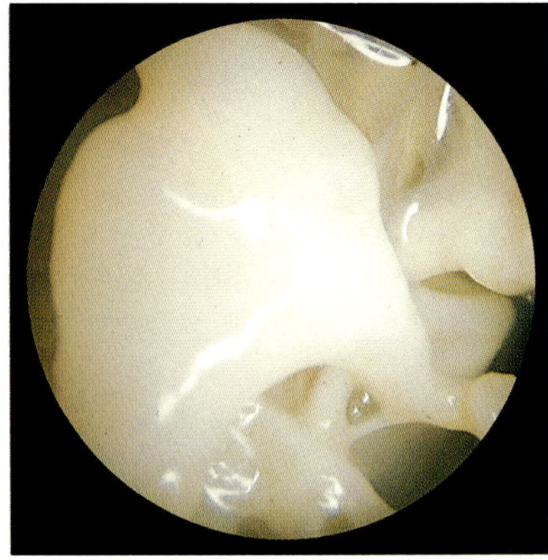

Fig. **30**   **Endoscopic view of the medial surface of the ossicular chain, the diaphragm with the tensor fold and the entrance to the lateral epitympanic air cushions.**

The following conclusions can be drawn from the above findings:

The air accumulating in front of the tympanic diaphragm is conducted in several directions for aeration of the posterior segment as shown in Figure **23**:

1. The most superior current of air branches off the upper aeration pathway and leads around the cochleariform process and the tensor tendon through the anterior isthmus in a medial and frontal direction to the protympanic recess and to the medial side of the head of the malleus, depending on the anatomy of the malleoincudal fold.

2. Part of the air flows past the anterior isthmus inferior to the neck of the malleus, the posterior fold of von Tröltsch and inferior to the long process of the incus. Here it is deflected by the chorda tympani and its folds, and reaches the entrance to Prussak's space and aerates this cul-de-sac from behind.

3. Part of the air which reaches the diaphragm comes along the facial ridge via the superior aeration pathway and mixes with air from the lower aeration pathway leaving via the sinus tympani at the exit from the oval niche. This mixed air flow passes the second narrowing mainly through the posterior tympanic isthmus. Together the airstreams envelop the ossicles from the medial side and refill the antrum, where air is lost due to absorption by the extensive mucosal surfaces.

The term "tympanic diaphragm" is of long standing. The accumulation of mucosal folds in the space between the tympanic segment of the facial nerve and the long process of the incus, the stapes and the tensor canal was described for the first time as "le diaphragme inter-attico-tympanique" by Chatelier and Lemoine in 1946, and they comment that it was known to Sexton in 1888. Stimulated by the problems of acute otitis media in neonates and infants, Chatelier and Lemoine prepared sections from the temporal bone of patients of this age group and viewed them serially by stereoscopy. In patients this young they

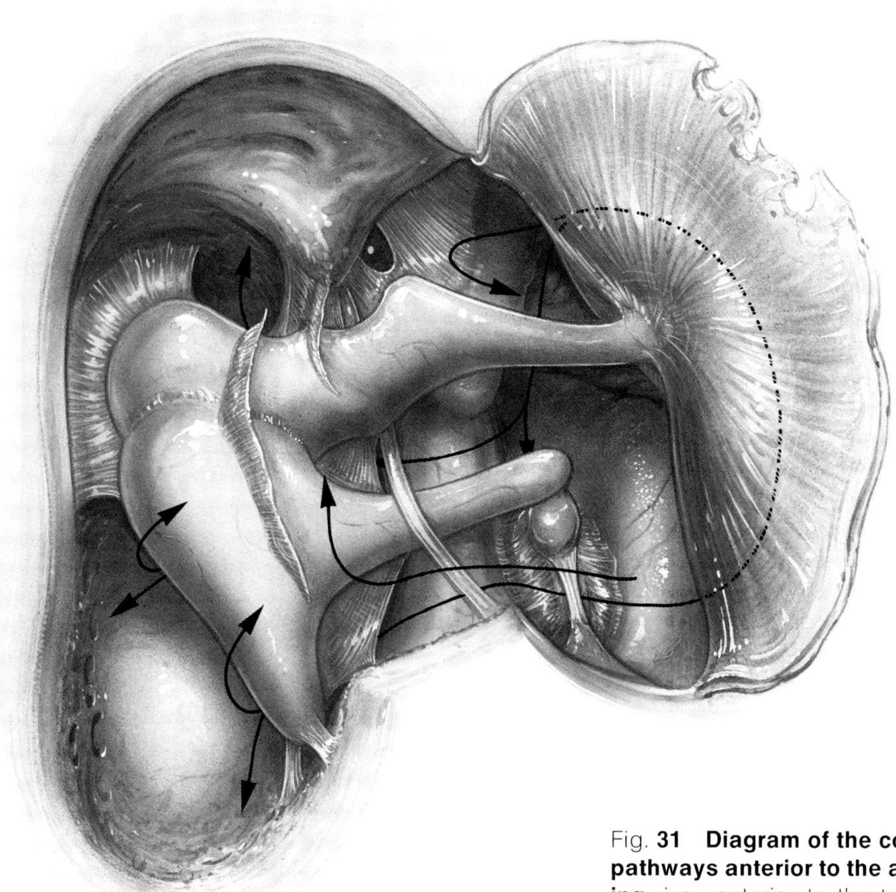

Fig. **31   Diagram of the composition of the aeration pathways anterior to the area of the second narrowing**, i.e., anterior to the tympanic diaphragm and its prolongation to the epitympanum

could only observe one opening through the folds passing to the epitympanum, i.e., the anterior tympanic isthmus bounded by the long process of the incus, the stapes and the cochleariform process with the tensor tendon. A posterior tympanic isthmus is absent at this age. The mucosal folds of the diaphragm are thick in the neonate because a lot of embryonal mesenchyme is still retained within the stroma. *Ossification* and the formation of an air-containing space are not yet complete, and the entire posterior segment is aerated solely via the anterior isthmus. The antrum is still larger than one cell, and pneumatization is almost absent.

Although the system of folds has been known to anatomists since Hammar's description in 1902, it was scarcely mentioned in otological textbooks until the last decade. The epithelium of the middle ear is sometimes said to consist only of flat endotheliod cells, and sometimes of a thin single layer of cuboidal epithelium, with ciliated cells only in the tympanic ostium of the eustachian tube. The high degree of structural differentiation of the mucosa in the various segments of the middle ear cavity and its functional significance were not recognized in earlier years. Interest was stimulated by the increasing frequency of

middle ear effusions and their sequelae, by the unsatisfactory antibiotic treatment of otitis media, and especially by the increasing interest in immunological and allergic disorders of the mucosa of the upper airways, including the middle ear. Proctor (1964), Bollobas (1972) and now also Aimi (1971) have stimulated interest with their impressive illustrations.

The diaphragm may be well or poorly developed, and the apertures of the tympanic isthmi may be of various widths. They are subject, like all other regions of the middle ear, to the factors which are decisive in the shaping of the outline of the middle ear.

The following is an example: If the sigmoid sinus is displaced far forward and the bulb of the internal jugular vein lies high within the floor of the middle ear, the curvature of the external meatus is more marked because the free development and shaping of the tympanic bone are prevented. Accordingly, the superior ends of the tympanic ring which form the anterior and posterior tympanic spines are closer together, and the tympanic notch between them is smaller. The cochleariform process and the tensor tendon lie closer to the posterior wall of the middle ear and its incudal fossa, the pyramidal process and the eminences (pyramidal, chordal and styloid). The space in which the mucosal folds belonging to the tympanic diaphragm extend is much narrower. In such cases a low middle fossa dura is to be expected, and the ossicular chain is smaller in size.

The *anterior tympanic isthmus* is the earliest air space connecting the mesohypotympanum and the epitympanum. It is bounded by the tensor fold and the tensor tendon anteriorly and by the anterior crus of the stapes and the long process of the incus posteriorly. It thus belongs to the zone of the saccus medius. From the point of view of development, it is the oldest, and often the only, connection of the epitympanum and the retrotympanic space with the anterior segment.

The *posterior tympanic isthmus* is bounded by the stapes, the stapedial tendon and the posterior part of the sinus tympani, and forms an important section of the lower aeration pathway. It opens into the facial recess and the incudal fossa. It is the portal of entry to Prussak's space and to the air cushions (vibration dampers) lateral to the ossicles, which can only be aerated from this point.

In some cases, however, if *ossification* and the formation of the air space do not proceed uniformly, and resorption of the mesenchymal tissue is delayed, several mucosal folds may persist so that the posterior isthmus is not open. The air can then only reach the posterior segment through the anterior isthmus. In others, the formation of the air-containing space may proceed smoothly, and a broad connection develops between the two segments. It is not possible then to speak of an anterior and a posterior isthmus, but only of a wide opening in the diaphragm. Aimi (1971) claims that there is only one tympanic isthmus.

Relation of the Sigmoid Sinus and the Jugular Venous Bulb to the Tympanum and the Retrotympanic Spaces
(Figs. **32–36**)

The size of the air-containing space of the anterior segment of the middle ear space is mainly determined by the formation of its posteroinferior part, i.e., the depth and breadth of the hypotympanum, the internal and posterior tympanic sinus, the facial recess and the posterior tympanic isthmus. The configuration of these walls depends on the growth of the tympanic bone, and on the position of the bulb of the internal jugular vein. The sigmoid sinus can be displaced far forward and join a high jugular bulb at an acute angle. The hypotympanum is then absent (Fig. **36**), and the entrance to the round window niche is obstructed.

The forward displacement of the sinus leads to rotation of Trautmann's triangle from an almost sagittal to a more inferior plane, which then makes postaural access to the middle ear difficult. The danger of damage to a high jugular venous bulb at

paracentesis, tympanoscopy or even tympanoplasty is great, and the eradication of sublabyrinthine cells or cells in the sinodural angle is very difficult.

Evaluation of the lower part of the middle ear through the facial-chordal angle, clearance of adherent matrix from the tympanic sinus and the facial recess under vision, and introduction of an allogenic en bloc middle ear transplant via an extended posterior control window at posterior tympanotomy are all difficult or impossible.

Such ears are very susceptible to slight variations in air pressure due to the reduction of the air-containing volume of the anterior segment of the middle ear system. If, in addition, the middle ear mucosa is inflamed, producing edema, infiltration, hyperplasia and exudate, then the air-containing volume of the middle ear cavity is even less, and the danger of damage to the tympanic membrane (the only wall of the middle ear which can compensate for changes in air pressure) is great. The inflammation rapidly extends to the system of folds in the tympanic diaphragm, so that the epitympanum and antrum are cut off from their aeration and drainage systems, and mucociliary clearance is paralyzed. Herein lies the genesis of recurrent middle ear effusions leading to atelectasis, adhesive processes, tympanosclerosis and even cholesteatoma.

Anteromedial displacement of the sigmoid sinus with a high jugular venous bulb brings the jugular fossa close to the cochlear canaliculus, and in a superomedial direction, close to the aperture of the endolymphatic sac, the subarcuate fossa and the entrance to the internal auditory meatus. The two latter anatomical relationships narrow the translabyrinthine access, whether for diagnostic endoscopy of the cerebellopontine angle or for the removal of an acoustic neuroma. The danger of bleeding from the accessory veins is increased because the opening of the inferior petrosal sinus can be displaced.

The most serious results of a high jugular bulb are:
1. obstruction of the inferior aeration pathway;
2. narrowing of the tympanic diaphragm and the posterior tympanic isthmus, which is the pathway for air to the epitympanum and antrum.

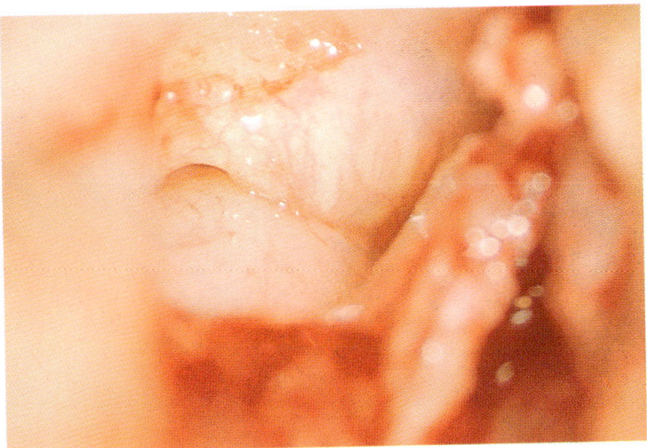

Fig. 32 Osteoplastic epitympanotomy for a large cholesteatoma with deep retraction of the atrophic pars tensa into the facial recess and erosion of the epitympanic wall. A view of the hypotympanum is shown. There is obstruction of the lower aeration pathway due to a high jugular bulb. The round window is slitlike, but open. These are the operative findings of the patient shown in Fig. **33**

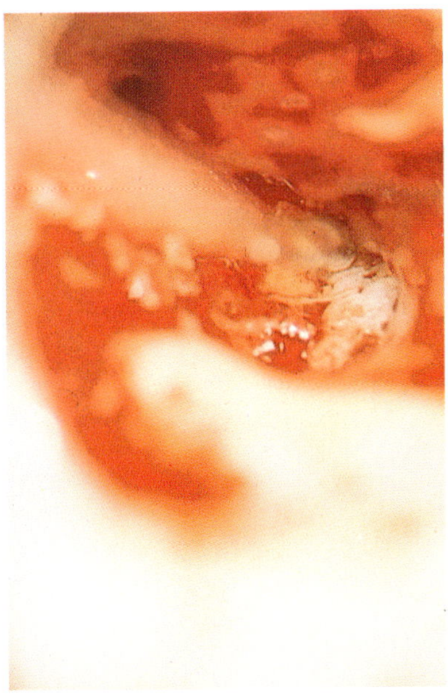

Fig. 34 Osteoplastic epitympanotomy. A high jugular bulb is covered only with thin connective layers, producing a blue transparent appearance. The operative findings are of the patient shown in Fig. **35**

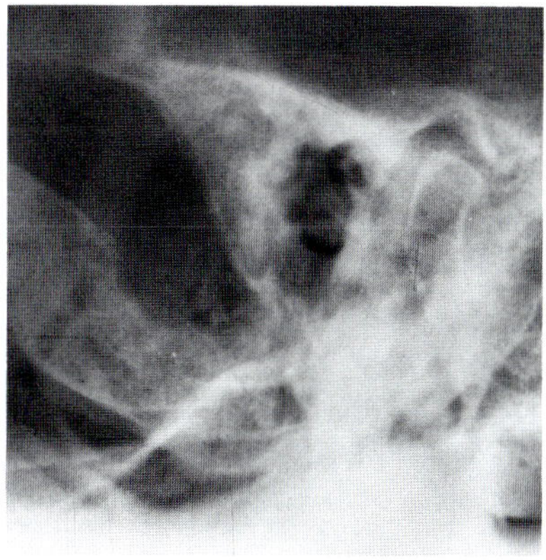

Fig. 33 Preoperative radiograph in Schueller's view with marked anterior displacement of the sinus and a high jugular bulb. The dura of the middle cranial fossa is low. the zygomatic arch is very narrow and the protympanum is low

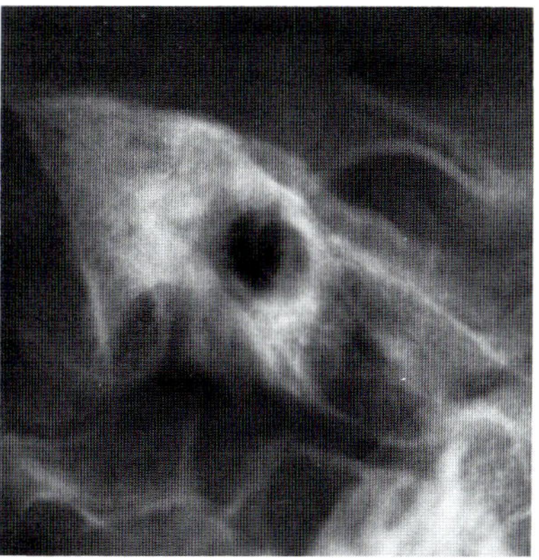

Fig. 35 Preoperative Schueller's view showing a high jugular bulb, and a nonpneumatized bone. An atrophic adherent tympanic membrane with a small defect in Shrapnell's membrane and a lateral tympanic cholesteatoma can be seen. The outline of the tympanic bone should be observed. The high jugular bulb prevented physiological displacement of the tympanic bone anteriorly and inferiorly in the phase of ossification and development

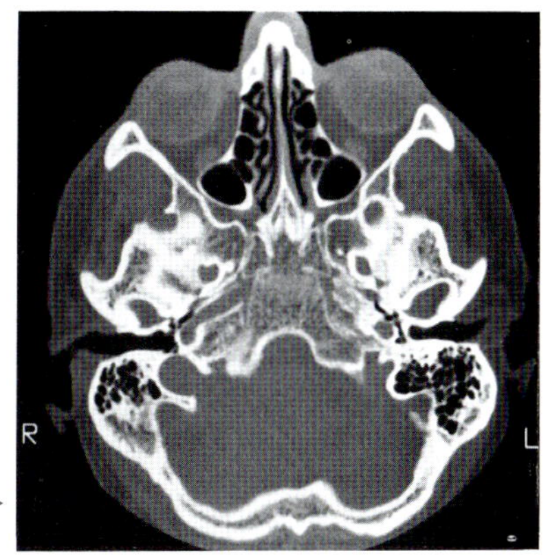

Fig. 36 Axial CT view of a high jugular bulb and ▷ narrow caroticobulbar angle

Epitympanic Air Cushions (Figs. 37–56)

In 1878 Politzer wrote in his textbook of otology that he had found a system of spaces in the ligaments running from the wall of the middle ear cavity to the malleus. Their arrangement is shown in Figure **37**. Furthermore he said that these spaces were limited medially by the neck of the malleus, inferiorly by the upper surface of the lateral process of the malleus (k), laterally by Shrapnell's membrane and superiorly by the superior mallear ligament. They consist of a very variable number of small and large cavities with round and oval boundaries which, like the large cavity(r) above the lateral process, have an epithelial lining and occasionally form the seat of a very obstinate inflammatory process, accompanied by perforation of Shrapnell's membrane. Politzer was thus one of the first to realize the anatomical significance of this part of the middle ear.

The mallear folds stretching between the internal surface of the lateral epitympanic wall and the lateral surface of the ossicles, the folds of von Tröltsch, the chorda tympani folds and Shrapnell's membrane together form the air-containing compartments arranged in two tiers, the so-called "epitympanic air cushions." Their size reflects the previous pneumatization processes. The outward displacement of Shrapnell's membrane when sound enters the middle ear and when the air in the ear is refilled is always accompanied by tension on the folds and

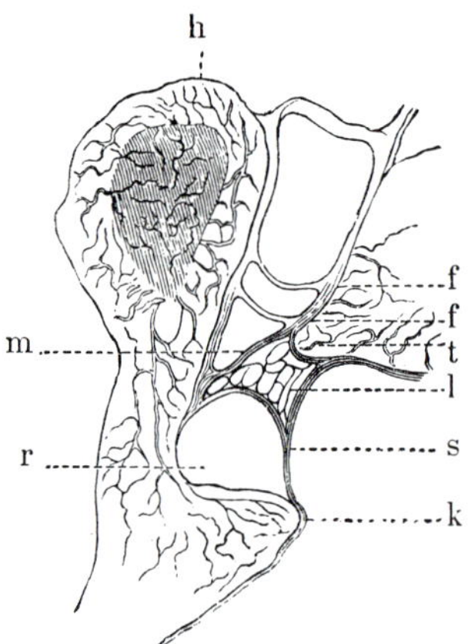

Fig. **37 System of cavities between the tympanic membrane and the neck of the malleus** (l). Inconstant mucosal folds (f, f), short process of the malleus (k), membrana flaccida (s) (Pollitzer 1878)

increase of internal pressure in the air cushions. A division of the tympanic membrane into pars tensa and pars flaccida in the calculation of the mechanics of the middle ear is inadequate. The action of Shrapnell's membrane should be considered along with its enclosed epitympanic air cushions.

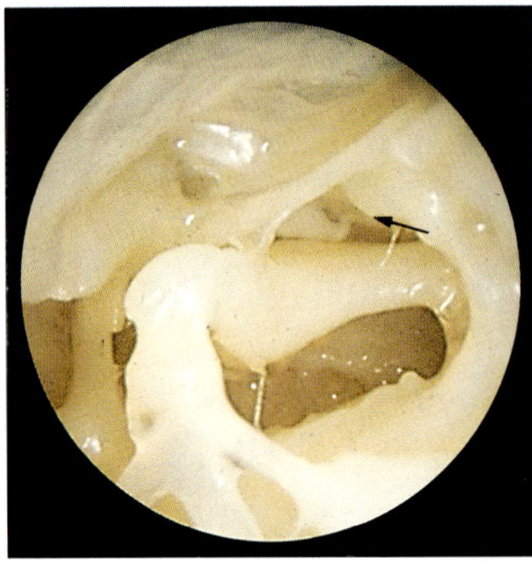

Fig. **38 The posterior tympanic isthmus.** The entrance to Prussak's space is marked with an arrow. Endoscopic view taken from the sinus tympani

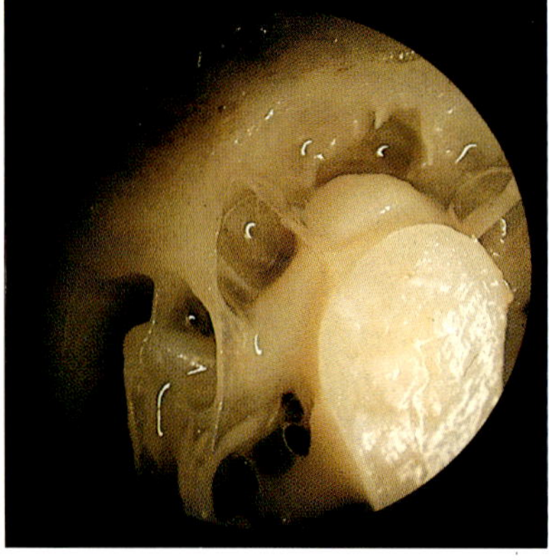

Fig. **39 Vertical serial section through the lateral epitympanic air cushions** (lateral to medial view of an illuminated 4-mm-thick serial section of the right temporal bone). The lateral mallear fold forms the roof of Prussak's space to the highest point of which the lateral mallear ligament extends. Above this lies the nearest air cushion, limited superiorly by the lateral malleoincudal fold. The floor of Prussak's space is formed by the anterior and posterior folds of von Troeltsch

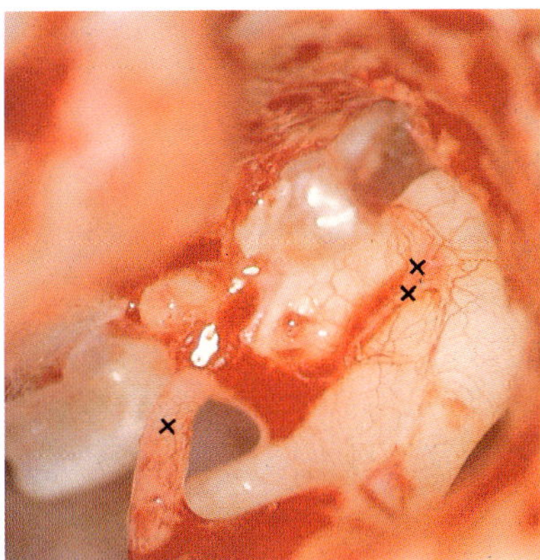

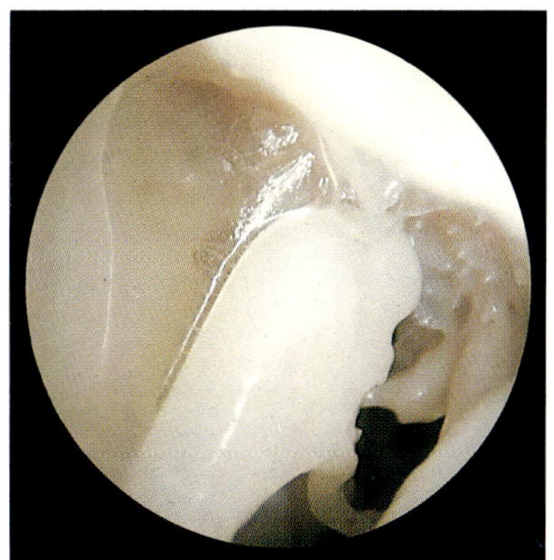

Fig. **40 Osteoplastic epitympanotomy.** Open epitympanum with intact ossicular chain after removal of a thick block of granulations in the tympanic diaphragm lateral to the ossicles. x = chorda tympani, xx = insertion of the lateral mallear fold which covers the superior layer of air cushions. The arrow shows the insertion of the lateral mallear folds which cover Prussak's space

Fig. **41 Posteroanterior view of the epitympanum taken from the aditus and antrum**. The protympanic recess lies anterior to the head of the malleus. In the depth and medial to the ossicles lies the tympanic diaphragm. The lateral malleoincudal fold is stretched lateral to the ossicles, and closes the lateral epitympanic space tightly. The space superior to this fold, extending to the tegmen tympani, is called the "recessus culiminis" by anatomists; it can only be provided with air from the medial side

The tympanic isthmus and the lateral epitympanic air cushions act as a one-way valve in the process of air exchange in the two segments against reflux and particularly against a sudden loss of gas and a fall of pressure behind the tympanic diaphragm; for example, during yawning. They function synchronously as a bottleneck through which pressure rises in front of the tympanic diaphragm when the air is refilled in the anterior segment of the middle ear when the eustachian tube opens, and through which gas absorbed in the posterior segment is continually replaced.

In this way, two systems arise for the aeration of the epitympanum, medial and lateral to the ossicles which interact in the maintenance of the internal pressure. In the horizontal plane the diaphragm also divides the middle ear into two systems which lie on both sides of the vibratory axis, one fixed relatively firmly to the stapedial and tensor tendons, the other in the epitympanum, consisting of the incus and malleus supported only by the ligaments and the air cushions.

The number and arrangement of the mucosal folds finally determine how the air in the epitympanum is distributed further. In every case the air follows the developmental pathway of the sacs which were responsible for the formation of the air spaces of the middle ear. Later it is then possible to deduce from the position and number of the mucosal folds whether the two processes implicated in pneumati-

zation (ossification and formation of an air space) proceeded normally during the first postnatal phase. From the point of view of developmental biology, a third factor, which is critical in pneumatization, has to be considered; namely, the internal pressure and the filling with gas in the infantile phase. If the diaphragm is narrow, the isthmi will also be smaller. If they are bounded by numerous supplementary accessory folds, for example, the interossicular folds (see Fig. **16**), they close more quickly if the pressure in the middle ear cavity falls and the folds swell. The epithelium of the folds undergoes metaplasia and their surfaces produce more secretions. The vessels in their stroma dilate; an extravasate and a very vascular infiltrate are formed. The overloaded mucociliary clearance system breaks down, the folds adhere, the isthmi block and the air cushions disappear. This may be expressed alternatively as follows: if ossification and formation of the air space do not proceed uniformly and the resorption of the mesenchymal tissue is delayed because the continuous refilling with air in the sac system fails, the system of folds persists, and the posterior isthmus in the region of the diaphragm does not open at all. Air can then only reach the posterior segment through the anterior isthmus. Deficient refilling leads to reduction in the internal pressure, so that the pneumatization process slows down, and the posterior segment remains underdeveloped. The volume of the retrotympanum is

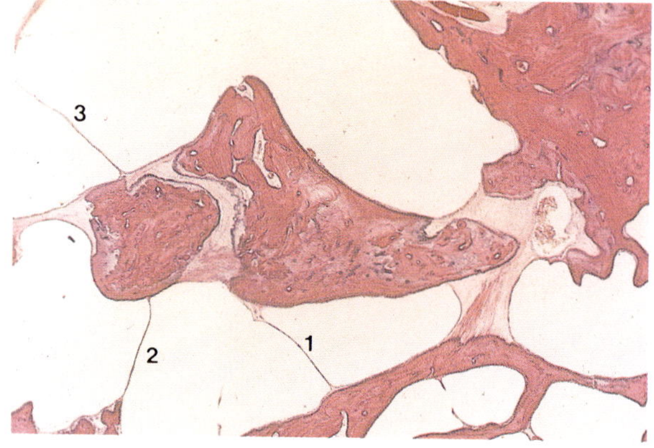

Fig. **42 Horizontal section through the epitympa-num of an adult human.** 1 = lateral incudal fold, 2 = lateral mallear fold, 3 = medial incudal fold

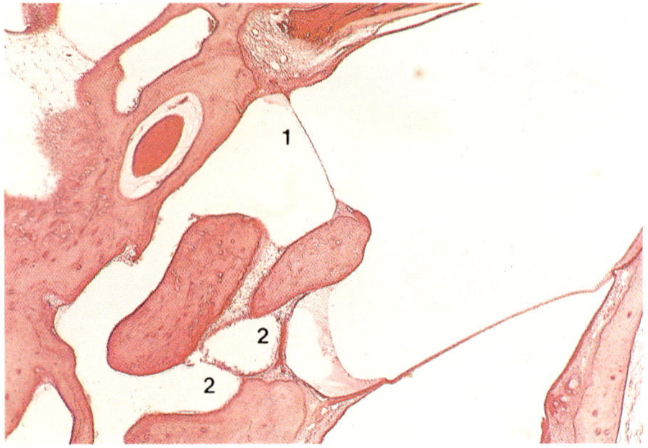

Fig. **43 Horizontal section through the epitympa-num of a squirrel monkey.** 1 = tensor fold, 2 = lateral mallear and incudal folds

small, and its access narrow; its later damaging effect is made even greater by marked variation in air pressure.

The body's powers of resistance develop during the important second phase of the three infantile developmental phases of the temporal bone and the shaping of the pneumatic middle ear spaces, when ossification and the formation of an air space proceed more slowly. The lining of the middle ear and the mucosal folds with their double epithelial surfaces and their loose stroma rich in blood vessels play a vital role in the degree of the response to internal and external stimuli.

If the tissues in the posterior segment have been in contact with each other and the potential space can be refilled with air because the isthmi are open again, scar tissue bands and adhesions can remain in the second narrowing, reducing the original size of the opening. The refilling of the epitympanum and the retrotympanic spaces with air remains at risk, even if the middle ear appears to be functionally normal. It now responds briskly to even smaller variations in air pressure. It becomes atelectatic; initially, with a very atrophic and indrawn tympanic membrane; later, with an adhesive process with pronounced retractions due to the folds, and all the sequelae, such as a retraction cholesteatoma.

We know from comparative anatomy that primates possess a very similar construction of pneumatic membranes in the epitympanum: their arrangement in the space lateral to the malleus and incus complex corresponds exactly to that in man (Figs. **42**, **43**). The malleus and incus are formed from the primary mandible during the developmental phases of the infant so that they can vibrate freely at every frequency which the infant needs for acoustic perception of its environment.

Parallel with this development, the axis of rotation of the ossicles is displaced further and further from their center of mass. The air custions are formed in this lightweight construction at the points where the greatest weight and vibrations are received. These are:

1. on inward movement of the handle of the malleus anchored within the tympanic membrane;
2. on inward rotation of the mass of the ossicular chain in the epitympanum.

Fig. **44 Schüller's view of a well-pneumatized middle ear.** The series of small pneumatized cells arranged like a chain of pearls surrounds the outline of the base of the pyramid and defines the superior and posterior surfaces of the pyramid

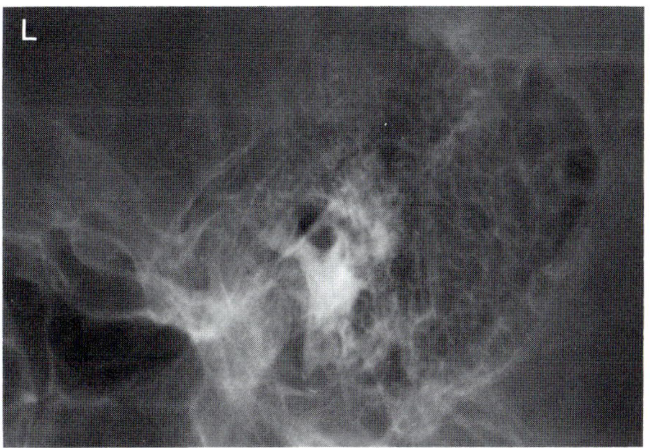

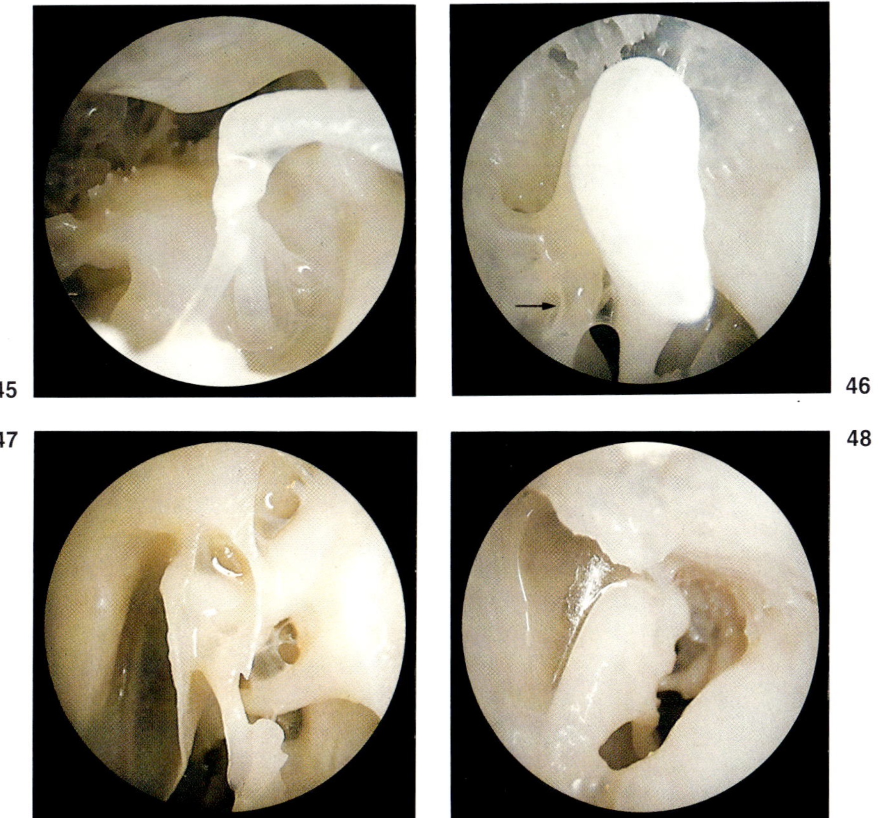

Fig. **45 Endoscopic view of a well-pneumatized middle ear**, as in Fig. **44**, with large air volume, a wide tympanic diaphragm, and ideally sculpted middle ear outline. The free space in the oval window and the well-shaped stapes with its tendon should be observed

Fig. **46 Endoscopic view of the same ear as in Fig. 45.** The epitympanum is wide open. On the right and below, the chorda tympani is shown by an arrow, and its folds and the lateral mallear fold which cover Prussak's space form the floor of the second upper level of the lateral air cushions. A small accessory fold stretches between the chorda tympani and the long process of the incus

Fig. **47 Posteroanterior endoscopic view of Prussak's space.** This is the same specimen als Fig. **46**. The anterior fold of von Troeltsch stretches anterior to the short process of the malleus and leads directly laterally into the anterior tympanic stria and the fibrous annulus, and medially into the anterior mallear fold. A fine interossicular fold stretches between the neck of the malleus and the long process of the incus

Fig. **48 Endoscopic view of the same ear as in Fig. 47.** The upper layer of the lateral air cushions is covered by the stretched and well-formed malleoincudal fold. Filling by air is only possible via the posterior tympanic isthmus. The tympanic diaphragm is wide open, with a deep protympanic recess in the fundus of which the tensor fold is stretched

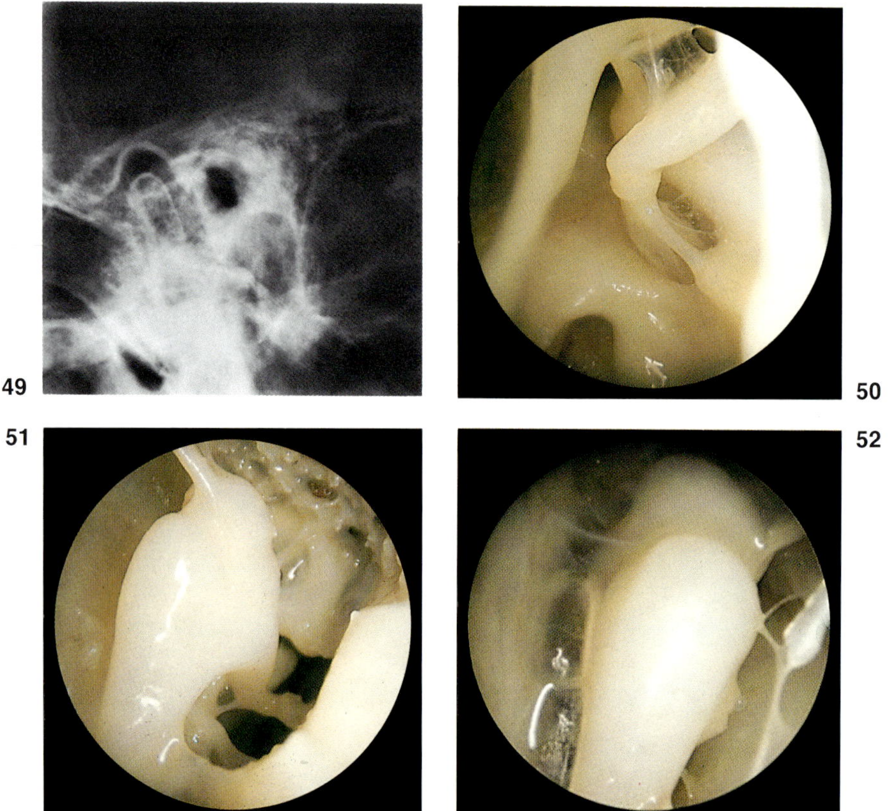

Fig. **49 Schüller's view of a middle ear with minimal pneumatization, a high jugular bulb, and a clear contour of the inferior surface of the base of the petrous bone,** a bony scar as an indication that there was disturbance of aeration and drainage in the development phase and that ossification and the formation of the air containing space did not proceed evenly but were interrupted

Fig. **51 Endoscopic view of the same ear as in Fig. 49 looking from the aditus into the epitympanum**. The tympanic diaphragm is indeed open, but obviously narrower, compared to Fig. **48**. The compartments lateral to the ossicles are smaller, so that the air content of these lateral epitympanic air cushions is less

Fig. **50 Endoscopic view of the same middle ear as in Fig. 44.** A small interossicular fold between the long process of the incus and the neck of the malleus divides the diaphragm into an anterior and a posterior isthmus. There are several delicate stapedial folds, particularly leading to the facial canal. The space is narrower than in Fig. **45**

Fig. **52 Endoscopic view of the same middle ear as in Fig. 51**. Here, seen from above downward, in the direction of the lateral epitympanic air cushions. At this point they are very small and offer less protection as a shock absorber against variations in air pressure

In this way the lateral air cushions act as a vibration damper for the bodies of the malleus and incus. They have a double function: They intercept the vibrations and dampen the after-vibrations at their own frequency.

The topography thus assists the transmission system in becoming more quickly receptive to successive sounds. The system of folds is the last biological developmental phase in the acoustics of the middle ear, intended for damping of after-vibrations and fine tuning of sound.

The folds and air cushions thus have many physiological functions: they compensate for variations of the bony outline, for the size and position of the tympanic membrane, and for the ossicles in relation to the size of the air space in the anterior and posterior sectors. Even in early childhood they form a regulator for the fine tuning of the middle ear over all frequencies of the tonal range, for the constant auditory threshold, as well as for suprathreshold sound. They achieve this despite the very variable form and extent of the compartments of the middle ear, the air cushions and the relations of the vibrating parts of the *anterior* segment (the taut tympanic membrane, the handle of the malleus and stapes)

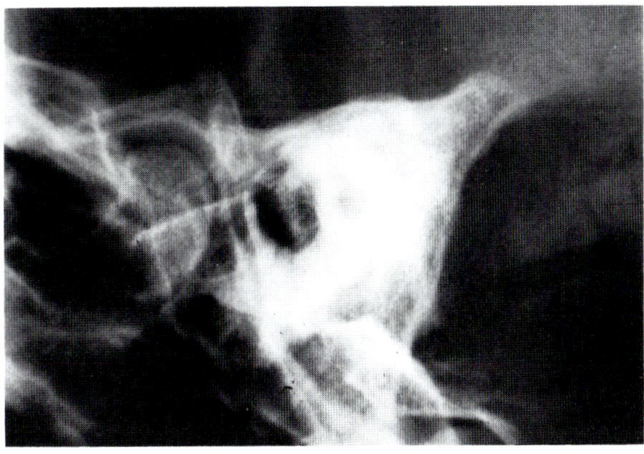

Fig. **53   Schueller's view of a middle ear with poor pneumatization.**

and of the *posterior* segment (the head of the malleus and the incus with their joint).

It is indeed very difficult to understand how similar auditory thresholds are achieved in this part of the middle ear, which varies enormously not only between one person and another, but even between the right and left ear of one individual, and in which the spatial and tissue conditions can vary markedly during childhood.

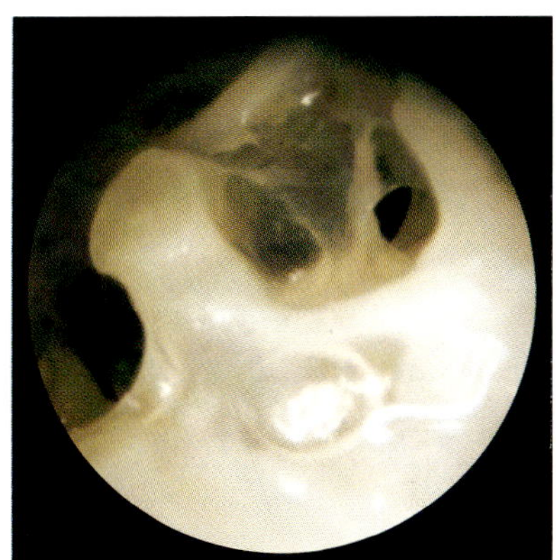

Fig. **54   Endoscopic view of the same middle ear as Fig. 53, showing a view of the tympanic diaphragm from the tympanic sinus.** The posterior isthmus is obstructed by numerous stapedioincudal folds. The fine structure of the stapes is not recognizable. Aeration of the posterior segment is only possible via the anterior tympanic isthmus. The entrance to the lateral epitympanic air cushion is blocked

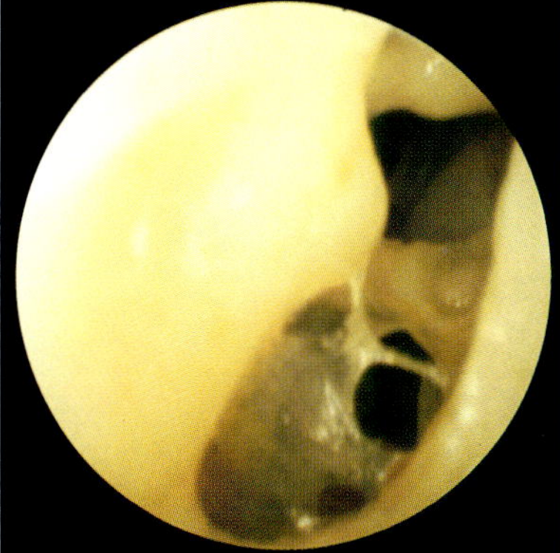

Fig. **55   Endoscopic view of the same middle ear as in Fig. 54, showing a view of the tympanic diaphragm from the tegmen tympani.** Only the anterior tympanic isthmus is free to form the air pathway to the posterior segment

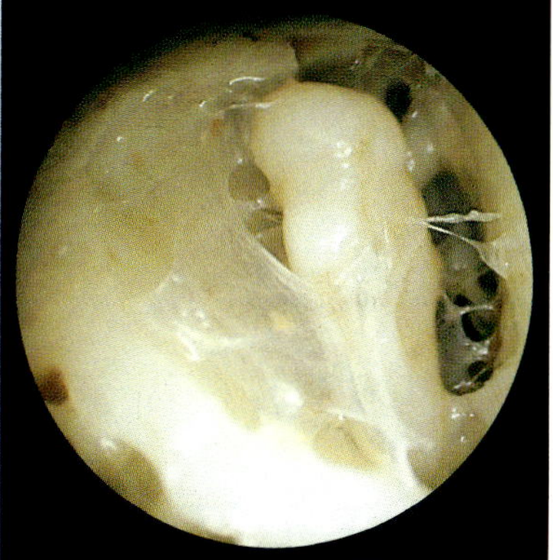

Fig. **56   Endoscopic view of the same middle ear as in Fig. 55, showing blockage of the lateral segment of the epitympanum.** The air cushion is not recognizable and is no longer present as such

Principles and Definition of Tympanoplasty

Air permeates the floor of the three cranial fossae from the viscerocranium through the entire base of the neurocranium. Beyond the tubal torus, its only purpose is to compensate for the loss of auditory threshold in the middle ear arising at the interface with the perilymph due to the sound wave resistance. The only functional reason for continuity between the air in the temporal bone and the air in the middle ear (including the antrum) is to prevent standing waves in the middle ear cavities, an air space open in one direction only.

The epitympanum forms the greatest problem in middle ear inflammation. Loss of this area robs the complex middle ear structures of their function. The epitympanum is the point at which the aeration pathways divide in a sagittal direction towards the occipital bone, and in a sphenoclinoid direction toward the pyramidal apex. To describe the reconstructive procedure, the surgeon had to create anatomical and functional terms which were not familiar to the anatomists and physiologists.

Embryology plays such an important part of planning an individual operation that it will be discussed along with the explanation of the operative method in the next chapter.

Tympanoplasty

This term was coined by H. L. Wullstein in 1952. Much earlier, Berthold (1878), Ely (1881) and Tangemann (1883) had tried to close central perforations in dry ears by a form of myringoplasty, without any knowledge of the state of the middle ear. Fifteen years later, in 1893, Berthold reported the failure of these attempts.

Tympanoplasty is defined by the author as an operation whose goal is absolute healing of the aerated spaces of the otobase, from the eustachian tube to the cells in the occipital bone and pyramid. It is applicable to any inflammation, trauma or benign neoplasm, and includes reconstruction (or primary construction, in the case of congenital anomalies) of the optimal system for middle ear function

in one operation. It is tailored therefore to the type and extent of the middle ear disease.

H. L. Wullstein in 1952 divided tympanoplasty into types I–V, based on the type of reconstructive operation used and the audiologic system which was constructed (Fig. **57**).

Types with Sound Pressure Transformation
(i. e., increased sound pressure of one window, usually the oval window)

Type I – Hearing is achieved via an anatomically and functionally intact lever mechanism of the ossicular chain.

Type II – Hearing is achieved via an abnormal but reconstructed lever mechanism of the sound-conducting chain.

Type III – Hearing is achieved *without a lever mechanism but with sound pressure transformation of the tympanic membrane*. This requires a columellar system in the reconstructed epitympanum (i. e., with a "deep middle ear") provided by either: (a) a raised stapes or a stapedial replacement or (b) a stapes in a middle ear consisting solely of the mesohypotympanum, i. e., a "shallow middle ear."

In the following discussion Type III tympanoplasty is always subdivided into Type III "deep" or Type III "shallow."

Types with Sound Protection

Type IV – Hearing is achieved by sound protection of one of the windows (usually the round window) through the lower aeration pathway. The middle ear is reduced to only the hypotympanum, and the resulting small space is called a cavum minor.

This method of hearing, in the presence of a perforation of the tympanic membrane, can be produced spontaneously by secretions in the hypotympanum or by patches on the tympanic membrane. It was known 100 years ago and was used by many deaf patients.

A *physiological exchange of the round and oval windows*, i. e., *sonoinversion*, was first demonstrated by H. L. Wullstein in 1950, using the transtemporal route for endocranial extradural fenestration of the arcuate eminence for fixation of the stapes by otosclerosis or tympanosclerosis. The round window replaces the oval window after iatrogenic eardrum perforation. The scala tympani is accessible from the external auditory meatus in place of the scala vestibuli.

Type V – The middle ear cavity is closed, and hearing is achieved by *sound protection for the round window with Simultaneous obstruction of the oval window, via a replacement window in the scala vestibuli.* This is the method of hearing after fenestration of the lateral semicircular canal for otosclerosis ("fenestra novovalis", Lempert 1945).

This classification is based on a mechanicophysiological view of the middle ear, and the types of reconstruction that can be achieved surgically by tympanoplasty. It is therefore permanently valid and attempts to rename each individual type, for example, tympanostapediopexy, have not become established because of their lack of clarity.

The theoretical amplification due to sound pressure transformation was calculated to lie between 1:14 and 1:17 by Dahmann (1929, 1930), based on the ratio of the functioning area of the tympanic membrane to the size of the stapes footplate. The lever effect of the ossicular chain was calculated as only 1:1.3. Both effects combined produce an effect between 1:18 and 1:22. Calculated in decibels, the gain due to sound pressure transformation is between 23 and 27 decibels, which is similar to the average threshold of 25 to 30 decibels after fenestration of the lateral semicircular canal, when hearing is achieved only by sound protection of the round window. These values were later confirmed by calculations by Bèkèsy and others (1942).

Tympanoplasty reconstructs a hearing system which is no longer natural but is of variable quality due to different pathological conditions. Variable hearing results must therefore be expected for each type. Accordingly, hearing results for a total defect of the tympanic membrane were calculated by our former colleague, H. G. Schmitt (1958). The graph (Fig. **58**) shows the results over the various grades of hearing improvement using sound protection (the theoretical maximum hearing level is 26.88 db) up to normal sound pressure transformation (the theoretical maximum is 1:22). Phase displacement,

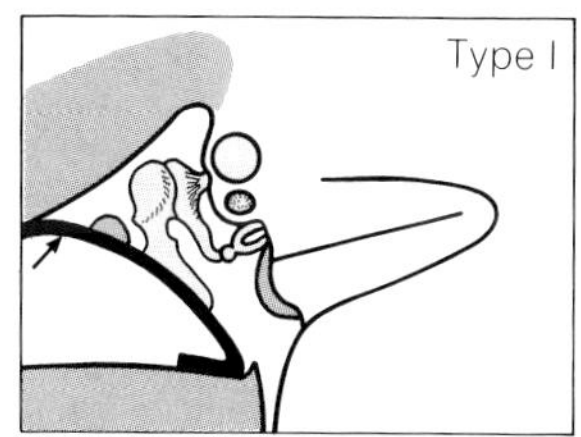
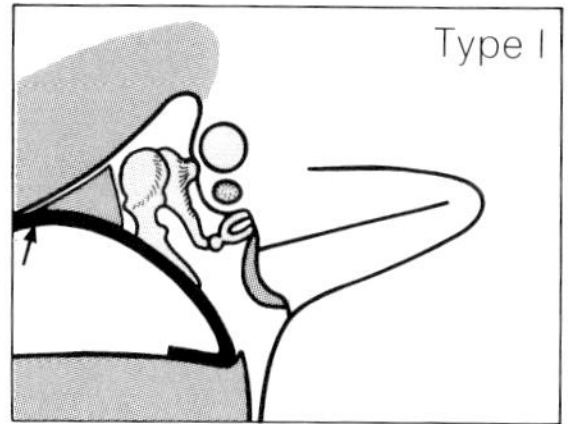

Sound pressure transformation by the lever action of the ossicular chain

Old technique
with antral inspection (—▶)

Osteoplastic
epitympanotomy
Incision for the bone flap (—▶)

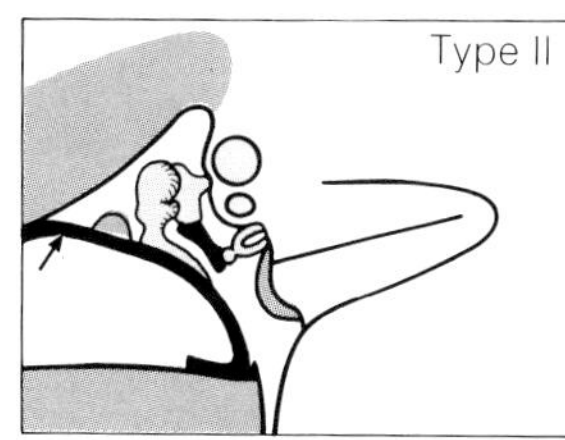
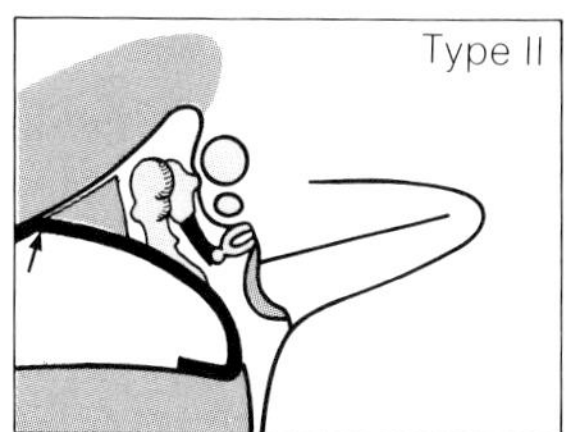

Sound pressure transformation by bridging of a localised defect of the ossicular chain

Old technique
with antral inspection (—▶)

Osteoplastic
eritympanotomy
Incision for the bone flap (—▶)

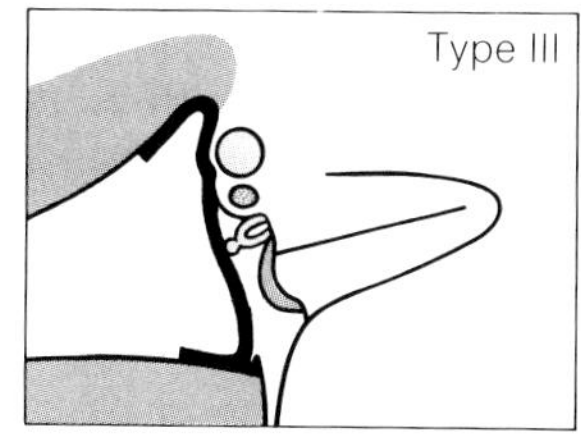
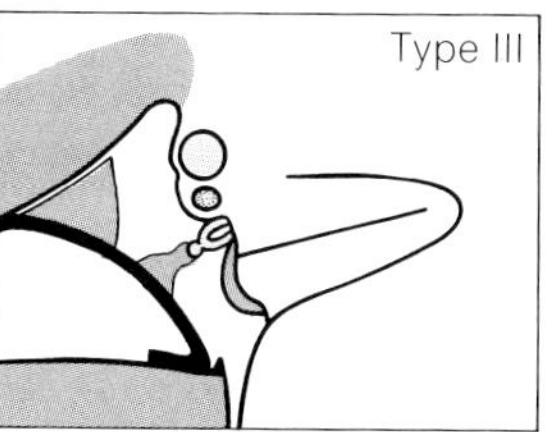

Shallow tympanic cavity with a low columella

Old open technique

Osteoplastic technique
with high columella

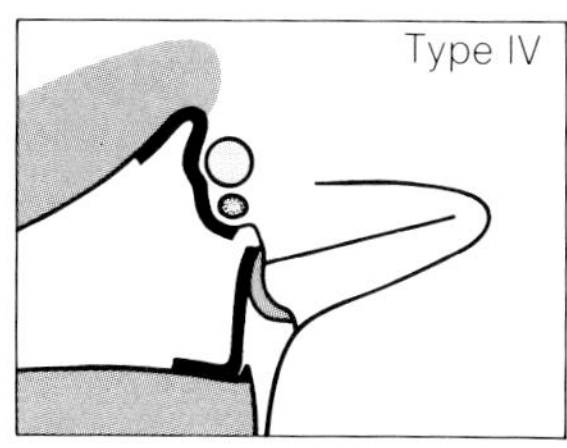
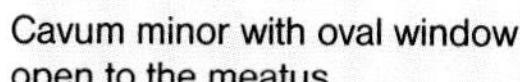
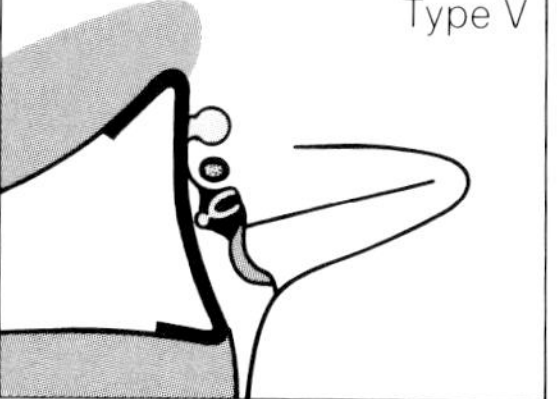

Cavum minor with oval window open to the meatus

Blocked oval window

Sound protection at the round window without sound pressure perforation

Fenestration of the semicircular canal

Fig. **57**   **Types of tympanoplasty (1953)**

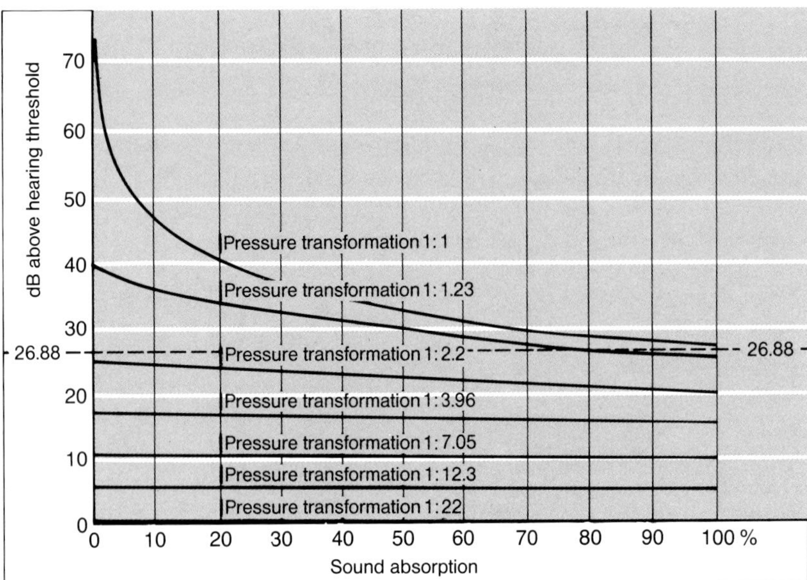

Fig. **58 Dependence of the hearing threshold on sound pressure transformation.** Sound absorption is shown as the abscissa, and the ordinate is the hearing loss in dB above normal thresholds (Schmitt 1958)

resonance of the external meatus, sound insulation and absorption by the tympanic membrane are not expressed in this figure.

The types therefore make mathematically predetermined demands on the impedance of the middle ear by sound pressure transformation or sound protection, provided that the impedance of the external meatus is not changed by the operation. Removal of the posterior meatal wall and the creation of a meatal cavity with the antrum and even a wide-open mastoid alters the natural resonances of the meatus.

The duty of the surgeon is to eliminate any pathological and anatomical impedance disorders which may be present; such as: obstructions of the middle ear, fixation by fibrosis or osteophytes, tympanosclerosis, mucosal edema and granulations, which all may increase or reduce the sound reflection and absorption, and alter impedance.

The tympanic space is wide open to the antrum through the anterior "sound-hard" wall of the protympanic recess on one side and the end of the inferior aeration pathway, i. e., the sinus tympani in the aditus, on the other side, to prevent standing waves from becoming a disturbing factor in the middle ear (Lehnhardt 1978). A large irregular antral space should therefore be created at the end of an operation with wide clearance of the mastoid process and obliteration by plasticine (see p. 99). The fact

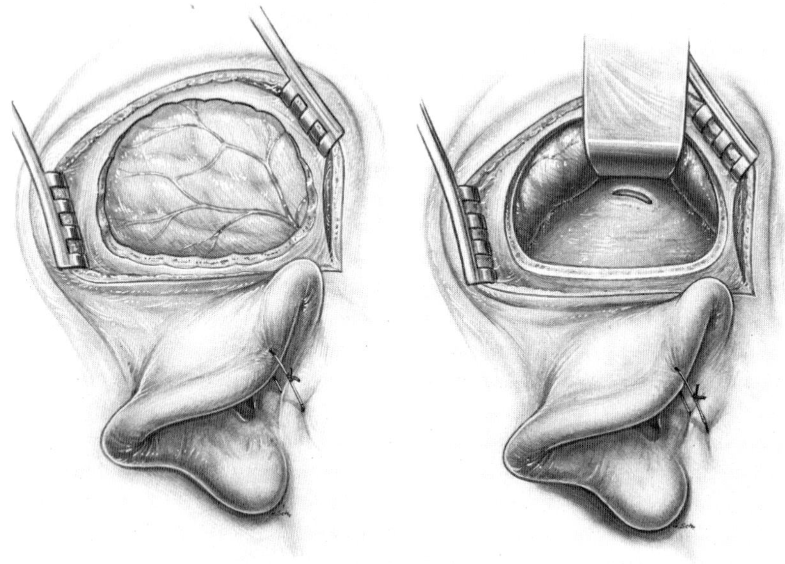

59   60

Figs. **59—60 Extratympanic endocranial fenestration for chronic otitis media and labyrinthine pressure disturbance** (H. L. Wullstein 1951)

that patients with middle ear disease are mostly satisfied with any improvement of their ability to understand speech rests on the fact that they have long forgotten their earlier tonal sound quality.

The repercussions of phase displacement in the middle ear will not be discussed here because they are too confusing and are still partially under discussion.

Aeration Pathways

Various structures partake in effective aeration of the middle ear. The two aeration pathways from the eustachian tube to the oval and round windows play a decisive role (Fig. **61**). Both lead around the promontorium, which is thus a *functional* unit of the *middle ear*. The conus of the eardrum comes close to the promontorium, increasing the effect of the air currents.

Research and definition of the "upper and lower aeration pathways" (H. L. Wullstein 1952) developed from the clinical observations during individual tympanoplasties carried out by the author.

The *upper aeration pathway* begins at the tympanic osteum of the eustachian tube and is directed beneath the canal of the tensor tympani muscle straight to the anterior part of the oval window and then around the processus cochleariforms into the epitympanum.

The *lower aeration pathway* is directed around the promontory through the hypotympanum to the round window and from there on through the tympanic sinus to the recessus facialis, the posterior part of the oval window and to the aditus ad antrum.

Restoration of function of the superior and inferior aeration pathways was from the beginning the most important goal of tympanoplasty. Both must be freed carefully so that their mucosa and that of the deep hypotympanic cells recovers completely.

Control Windows

As soon as tympanoplasty had reached the stage where it was a reliable method to create a new tympanic membrane to partition the internal air-containing space in the temporal bone from the external air in the meatus, the next development was to ascertain the type and extent of the chronic disease in the middle ear system so that the operation cound be better planned.

The critical region is always the epitympanum. Its health and capability of function, and the nature

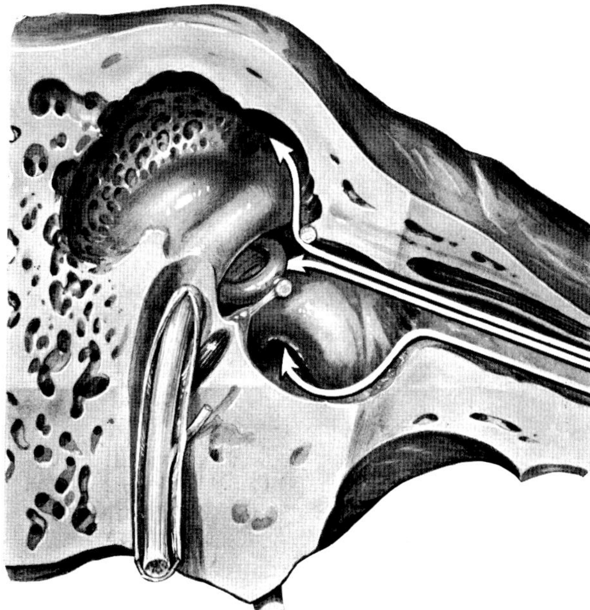

Fig. **61**   **Aeration pathways** (H. L. Wullstein 1968)

and severity of the dangers of complications arising at this point are significant. From the very early days of tympanoplasty it was important therefore to decide what was concealed in the epitympanum: whether it must be sacrificed with the ossicular chain or whether it could be preserved using sound pressure transformation.

H. L. Wullstein (1952) created three control windows to allow the state of the pathology in the middle ear to be assessed correctly (Figs. **62–69**):
1. upper;
2. antral;
3. lower:
   a) meatal along the bony annulus:
   b) retromeatal through the facial-chordal angle.

An *upper control window* in *the middle ear* is created by elevating Shrapnell's membrane at the bony edge of the tympanic notch. Granulations, polyps and cholesteatoma, especially at the entrance to the epitympanum, can thus be exposed, and the parts of the ossicles which are at most risk (i.e., the long process of the incus and the crura of the stapes) can be assessed. Nowadays, an upper middle ear control window is always the first step in disclosure of the epitympanum at osteoplastic epitympanotomy.

Any type of inflammation must pass from the epitympanum into the mastoid spaces through the aditus. Therefore an *antral control window* (pre-

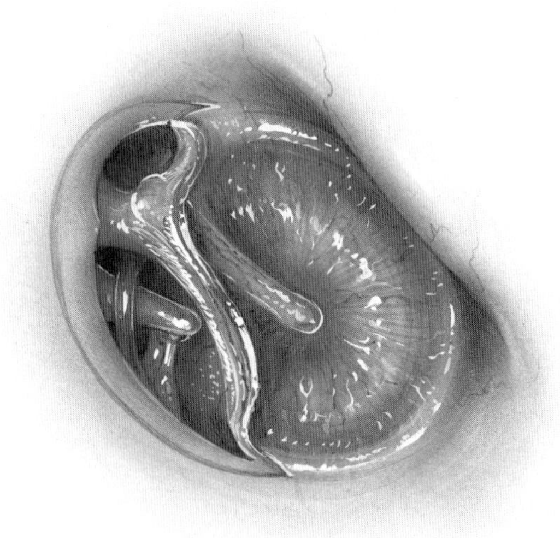

Fig. **62**   **Upper middle ear control window.** The tympanic membrane and its fibrous annulus, posterosuperiorly, are released with the elevator from the bony annulus after elevation of Shrapnell's membrane. 1 to 2 mm is removed from the edge of the lateral epitympanic wall with a suitable diamond burr. Both the epitympanum and the round window can be seen with the angled endoscope (H. L. Wullstein 1952)

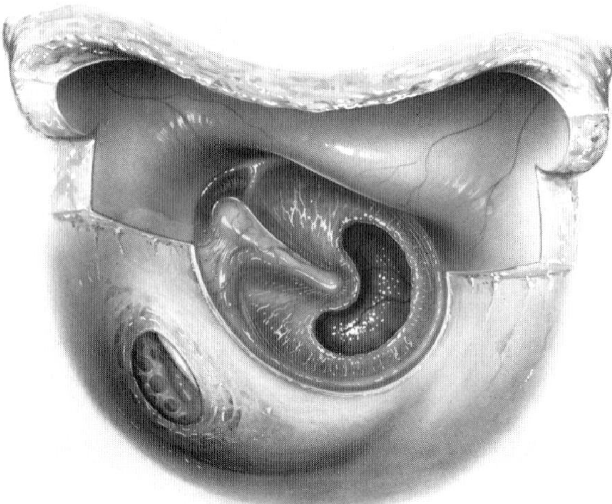

Fig. **63**   **Antral inspection window.** Depending on the bulging of the meatal wall superiorly and posteriorly, the thin bony lamella leading to the aditus is perforated with a suitable diamond burr, and the access is widened until the tegmen lying over the aditus ad antrum and the posterior edge of the short process of the incus become visible (H. L. Wullstein 1952)

viously carried out through a postaural or endaural incision) is advised after opening the area immediately below the tegmen antri through a burr hole posterior to the aditus.

If it is unlikely that the epitympanic wall is to be temporarily resected, the epitympanum can nowadays be inspected using an angled endoscope. The opening of the antrum lies so far posterior that a bony lid can be constructed, should exposure of the epitympanum become necessary.

The *posteroinferior inspection opening* is morphologically and functionally significant in patients in whom the two physiologically important posterior quadrants of the pars tensa are preserved. In large kidney-shaped defects extending into the anteroinferior quadrant, the pars tensa loses valuable tension and position if the fibrous annulus is released from the bony annulus as far along the meatal floor as is necessary to inspect the hypotympanum and the round window niche. For this reason the posteroinferior inspection window is created posterior to the bony framework of the tympanic bone *through the facial-chordal angle between the facial nerve and the branching chorda tympani.* If pneumatization is very well developed, a fine track of cells leads here into the tympanic sinus, limited superiorly by the ponticulus. The ligament of the short process of the incus is anchored in the incudal fossa at this point. This access originated with fenestration for otosclerosis (Fig. **65**) to allow the ankylosed stapedial crura to be fractured behind an undisturbed tympanic membrane with its bony work intact.

Only too often the replaced Sourdille-Lempert flap led to degeneration of the elastic fibers of the tympanic membrane, loss of sound protection and thus a conductive deafness of about 10 dB. Furthermore, the meatal flap was usually too small for total cover of the exposed cells, often leading to infection. The aditus, the window in the semicircular canal and the cells then needed to be covered with a free full-thickness skin graft. Finally, this access via the facial-chordal angle for the first time made it possible to decompress the facial nerve in its entire mastoid and tympanic course almost to the geniculate ganglion, preserving the middle ear (Fig. **69**). This obviated the decision to either decompress the facial nerve with sacrifice of the middle ear or to preserve the middle ear but abandon access to the tympanic part of the course of the facial nerve.

The view through this lower control window, as far as the origin of the chorda tympani from the facial nerve, allows the entire hypotympanum and the tympanic sinus to be inspected. If offers a direct view of the round window membrane in the depths

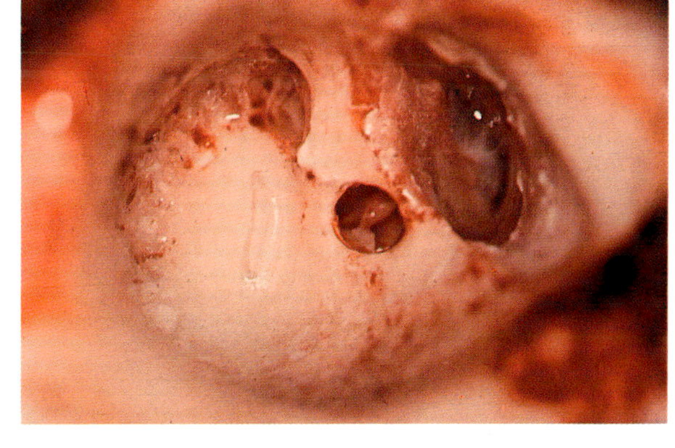

Fig. **64** **Lower control window.** Variation of the fenestration of the lateral semicircular canal as described by H. L. Wullstein. The ossicles and the tympanic membrane are preserved in the undisturbed space in order to prevent a significant loss of hearing (6–10 dB) due to reduction of sound protection of the tympanic membrane. Fixation of the stapes due to otosclerosis is assessed. The cupola of the semicircular canal is drilled down (Leica camera, Zeiss microscope, Opmi 1 1954). **This is the first photograph ever taken during an operation using an operating microscope**

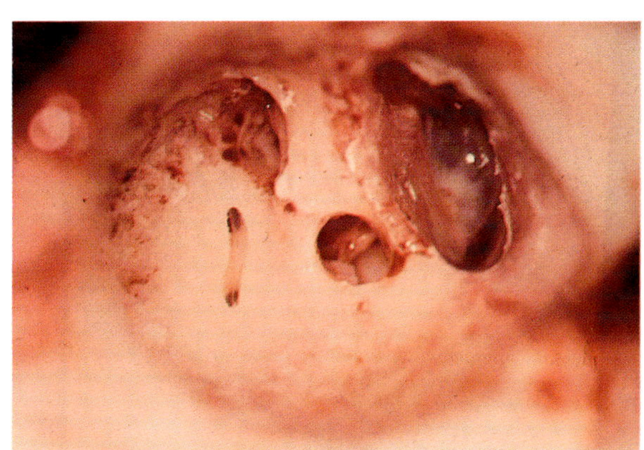

Fig. **65** **Lower control window.** An open window lying posteriorly, far removed from the crista ampullaris, scarcely causes any dizziness. The endolymphatic and perilymphatic spaces are visible (Leica camera, Zeiss microscope, Opmi 1 1954). The fenestration is furthermore indicated for certain congenital anomalies, and possibly for complete obstruction of the oval window with functional loss of the malleus and incus. The length of the window is 6 mm, and its width 0.6 to 0.7 mm (0.9 mm over the ampulla). The thickness of the bony wall is 0.1 to 0.2 mm

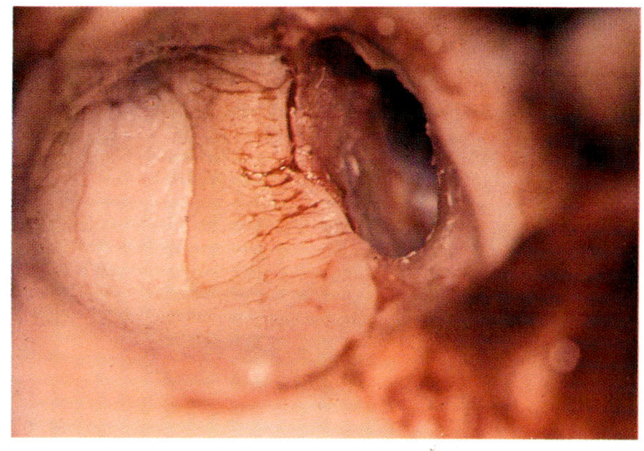

Fig. **66** Removal of the posterior meatal wall is always necessary to allow access of sound to the labyrinthine fenestration in this indication. Because a variation of Sourdille's flap is too small, a free full-thickness skin graft has been placed over the aditus, the open inner ear and the entire pneumatic spaces (Leica camera, Zeiss microscope, Opmi 1 1954). Normal healing without reaction in the open inner ear (see the healing phase of free full-thickness skin grafts)

of the round window niche and of the posterior crus of the stapes. The removal of the ponticulus does not constitute an appreciable audiological loss *with good sound pressure transformation* of a healthy tympanic membrane.

The combination of interior inspection behind the bony meatus with antral control window up to the tegmen tympani became available as a direct result of the introduction of diamond burrs into microsurgery. This provided a view from behind of the round window membrane, including the ampullary crus of the anterior semicircular canal, during de-

compression of the facial nerve and dissection of its sheath (H. L. Wullstein 1952–56). Granulations may be removed directly from the round window membrane by this approach.

Anterior and Posterior Paralabyrinthine Points of Danger

An *intracranial* cholesteatoma may on occasion be very large. It has been known for a long time that cholesteatomas at this location are very dangerous.

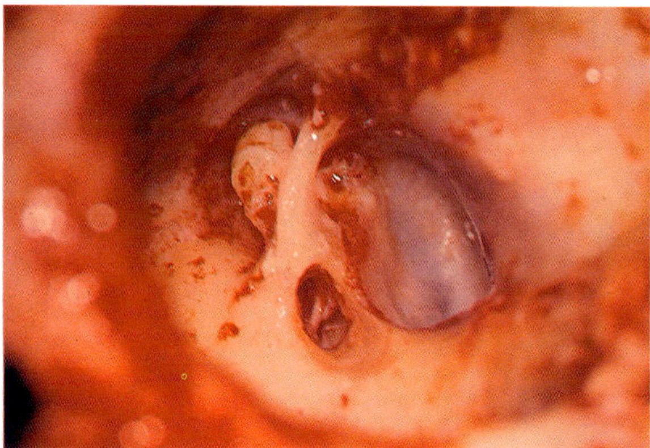

Fig. **67** **Lower control window.** Mucoperiosteal chronic otitis media with preservation of the bony bridge and the entire pars tensa (Leica camera, Zeiss microscope, Opmi 1 1954)

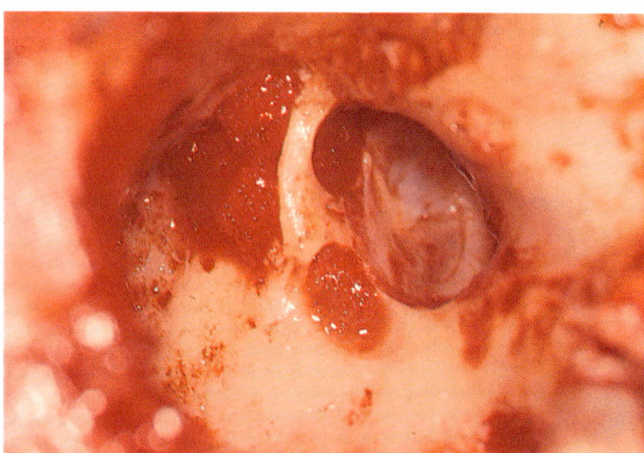

Fig. **68** **Lower control window and epithympanum filled with compressed gelatin sponge (shaped drop).** Thereafter covered as for fenestration and continued with closure of the partial tympanic membrane defect (Leica camera, Zeiss microscope, Opmi 1 1954)

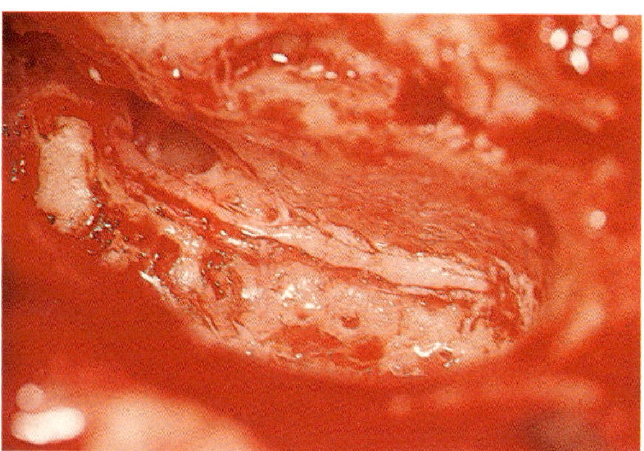

Fig. **69** **Decompression of the facial nerve medial to the ossicles using a lower control window.** The sheath is slit from the first genu at the crus of the anterior semicircular canal (the junction of the labyrinthine and tympanic segments of the facial nerve) as far as the stylomastoid foramen. The middle ear and the posterior meatal wall are closed and undisturbed (Leica camera, Zeiss microscope, Opmi 1 1956). The operation was demonstrated as a film in 1957 during the International E.N.T. Congress in Washington. It was the first neurosurgical operation under the microscope using the diamond burr

On the other hand, their origin and early forms have not been satisfactorily explained and differentiated. After the introduction of microsurgical tympanoplasty, H. L. Wullstein (1953) was able to trace the penetration of *primary inflammatory cholesteatoma* into the middle cranial fossae. *Careful direct inspection of the two points of danger is therefore mandatory when assessing an epitympanic cholesteatoma.*

The anterior paralabyrinthine point of danger leads into the loose spongiosa of the *antelabyrinthine trigone* between the labyrinthine course of the facial nerve, the ampullary crus of the anterior semicircular canal and the cortical bone of the floor of the middle cranial fossa. If the bone is well pneumatized, the anterosuperior cell track leads from here through the paralabyrinthine narrowing to the pyramidal apex.

The *posterior labyrinthine point of danger* lies deeply in the spongiosa bounded by the posterior crus of the anterior semicircular canal and the superior crus of the posterior semicircular canal (at their confluence, to form the crus commune), as well as by the cortical bone of the middle and posterior cranial fossae. This is the *postlabyrinthine rhomboid*, through which the space over the internal meatus is reached.

Anterior to this rhomboid lies the *tractus niche* (H. L. Wullstein 1948), a three-dimensional space located over the lateral semicircular canal, between the two vertical semicircular canals. The obliterated subarcuate tract of the embryonal vascular cord from the subarcuate fossa to the inner ear capsule opens in the depth exactly at the center of the anterior semicircular canal. On a radiograph it looks like a garland, and is a reliable diagnostic landmark (see pp. 121–5). The cholesteatoma, in particular the large infants' cholesteatoma, often erodes the tractus niche dramatically. A labyrinthine fistula, i. e., a *chronic* localized osteitis, at this point is rare. On the other hand, an *acute total* osteitis of the bony inner ear often starts at this point (see p. 129). In radiographs, and in CT scans, if the chlolesteatoma has not extended beyond the aditus, it can be confused with a healthy *macroantrum*. Their appearance is similar, with a prominence of the three semicircular canals.

Gelatin Sponge (Wullstein's Shaped Drop) — Electrolytic Exchange for the Healing of a New Tympanic Membrane

The creation of a new middle ear demands that the membrane heal, and that its two surfaces be free on either side and be bounded by air ("free skin graft," Wullstein 1952). For this reason, Moritz (1952) and Zoellner (1952) created two pedicled skin flaps to provide internal and external covering to prevent adhesions forming within the middle ear. The meatal skin was pedicled on the tympanic ring and rotated over the mesotympanum to form the internal surface of the new eardrum. A second long, narrow pedicled skin flap as outer cover was introduced from the mastoid over the sinodural angle of the radical mastoid cavity and laid over the internal skin flap. Because of the relation of the length and breadth of the flap, it was not nourished by its pedicle but by its contact with bone. This demanded the creation of a wide radical cavity. On the other hand, it was impossible to preserve the epitympanum. Mainly because of the transplantation of skin to the inner surface of the middle ear, this technique was not generally accepted (Figs. **70–73**).

A free graft, as described by H. L. Wullstein (1952) offers a 2-mm overlap around its entire circumference as a contact for blood supply and for adhesion to the surrounding area. Free tissue of this type dies rapidly, not from an insufficient blood supply but because of a lack of fluid and an electrolyte exchange imbalance. It became clear that it was necessary to retain the blood supply until the very first circulatory exchange, i. e., by preparing the way for a longitudinally directed capillary system extending over the surface.

The correct provision of electrolytes for the open wound surface of the free graft and a high antibiotic activity are achieved by filling the middle ear cavity after careful cleaning, using Ringer's solution with an antibiotic added. Premature replacement of this solution by air due to the activity of the eustachian tube when the patient swallows must be prevented. Care must be taken to ensure that the watery solution be retained for three to five days postoperatively without blocking the eustachian tube.

From the early days to the present the most suitable material has been *gelatin sponge* (H. L. Wullstein 1952). Its pores become saturated with the watery solution, but furthermore, after *1–2 hours of preoperative saturation*, the gelatin itself takes up more than 20 times its own weight in water. It becomes so saturated that the water can be drained off and also resorbed. This occurs more quickly in brisk leucocyte inflammation, due to the enzymes. This fully saturated piece of *gelatin sponge* (the shaped drop) can be placed with forceps or a needle into the middle ear to provide an arbitrarily shaped (not necessarily horizontal) supporting surface for the graft.

Penicillin is very active, and originally was seldom allergenic. Streptomycin and some antibiotics have never been used. New antibiotics must be tested for their toxicity, compatibility, allergenic effect and resistance to bacteria. Ringer's solution was for a time replaced by nutrient tissue fluids to encourage healing, but these fluids also stimulate the growth of bacteria. The authors have resumed the use of Ringer's solution with an appropriate antibiotic added, because only the electrolytes, not the supplementary nutrients, are necessary.

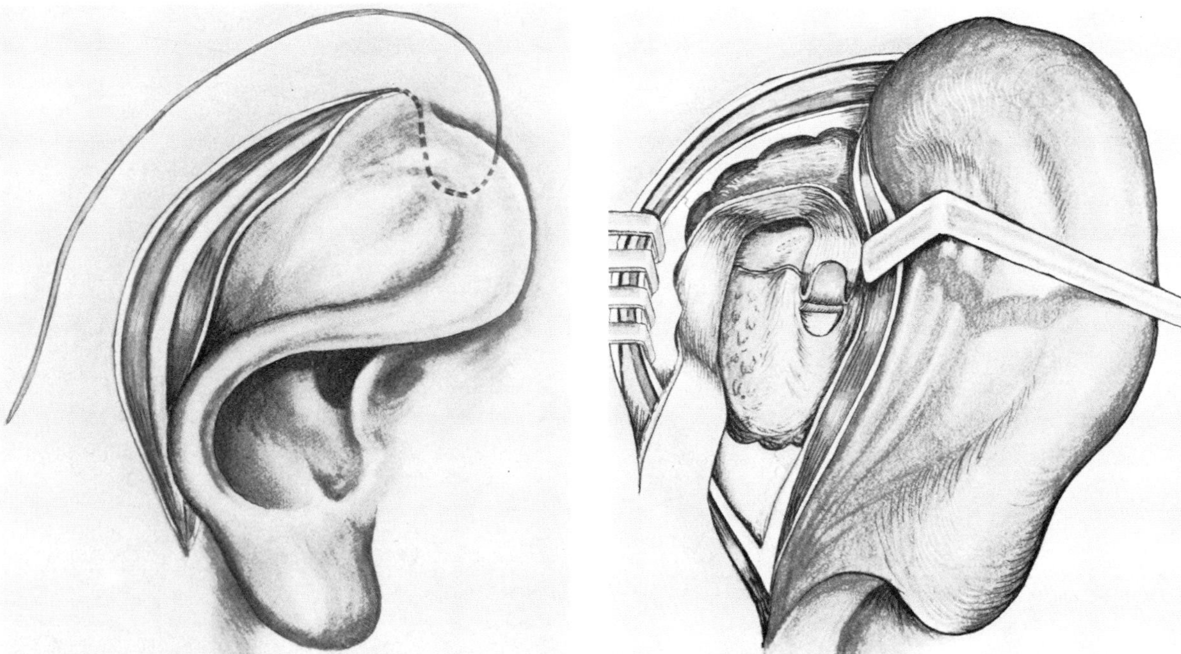

Figs. **70–71** **Rotation and folding of a pedicled skin flap to close the mesotympanum using a wide radical mastoid cavity** (Moritz 1952)

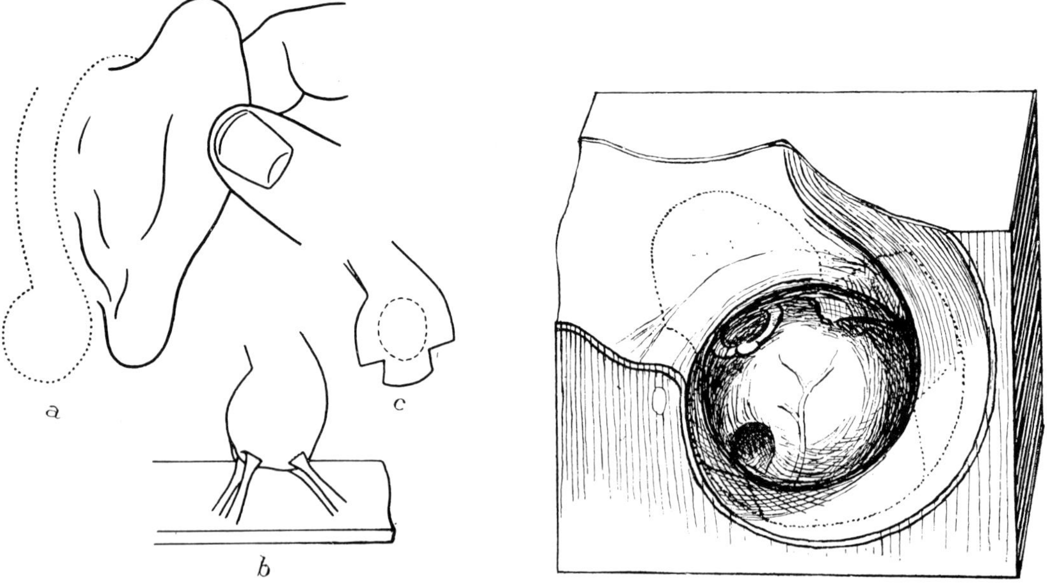

Figs. **72–73** **The technique proposed by Zoellner** (1952)

Activity of the Middle Ear Mucosa

Complete healing of the *mucosa* over all wound surfaces of the middle ear, the tympanic membrane graft and the ossicles is a basic prerequisite for the success of tympanoplasty. Small, and even medium-sized mucosal defects and superficial necrosis of cortical bone are immediately overgrown by surrounding mucosa. The middle ear mucosa demonstrates an enormous capacity for regeneration. The authors have repeatedly shown that the middle ear mucosa is a good friend to the otologist if he provides the correct prerequisites for rapid healing, i. e., immediate ventilation and drainage along the aeration pathways. On the other hand, extensive mucosal defects cannot be covered quickly enough by the regenerating mucosa to prevent adhesions or granulations. Healthy capillary buds on the surface, and restitution of mucociliary clearance are necessary prerequisites for growth of the mucosa, whereas granulations hinder epithelialization.

Healing of Free Grafts
(Figs. **74–83**)

Animal experiments and tissue biopsies have shown that the healing of the free-standing graft follows the same phases as that of a graft on a bed:
1. a phase of plasmatic circulation;
2. a phase of capillary sprouts and revascularization;
3. a phase of reorganization.

Graft survival depends on the following factors:
– initially, on the resumption of the exchange of electrolytes, oxygen and water;
– continuation of metabolism, particularly of glycogen, and of protein exchange in the cells via revascularization and thus
– the resumption of mitoses.

Electrolyte exchange and tissue respiration must be rapidly resumed at the beginning of the first phase of plasmatic circulation. Under the correct conditions for tympanoplasty (see Fig. **74**), a full-thickness skin graft takes part in water and electrolyte metabolism on the wound surface within 15 minutes of transplantation. Scarcely an hour later, maximal fluorescence is reached as evidence of this activity. In contrast, any resorption from the keratinized side is slow and inadequate. The same results have been shown by in vivo experiments in animals (see Fig. **75**).

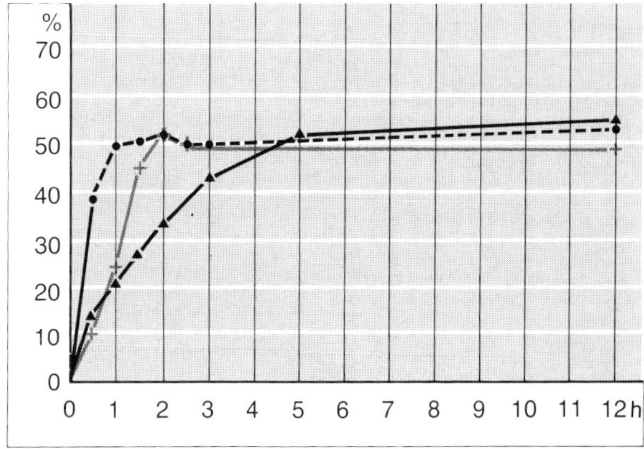

Fig. **74   Diffusion speed in maximally saturated gelatin sponge** measured by light emission of a watery penicillin solution diluted with sodium fluorescine 1:1000: ● Temporalis fascia (13 measurements); + + full-thickness skin (15 measurements); ▲ full thickness skin and temporalis fascia (11 measurements) (Bandtlow 1967)

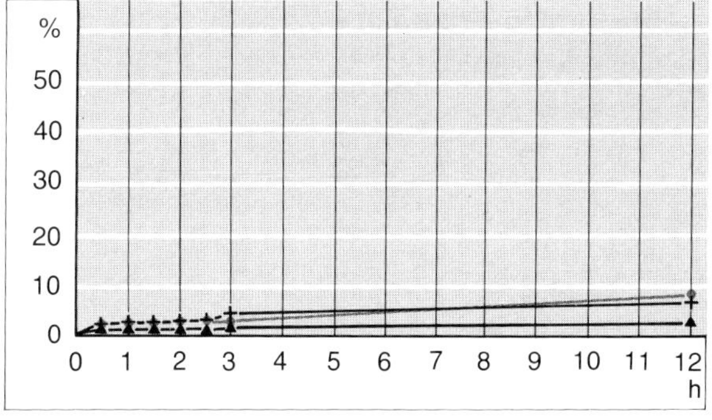

Fig. **75   Diffusion speed over the surface of human skin.** Measured by light emission of fullthickness skin diluted with sodiumfluorescine 1:1000, introduced onto the skin surface. Gelatin sponge maximally saturated with watery penicillin solution (6 measurements); + gelatin sponge maximally saturated with synthetic nutrient medium (5 measurements); ▲ gelatin sponge half saturated with watery penicillin solution (5 measurements) (Bandtlow 1967)

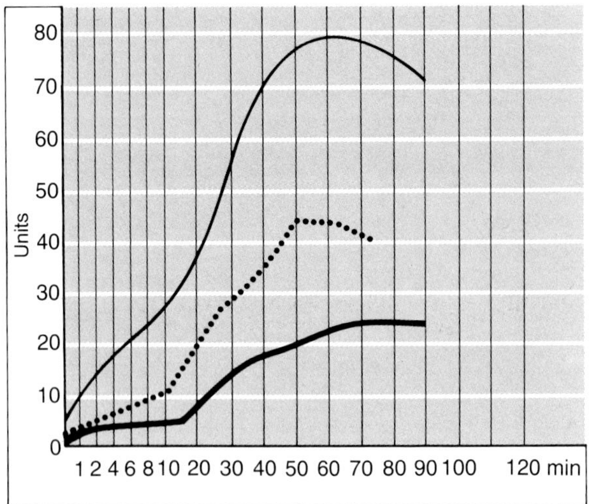

Fig. **76   The speed of exchange of fluorescine dye via the periosteum from the local blood circulation.** A gelatin sponge saturated with physiological saline is introduced into the opened middle ear cavity and followed by intravenous fluorescine. The curves show the increase of fluorescence in the gelatin sponge: with a intact blood circulation in the mucoperiosteum (upper curve); after elimination of the local blood circulation (lower curve); with partial elimination of the local blood circulation (middle curve) (Gruenberg 1965)

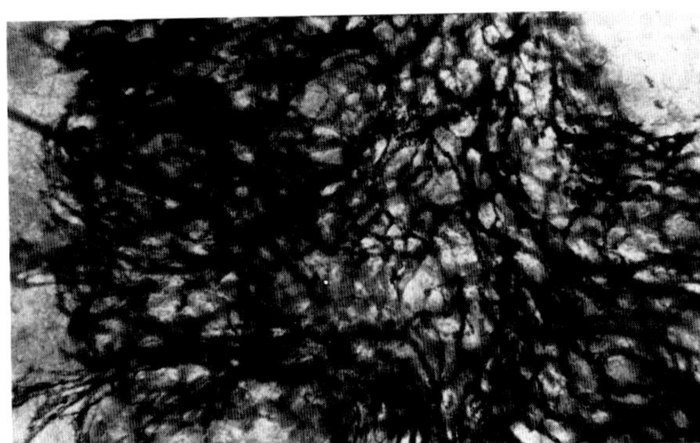

Fig. **77   A 6-day-old, full-thickness skin graft used as tympanic membrane replacement after injection of India ink into the common carotid artery in vivo.** Complete circulation of the entire graft with a thick marginal zone and a central area of vessels of small calibre. The specimen has been treated in wintergreen oil (150 ×) (Bandtlow 1967)

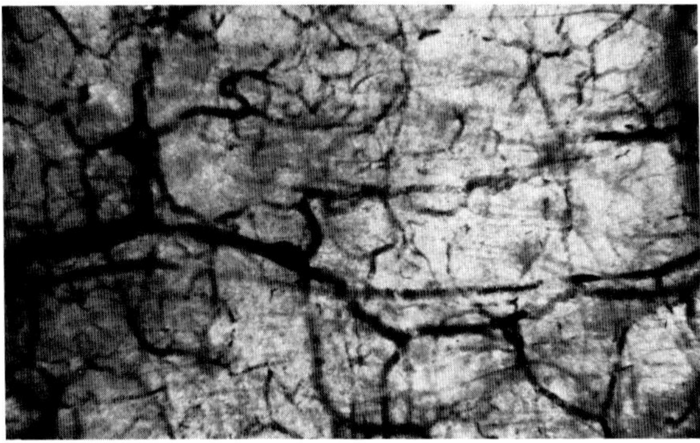

Fig. **78   Vascular picture of masseter fascia of rabbit 16 days after transplantation as a double graft.** The vascular arrangement in the transplanted fascia corresponds to that in the nontransplanted. Injection of India ink into the common carotid artery in vivo. Clearing in wintergreen oil. (6 ×) (Bandtlow 1967)

The minimum (about 10% of the normal) tissue respiration and hydrolysis necessary for survival is maintained with the help of the molecular oxygen dissolved in the watery solution. Interruption of tissue metabolism in this early phase which does not lead to partial or total necrosis can cause infiltrates in, and resorption of, the free graft that persist for many years and can be demonstrated by histology. They are only slowly overcome by the tissue, even if the graft heals normally and appears normal.

The next condition for survival of the free graft is rapid resumption of cellular metabolism. The beginning of capillary sprouting and tissue organization coincide almost exactly. Capillaries can only sprout in a longitudinal direction from the edge of the graft. From the sixth day onward, injections of India ink show that the capillary buds have established connections with the existing vascular network of the free graft and developed a perfusion almost identical to that before the excision.

The collagenous fibers have a biological half life of only 20—40 days, and as little as 9 days in a wound, and their protein metabolism is certainly not inert. Like the mucopolysaccharides, they tend to absorb water into the fiber and to swell; the pH falls from about 7.0 to 3—4, due to an inflammatory acidosis. The collagen is dissolved by collagenase and, by intermediate steps, by protease, to form a precursor of gelatin. A skin graft as a free-standing tympanic membrane demonstrates the principles of healing much more clearly than an inert tissue like fascia does.

A serious disruption of the energy metabolism in the cells, i.e., of the activity of the mitochondria, prevents the maintenance of the electrolyte gradient of the cells and of the protein metabolism. Lysosomes cause autolysis and necrosis, leading to liquefaction and coagulation of the graft. Even more fluid is absorbed during liquefaction, for example, by the collagenous fibers. Total or partial necrosis should no longer occur under present operative standards.

The newly formed vessels demonstrate an increased enzyme activity, especially from the twelfth to the twenty-fourth day, with involution after thirty-five days. Phosphatase activity is not found in necrotic zones but is found in excess in the capillaries and cells of the demarcation zone. If necrosis occurs in a damaged autogenous graft or a previously untreated allogenic transplant after the first apparent growth, both types of graft have passed through the phase of plasmatic circulation, but have not successfully acquired capillary formation. This correlates with the clinical appearances, in which initially normal healing is followed a few weeks later by liquefaction or even coagulation.

There are critical, but not extensive, *mucosal defects*; for example, on the facial canal ridge on the promontory and in the entrance to the oval niche, where adhesions to the stapes must be avoided at all costs. Orthotopic mucosal grafts from the surrounding area should be considered for small areas. Osteoplastic epitympanotomy has taught us that the mucosa posterior to the aditus is often quite healthy. Enough mucosa can be obtained from the surface of the semicircular canals or from the tegmen antri to cover the entrances to the round and oval window niches on both sides of the stapes.

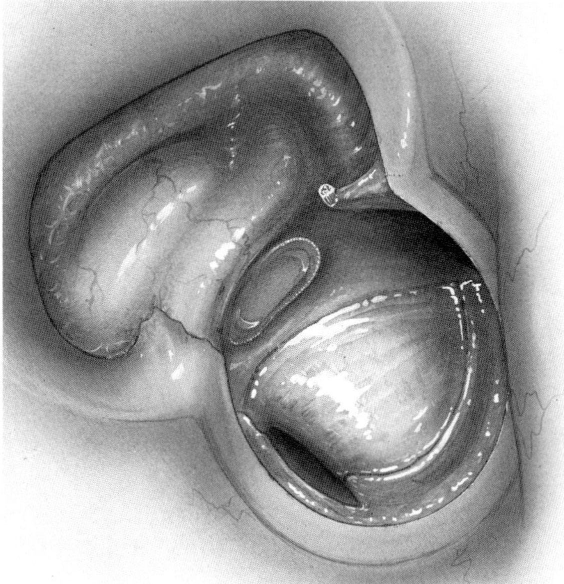

Fig. **79 Mucosal graft in the middle ear in a patient undergoing Type IV tympanoplasty.** Mucosa was taken from the lip 0.1—0.2 mm thick, to cover the hypotympanum and the promontory. Careful step-by-step adaptation of the graft with the middle ear mucosa is to be achieved. The round window niche and membrane can only be covered with mucosa after flattening of the overhanging edge (H. L. Wullstein 1952)

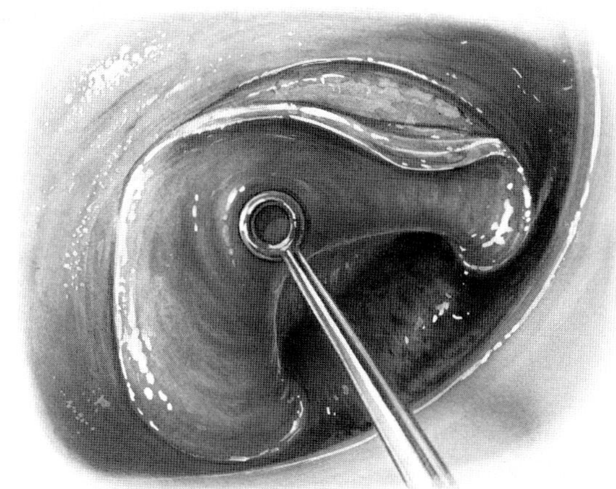

Fig. **80 Mucosal cover of the round window membrane.** The mucosal graft is moulded into the flattened round niche and onto the promontory. Because of the danger of later scar tissue, all blood clots between the graft and the round window membrane must be carefully aspirated. As little as possible should be removed from the subiculum, in order to preserve its function of diversion of the air stream anterior to the round window (Wullstein 1952)

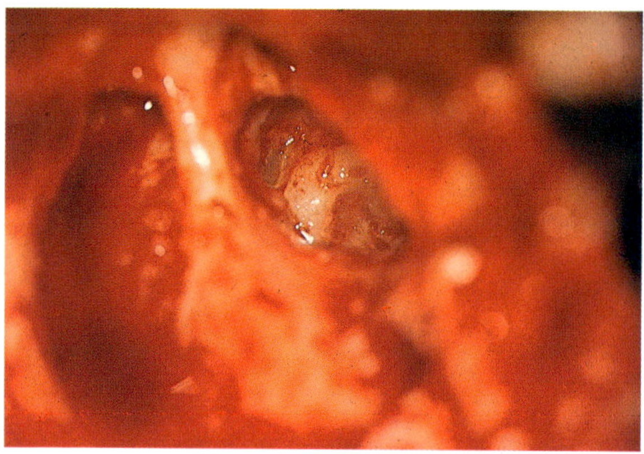

Fig. **81   Chronic middle ear inflammation with cholesteatoma.** Type III tympanoplasty. The bony pillar over the aditus is the only remaining part of the posterior meatal wall. The oval window niche is empty, and there is a large mucosal defect in the hypomesotympanum. The subiculum is flattened as necessary in order to be able to remove the cholesteatoma matrix from the deeplying round window niche (Leica camera, Zeiss microscope, Opmi 1 1954)

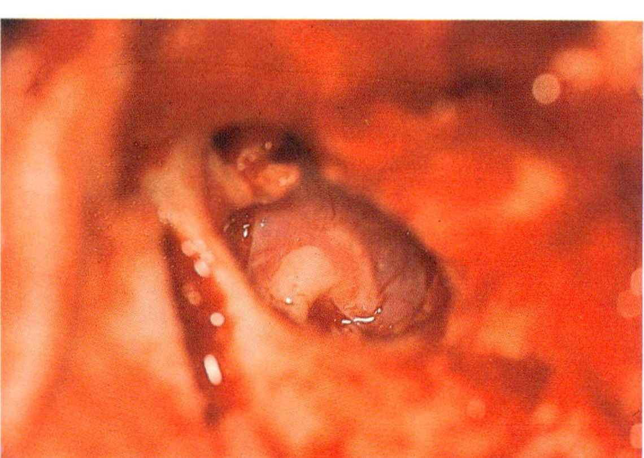

Fig. **82   Chronic middle ear inflammation with cholesteatoma.** Type III tympanoplasty. The same site as in Fig. **51**. The denuded bone on the promontory is covered with an amnion graft (Leica camera, Zeiss microscope, Opmi 1 1954)

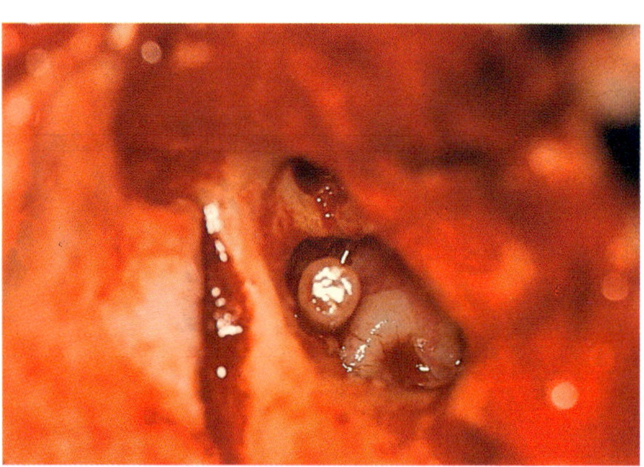

Fig. **83   Chronic middle ear inflammation with cholesteatoma.** Type III tympanoplasty. Same site as in Fig. **81** and **82**. A second amnion graft covers the flattened subiculum so that the amnion sinks back onto the round window membrane. The columella was made from Palavit, and rests in the oval window (Leica camera, Zeiss microscope, Opmi 1 1954)

Bone Grafts

Bone grafts can be considered for two purposes:
1. for reconstruction of the bony external walls;
2. for reconstruction of destroyed ossicles.

Sufficient autogenous bone, both cortical and cancellous, is available locally. The goal should be healing by *bone* as a replacement for the wall. In both cases, rapid re-epithelialization with mucosa is necessary; otherwise, it is inhibited by proliferating granulation tissue. Animal experiments have shown that autogenous bone grafts under or on the *periosteum*, which are completely embedded in tissue, demonstrate satisfactory vascularity after only six days, showing that bone reacts in almost exactly the same way as skin or fascia under satisfactory circumstances.

Extensive experience with osteoplastic epitympanotomy has proven that the *orthotopic* bony lid unites with the surrounding bone within four weeks, if it is in a correct position. Therefore, the original incision of the bony lid must be reopened with a conical diamond burr, if reoperation is needed (for example, to improve hearing).

Immediate bone healing *without* pseudoarthrosis due to interposition of connective tissue is only achieved by immediate firm contact of the two trephined or fractured surfaces, and is most likely with orthotopic bone with no large defects.

Contact points are often deficient when an autogenous but nonorthotopic bony posterior meatal wall is constructed. Union is then achieved only by connective tissue, and there is a danger that the graft will later prolapse into the mastoid cavity, due to scar tissue contracture. The meatal skin tube retracts into these broad clefts and forms a deep groove, sometimes causing a chronic bone infection. Healing can then only be achieved by complete removal of the bone. An *alternative* is to use a mortice and tenon joint (i.e., an *orthotopic* bone) with direct bony union when inserting the posterior and superior bony wall (Feldmann 1977). Unfortunately, this requires access through a mastoidectomy.

This method of reinserting the bony wall will fail if it later becomes necessary to expand the access by drilling down the temporal squama, owing to a deep middle cranial fossa with difficult access to the tegmen and the paralabyrinthine area.

Autogenous bone paste can be used to fill the bone cuts produced at osteoplastic epitympanotomy by drilling down the temporal squama. It is mixed with the plasticine mass (p. 51–3) for reconstruction of the walls. Despite its large pores, the loose framework of processed xenogenic bone (formerly lyophilized calf bone) does not absorb any fluid. It is unsuitable both for the walls and for filling of cavities.

The patient's own ossicles are preferred material for supplementing *ossicular defects*, provided they are not diseased due to osteitis or invasion by cholesteatoma. If they are healthy the mucosa over the ossicles must be retained, if possible. Struts between the ossicles and a columella are no longer formed from mastoid bone because spontaneous epithelialization over the marrow spaces is more difficult than with allogenic ossicles. Under the microscope it is technically easy to shape the ossicles as desired, to fit them to each other and then glue them together.

Autogenous diseased ossicles heated in an autoclave to 130° for 5 minutes produce an inert, dead material similar in weight and substance, which is very suitable for epithelialization.

Mucosal Grafts

Autogenous grafts should be considered for extensive *mucosal defects* but unfortunately, local material is not available. Such a graft must be very thin and easy to harvest. Mesothelium from veins or the mesentery are incapable of forming epithelium to cover a mucosal defect because they produce fibrocytes and, therefore, a wound surface rather than a tissue surface. Healthy antral mucosa is a good material for resurfacing.

A *split-thickness graft* can be taken easily with a small dermatome from the nonkeratinized part of the *inner surface of the lip*. The graft is ample in size and can be cut easily to the required shape.

Antral mucosa is taken by opening the anterior wall of the antral cavity with a conical diamond burr and turning back a flap. The mucoperiosteum is elevated from the incised bony flap. Care must be taken to use the correct surface when the graft is inserted.

Cartilaginous Grafts

Cartilage is easy to take. A thin slice or a piece with a markedly curved edge may be taken from the conchal fossa or from the dome of the tragus. It is taken in one of two ways: firstly, without perichondrium, for interposition between the lentiform process of the incus and the head of the stapes; or, secondly, with the adherent, relatively thick perichondrium that is laid on a columella system for union with a tympanic membrane graft.

Autogenous or conserved allogenic cartilaginous struts are used to stiffen tympanic membrane grafts which are in danger of retraction. The disadvantage is uncontrollable impedance. The correct permanent position of the tympanic membrane or tympanic membrane graft is best achieved by construction of adequate aeration and spatial relationships in the mesohypotympanum.

Autogenous cartilage is easy to cut and is often used for closing defects of the wall of the epitympanum or of the meatus. It does not possess the ability to change into bone or to enter into a firm cartilaginous or bony union with the surrounding tissue at the site of incision. During the operation it may appear satisfactory, but it does not form a fixed wall for a healthy epitympanum. It is doomed to prolapse into the epitympanum or the mastoid due to scar tissue retraction, and to undergo resorption. This is also true of allogenic cartilage, membranes of autogenous or allogenic periosteum and lyophilized dura, etc.

Surface Autografts

These may be ectodermal (full-thickness skin) or mesodermal (periosteum, fascia, etc.)

Surface- grafts *of mesodermal origin* was first used for repair of defects of the tympanic membrane at tympanoplasty by Bocca (1958). He removed periosteum from the temporal squama through the incision used for tympanoplasty. Later, temporalis fascia, an easily accessible, well-vascularized and very porous tissue, became more usual (Heermann 1960, 1961).

One of the important principles of tympanoplasty is that the entire internal surface of the free tympanic membrane graft must be overgrown by middle ear mucosa as rapidly as possible so that not the slightest defect remains. The internal surface of a tympanic membrane graft is not accessible for aftercare. Initially, we chose *full-thickness skin* for tympanoplasty, based on extensive experience with free full-thickness grafts for the antrum and mastoid

cells after fenestration. One of the two free surfaces could be observed undergoing normal healing or temporary local discoloration of the skin (Wullstein 1951, 1952). Furthermore, at that time, the traditional mastoid cavity with a retained epitympanum was still covered in the initial phase with the same full-thickness skin graft (Figs. **84–87**) because of the high risk of complications affecting the sinus and dura.

Thinning of the full-thickness skin graft at its edges to make it easier to adapt (Beickert 1957, 1958) caused oblique cuts through the skin appendages, leading to immigration of epidermis and iatrogenic cholesteatoma.

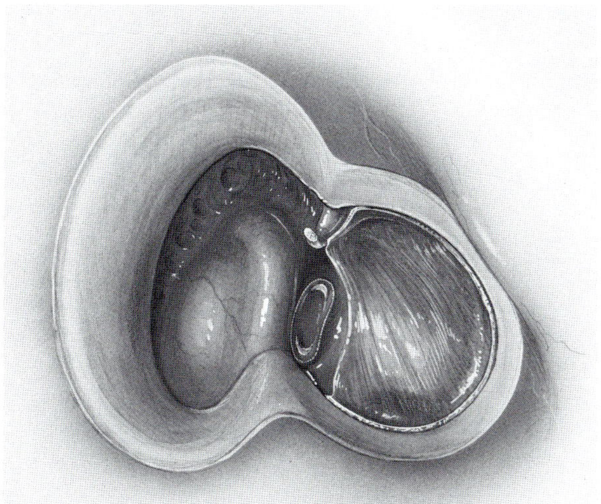

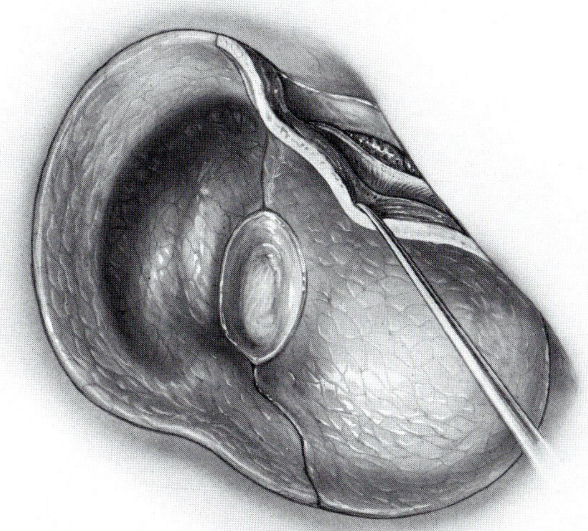

Fig. **84   Arrangement of the graft for a total defect in Type IV tympanoplasty.** The graft over the cavum minor consists of a double graft of fascia and skin. The fascia is laid on the fibrous annulus and is molded to the promontory along the oval window niche. Full-thickness skin is used to achieve massive sound protection, particularly with respect to the often necessary refilling of air in the cavum minor (H. L. Wullstein 1952)

Fig. **85   Arrangement of the graft in a total defect for tympanoplasty Type IV.** The problem is: 1. wide open oval niche; 2. well-aerated hypotympanum; 3. prevention of elevation o the graft from the oval window niche and the epitympanum by tubal inflation. For this reason, a split graft of full-thickness skin is used: 1. over the tubal ostium and the hypotympanum; 2. over the epitympanum and antrum; 3. thereafter, to cover the oval window niche with the thinnest split skin (H. L. Wullstein 1952)

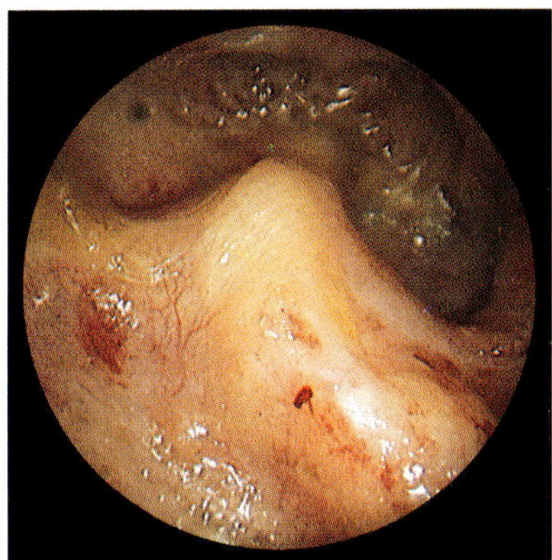

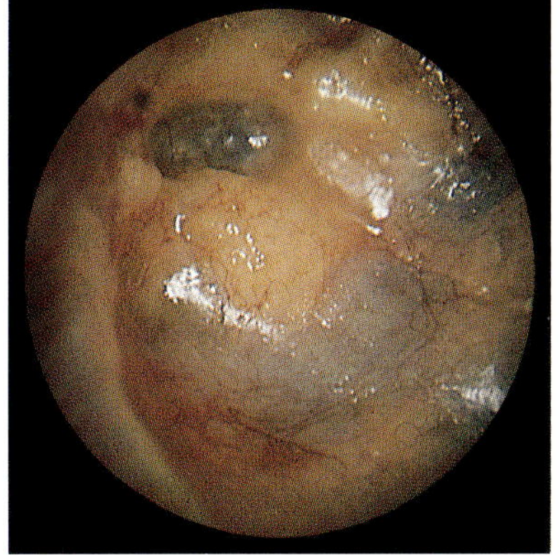

Fig. **86   Tympanoplasty Type IV in contralateral deafness, carried out on 3rd October, 1953.** Chronic middle ear inflammation with cholesteatoma, total defect of the tympanic membrane and ossicles. Full-thickness graft of the middle ear. Amnion graft on the promontory. Endoscopic picture on 8th July, 1990, over 35 years later

Fig. **87   Tympanoplasty Type IV on 3rd October, 1953, with contralateral deafness.** Cavum minor only with the inferior aeration pathway from the tube to the round window. The oval window niche is empty and covered with a split skin graft. Endoscopic view on 8th July, 1990. The audiological results in Type IV tympanoplasty are similar to those obtained in fenestration surgery

Allogenic and Xenogenic Tissue

Ossicles, Tympanic Membrane and En-Bloc Grafts

Allogenic and xenogenic tissue grafts used in ear surgery are very much simpler than other organ transplants. In the latter, the function of the living tissue must be retained and restored immediately after the transplantation. However, immunosuppression, with its enormous attendant risks, is unnecessary in ear surgery: the donor tissue is deprived of its immunological property of rejection so that healing proceeds smoothly.

In middle ear surgery all previous investigations have concerned immunological compatibility. Conservation and removal of immunogenicity can be achieved by chemical means, by lyophilization, deproteinization, irradiation or deep freezing. These methods are subject to constant change, and there is therefore no point in a surgical text in going into details. Suitably prepared specimens are universally available from a tissue bank, but are expensive. Many methods of preservation are simple; for example, that first described using cialit (Marquet 1967) or with previous stiffening of the tympanic membrane by brief immersion in formaldehyde (Smyth 1971 and Perkins 1970). Every otological microsurgeon can therefore prepare the ossicles and an en-bloc graft of the entire middle ear system himself (Marquet 1967). The most logical step was the use of xenogenic tissue such as deproteinized collagen of calf vein (Zini and Sana 1976), or protein cross-linked pericardium, which has the advantage that it has endothelium on both surfaces (Pfaltz 1984).

Allogenic stapes, incus or malleus are suitable materials for bridging defects of the *ossicular chain* if the patient's own ossicles are not suitable for this purpose. Their nontraumatized, nonreactive cortical bone, or the smooth surface produced by sculpting, offer a good base for overgrowth of middle ear mucosa.

Kelemen possessed a histological preparation of this type from a patient with two stapes footplates: the allogenic stapes ossified on the patient's own footplate and the two were entirely covered by mucosa. The value of allogenic ossicles is compared with bioinert alloplastic material below.

Replacement of the Tympanic Membrane with Allogenic and Xenogenic Tissue

The same tissues which are used for autogenous grafting (skin, periosteum, fascia, perichondrium, thin slices of cartilage and dura) have also been used as xenografts. Allogenic sclera was also used previously, but has now been abandoned because of the excessive retraction due to its elastic fibers.

The use of these grafts will be discussed under three headings:
1. for closure of defects of varying size.
2. for aeration disorders (atelectasis, retractions and adhesions), as tissue with the stiffest possible structure;
3. as the tissue of choice to improve hearing, both to close the perforation and to provide differential sound transport.

In the course of time, allogenic and xenogenic denatured tissues change into robust scar tissue. They are unable to heal like an autogenous living graft in the first active phase of plasmatic circulation because there is no immediate electrolyte exchange. The second phase of ingrowth of vessels, and the third phase of reorganization are accomplished very slowly in dead tissue lacking active metabolic processes.

Overgrowth with the patient's own mucosa must lead to a nonreactive incorporation on both surfaces to form a new free-standing tympanic membrane. This requires the development of a capillary system lying parallel to the surface in the shortest possible time, as has been demonstrated experimentally for autogenous skin and fascial grafts. This capillarization of the surface is achieved most reliably by covering the allogenic or xenogenic tissue with a thin layer of autologous fascia pushed under the edge of the healthy epidermis of the tympanic membrane or the neighboring meatal skin. This foreign tissue can also be covered by thin, pressed-out fascia on its inner surface before the new tympanic membrane is replaced. The two fascial surfaces in the tympanum, and those in the meatus, are embedded in the compressed gelatin sponge, so that both sides of the foreign tissue are covered by active autogenous fascia with its rapid vascularization.

Allogenic en-bloc grafts offer three properties which other tissues used to replace the tympanic membrane do not possess:
1. a human collagenous fiber structure;
2. a flat funnel shape;
3. firm fixation to the handle of the malleus and thus to the malleus itself and the entire ossicular chain.

Whereas the first two are not necessarily permanent, the third has the decisive advantage of the en-bloc graft. It provides the ideal solution for the empty middle ear without ossicles and only a small remnant of tympanic membrane. There are, however, two prerequisites: there must be enough mucosa in the host tissue from which re-epithelialization of the large wound of the middle ear and the en-bloc graft can originate; the epitympanum must be wide open, so that accurate positioning of the graft ensures function of the sound-conducting system and aeration with drainage. Osteoplastic epitympanotomy is therefore the preferred method.

The disadvantage of the en-bloc graft is that neither tendons nor folds are available to suspend the bodies of the malleus and incus in the epitympanum to form a functional unit. To our great surprise we found *a broad mucosal overgrowth when the epitympanic wall of an en-bloc graft was reopened* if the upper malleoincudal fold leading to the tegmen tympani had regrown (see Fig. **192**).

Follow-up of the long-term conversion of the collagen fiber system into the body's own tissue would require phased animal experiments, using collagen marked by isotopes, a difficult task with the thin tympanic membrane of experimental animals. In any case a largely connective tissue sheet of scar tissue forms slowly. It is not possible to rely in the long term on the specific function of the collagen fiber network that merges into a ground substance and possesses a true transformer property. The funnel shape is preserved by firm fixation to the handle of the malleus, but in an en-bloc graft, where the malleus is not fixed by mallear ligaments in the epitympanum, the scarred tympanic membrane contracts and luxates externally. For this reason an allogenic en-bloc graft is of limited value and is used mainly for total defects of the middle ear system because of the attached annulus and meatal skin.

Autoimmunological Processes

Tissue tolerance has been important since the first free grafts were used in tympanoplasty. At that time there was no theoretical and experimental basis of immunology to draw upon, but the following conclusions of practical significance could be drawn from the first postoperative results:

Initially, total liquefaction necrosis of autogenous tissue was frequent. This and marginal necrosis were reduced as soon as the technique provided the transposed tissue with the necessary prerequisites for surviving the third healing phase (see above).

In decades of regular use, in thousands of tympanoplasties there have been no reports of rejection of *autologous* grafts.

Direct tissue union of bone to recipient bone and the development of an interposed connective tissue layer is determined exclusively by surgical technique.

The smooth surfaces of an *allogenic ossicle* are more easily overgrown by mucosa than that of au-

togenous mastoid cortex, which forms granulation tissue on the raw surface because of the marrow reaction arising in the spongiosa. This is then a purely pathological and tissue problem and not an immunological problem.

Because the allogenic ossicles do not transmit disease, due to the long prior bacteriocidal treatment with cialit, etc., they can be used without serological or other investigations of the donor. AIDS is discussed on p. 181.

Xenogenic ossicles can be used almost like allogenic material, but the inequality of shape and size of these ossicles is a handicap.

Allogenic tympanic membrane can be used if the patient's own material such as fascia, periosteum from the temporal bone, etc., is not available in sufficient quantities. Recently, xenogenic membranes rich in collagen fibers have been used successfully for parts of the tympanic membrane which need to be reinforced.

Amnion

Amnion is an allogenic tissue with a delicate stroma which serves as a *support for regrowing middle ear epithelium*. The middle ear mucosa demonstrates an extraordinary potential for regrowth in covering defects. Furthermore, epithelial and epidermal closure of a defect comes to a standstill if granulation tissue projects above the surrounding layer. If this granulation tissue is removed and if mucosa capable of regeneration lies close by, the defect can be covered with amnion. Mucosa from the surrounding area then grows under it, whereas the amnion itself undergoes autolysis. H. L. Wullstein has used this method for closing defects since 1952 (Fig. **83**). Operative checks have shown that the defects heal with an opaque, delicate, almost transparent middle ear epithelium. Animal experiments (H. L. Wullstein and Chang) have shown that implanted amnion grows beneath the epithelium of the middle ear cavity so that the amnion can be overlapped by epithelium. It is possible that some amnion cell units are incorporated during healing.

Amnion does not induce an immune response (Akle et al 1982). Indeed, it protects the fetus against the rejection reaction of its mother, who has a different genetic makeup. Fresh amnion adapts easily to all contours; formalin-dried material is less adaptable, but can be stored for an unlimited time.

Because the mother's serology is carefully tested before birth, there is now no objection to its immediate use. Amnion demonstrates an ectodermal epithelium lying over a delicate stroma. Fresh amnion can be used for about 4 days before it begins to decompose, but it keeps longer in 100 ml 1–2% formol Ringer's solution with 500 mg Cefotaxime added. The latter is active against pseudomonas aeroginosa, proteus and anerobes. The graft is washed before use.

Alloplastic Materials

Biomaterials may be divided into:
— *inert* materials such as metal oxides, polyethylene, polypropylene, polytetraflorethylene, vitrified silicone and aluminium ceramics, and crystallized pure carbon (graphite). These are tolerated by the recipient but are not converted into autogenous tissue;
— *bioactive materials* such as pentacalcium hydroxide triphosphate (hydroxyl apatite).
Early attempts were made to find an alloplastic material for a columella in complete defects of the ossicles, initially using acrylate (Palavit) (Fig. **81–83**). The material was sculpted with a narrow edge for the footplate and a broad dome for the tympanic membrane, ensuring that neither structure would be perforated.

Since then many different alloplastic materials have been introduced. Some are porous, soft and pliable such as proplast and plastipore; others are vitrified, such as acrylate and silicone-aluminium ceramics. The first group can be cut to shape, whereas the second must be drilled. They are permeated by connective tissue, although there is no evidence of healing and conversion to fibrous connective tissue. Indeed, in the course of the years, alloplastic materials become surrounded by foreign body cells and undergo resorption. The introduction of prosthetic artificial materials into all surgical disciplines has increased the risk of infection, especially with Gram-negative organisms.

The length of the columella must be able to be adapted to shallow middle ears and those of normal depth and, furthermore, into the angulations between the niches, so that the footplate lies opposite the tympanic membrane. The most reliable form of contact is a firm tissue union over a sufficient area, both at the stapes footplate and the tympanic membrane, but this is not achieved with alloplastic materials. The disadvantage of a bioinert columella is that the epithelialization of the fascia used to replace the tympanic membrane stops at the point of contact with the columella. A permanent defect remains at this point, forming the basis for slow atrophy, perforation, retractions and adhesions. This type of reconstruction is particularly jeopardized by the tendency of the middle ear to atelectasis.

Although the vitrified materials can be individually shaped in a similar manner to alloplastic ossicles, the danger of contact ulceration is much greater. Allogenic ossicles become biologically adapted in the long term and therefore offer better prospects of partial epithelialization. Extensive local resorption of an allogenic ossicle leading to interruption of sound conduction is unusual and can easily be restored.

Plasticine made of hydroxyl apatite and human biological glue (see below) has a high water content and offers favorable conditions for uninterrupted growth when covered by mucosa or in contact with the tympanic membrane. Before it becomes stiff, it can be easily modelled. There is as yet insufficient experience to show whether it is ultimately incorporated into the sound conduction system.

Tantalum and steel wire have proved useful as replacements for the stapes in otosclerosis. The wire heals without inducing a reaction, not only in the middle ear space but also when embedded in tissue, and therefore also in the sheet of connective scar tissue which seals the oval window. If a wire-teflon prosthesis is used, however, this is only achieved if the teflon piston is inserted into the perilymphatic space on a thin tissue layer such as a Shea (1958) vein graft. This provides a tissue seal and prevents a persistent perilymph fistula.

Human Tissue Glue, Hydroxyl Apatite and Plasticine

Foreign substances for use in epitympanotomy were introduced into tympanoplasty by S. R. Wullstein. They include the following:
1. A biological material, *human tissue glue*, was initially described under the name Tissucol. *Tissue adhesion* had been frequently attempted in tympanoplasty using inorganic substances such as acryl glues. Despite their adhesive effect, these substances acted in the long term as foreign bodies, and were therefore abandoned. The situation was changed completely with the successful development of the human tissue glue, Tissucol, which provided immediate, powerful adhesion. Adhesion was permanent and did not in any way inhibit the normal healing process. The glue has been used by S. R. Wullstein in rhinology and otology since 1977. It is used in septoplasty to avoid packing, which damages the cilia and goblet cells of the mucosa.
2. An inorganic substance, *hydroxyl apatite* (pentacalcium hydroxide triphosphate) is a nonvitrified powder. *Hydroxyl apatite is a ground substance for the formation of bone.*

3. *Plasticine* is a combination of 1 and 2. It guarantees a fixed contact with the bone, with no joint. Furthermore, it is continuously converted to autologous bone. If it is embedded in tissue with no bony contact, it is gradually converted into thick scar tissue. It is therefore suitable for obliterating mastoid cavities, for reconstruction of the meatal walls and for cover of dural defects associated with brain prolapse, etc.

The name "plasticine" for this bioactive material was chosen because the material is capable, for a short time, of being molded into any shape, which it then retains. This physical property is described as plasticity, in contrast to elasticity, in which the material returns to its original shape. Plasticine softens again in water after hardening and can then be molded into shape as before.

Free grafts of fascia, periosteum and even full-thickness skin heal as well on plasticine as on tissue, even if the surface is large. This astounding property can be explained by the fact that the healing process encounters the same biological prerequisites as in healing of a free-standing tympanic membrane graft.

Plasticine is prepared by the surgeon during the operation shortly before it is needed (see Figs. **88–91**). A bacteriocidal antibiotic, for example a cephalosporin, which is nonallergenic but which is active against pseudomonas aerogenosa, proteus and anaerobic organisms is also included.

1. The pentacalcium hydroxide triphosphate is first mixed with one or two drops of the antibiotic on a plexiglass plate.
2. It is then mixed with the fibrinogen part of the Tissucol.
3. Finally, the thrombin-calcium-chloride part of the Tissucol is added, and the mass is molded to the required shape while it remains malleable. The resulting plate is curved to form a new posterior or superior meatal wall, or to cover a bony defect in the middle or posterior cranial fossa. It may also be used on audiological grounds to obliterate a very large mastoid cavity which is free of mucosa up to the level of a wide but unevenly shaped antrum.

Plasticine also serves for fixing traumatized cortical fragments and fracture lines of the mastoid process, especially of the posterior meatal wall or of the temporal squama. It may also be used to fill the incision made by the diamond burr in the epitympanic flap if it is unusually wide after having had to be cut further and extended (see Figs. **92–95**).

Plasticine can be mixed with drilled fresh bone dust; for example, from the temporal squama. Bone paste alone without tissue glue is not rigid enough. On the other hand, it is very suitable for filling bone cuts; for example, of the epitympanic flap.

The composition of the plasticine has been determined by chemical analysis as follows (Schindler 1984):
- 75–80% water. This high water content indicates a marked porosity, which is appropriate for the electrolyte provision required for a free graft.
- 20–25% organic and inorganic materials (24–26% dry weight), of which 4.5% is potassium, and 34–36% calcium, of which 85–89% is calcium phosphate. The rest is hydrochloric acid and organic substances; for example, protein.

Bacteriological investigation of the porous material impregnated with a bacteriocidal agent showed that after implantation of a piece of this plasticine on an appropriate nutrient, there was initially a very effective zone of inhibition of bacterial growth. This fell to half after ten days but still demonstrated a significant effect after a longer period, i.e., the substance contained within it was still bacteriologically active. Because the bacteriocidal agent is only applied once, the question of resistance does not arise.

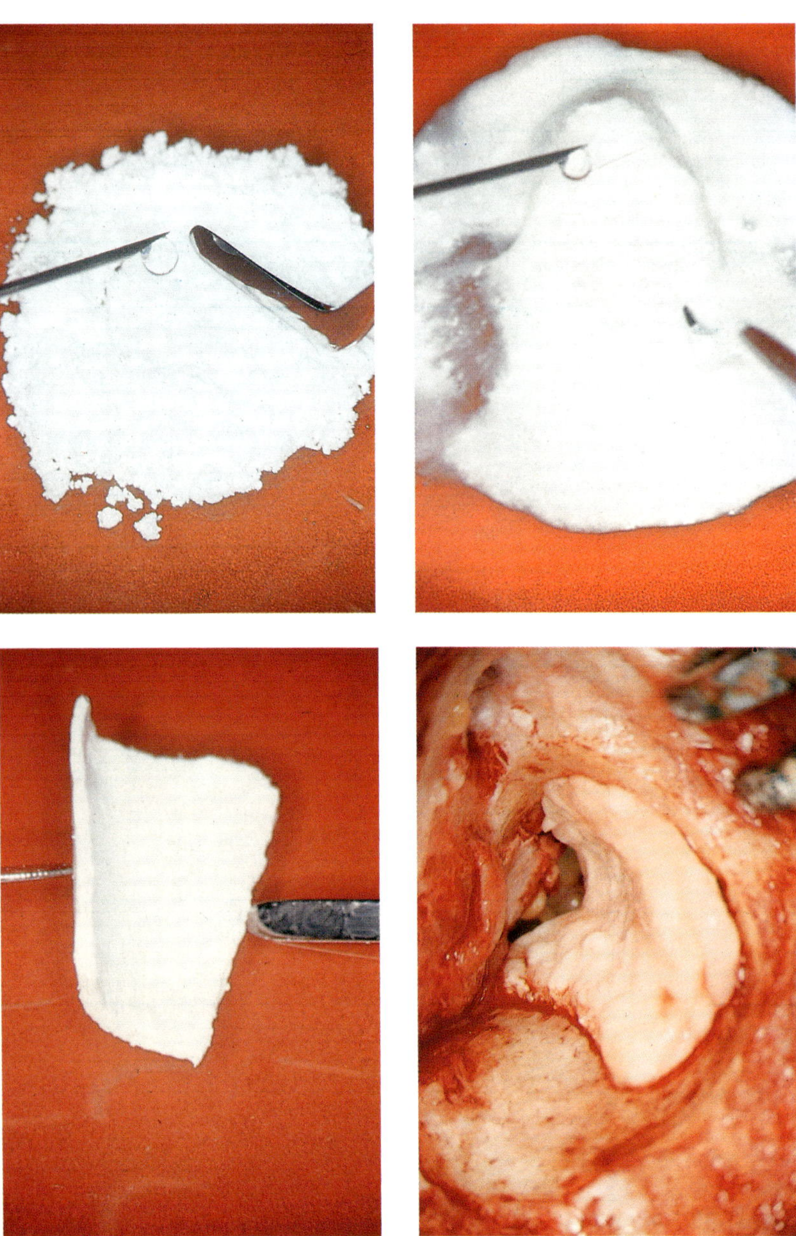

Figs. **88–91** **Preparation of the plasticine.** Shaping of the bony wall and its placement

Figs. **92–93 Osteoplastic epitympanotomy.** A large dural prolapse is exposed during clearance of a large cholesteatoma, replaced before reconstruction and sealed off with plasticine

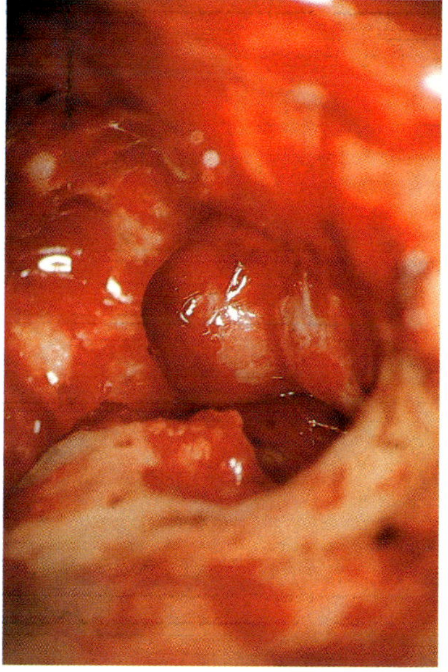
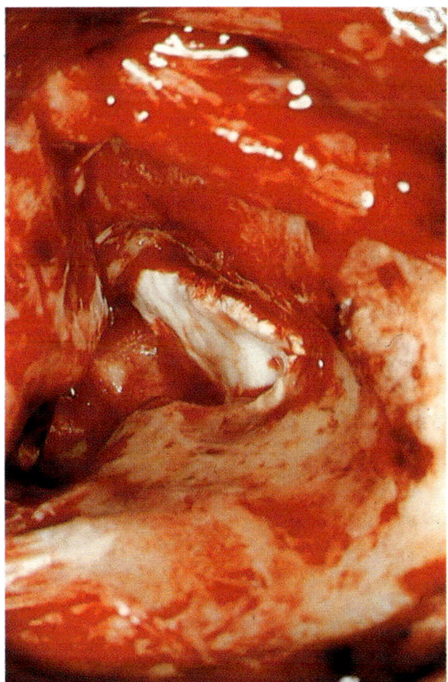

Figs. **94–95 Reduction of an old radical cavity with plasticine**

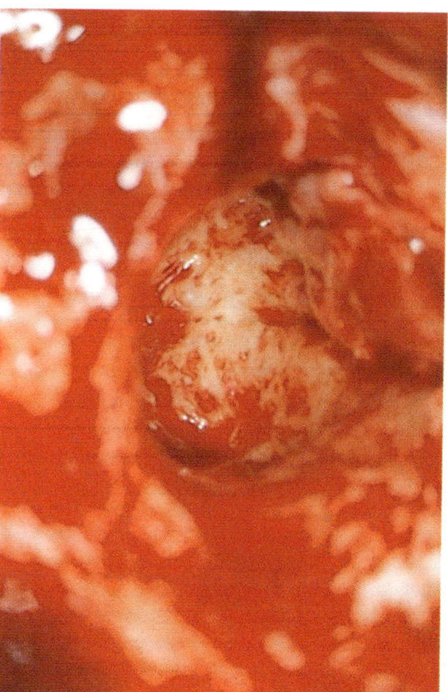
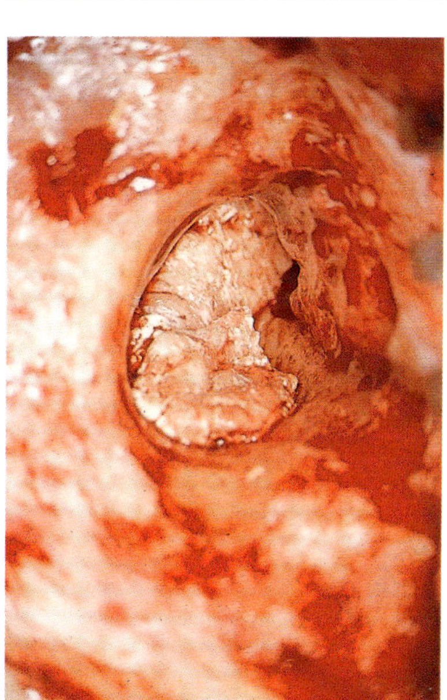

Evaluation of Autogenous, Allogenic and Xenogenic Tissues and Alloplastic Materials Both Bioactive and Bioinert

Autogenic Tissues

The ossicles lend themselves well to being reshaped and fitted. Cortical bone (from the mastoid process, for example) has the disadvantage that granulations sprout very rapidly from the marrow of the spongiosa on its internal surface and interrupt epithelialization. The result is a focus of chronic tissue irritation with secondary infection arising from the air spaces.

Allogenic Tissue

Reconstruction was revolutionized by Cialit treatment of inert tissue. Difficulties arise from different sizes of donor and recipient tissue. Healthy parts of the recipient tympanic membrane should be preserved. The introduction of a complete tympanic membrane with the annulus fibrosus is not always necessary or desirable, and partial replacement is often possible.

The unique advantage of the en-bloc graft is the natural congruity of the tympanic membrane and malleus. The correct positioning of the en-bloc graft in the "intact" canal wall technique was uncertain. With the introduction of osteoplastic epitympa notomy it immediately became a reliable procedure. A repeat osteoplastic epitympanotomy after an en-bloc graft to improve hearing demonstrated that a healthy middle ear epithelium had grown over the Cialit ossicles, leaving no defects. A regular broad fold had arisen, running from the summit of the malleus and the incus to the tegmen tympani. There is thus evidence that a suspension system can form when allogenic ossicles are used.

Marquet (1981) has demonstrated that the contact surfaces of the malleus and incus are shaped differently from lateral to medial. He concluded from his morphological findings that there is a functional fine tuning. He demonstrated the possibility of constructing an articulated columella system rather than a one-piece columella, using two fitted and glued allogenic ossicles.

The collagenous fiber system in the tympanic membrane is indeed not retained, but is converted into connective tissue. Nonetheless, sound transmission by the en-bloc graft remains worth striving for.

Xenogenic Tissues and Systems

The possibilities of control of immunological problems attending the use of such tissues is undergoing continuous development, as are operative techniques to ensure their rapid healing. The use of allogenic tissues and en-bloc grafts will remain difficult, because it is illegal to take them without the permission of the patient's relatives. Furthermore, serological tests must be carried out immediately after the donor's death.

Progress in immunosuppression and biochemistry have opened the way to abandoning the use of alloplastic transplant material because of difficulties of supply. Xenogenic tissue can often be used instead, and this can be obtained from young animals, under ideal conditions. The demand was originally created by vascular surgery. Zini and Sanna (1976) were the first to use calf jugular vein after enzymatic hydrolysis to construct a tympanic membrane (Xomed). Pflatz 1984 used calf perichondrium subjected to intra- and intermolecular cross-linking of the protein (Solco). This tissue has the great advantage of being covered on both surfaces by endothelium. It inhibits the budding of endothelial sprouts for a short time and thus facilitates the epithelialization of the neighboring surfaces; this is a prerequisite for smooth, rapid healing of a free-standing membrane. There are good prospects that xenogenic ossicles, which are easy to obtain, also could be used; in particular, ossicles of the same specific gravity and of similar materials (apatite) that are easily overgrown by mucosa.

The internal surface of the tympanic membrane is more likely to heal if mucosa capable of regeneration can be preserved in the tympanic cavity close to the edge of the perforation. Any persisting unhealed mass of granulations within the middle ear forms a source of continuing secretion. Reopening of healed middle ears since the introduction of tympanoplasty has repeatedly shown that the spontaneous healing capacity after the eradicating procedure is so great that a mucosal defect almost never remains within the cavity.

The external surface of a xenogenic tissue gives more cause for concern. The danger of abnormal healing of the external surface is great, because direct contact with the meatal epidermis is not reliably established around the entire circumference. However, even if a flat epidermis lacking in papillae slowly grows over the xenogenic surface, it does not adhere to the underlying layer. It is easily damaged by later manipulations; for example, cleaning by an inexperienced otologist. It has now become the rule to cover the meatal surface of an allogenic graft with thin autologous fascia. As shown on p. 42, chemotactic endothelial and capillary contact is established within hours, and the fascial vessels arranged longitudinally are reconnected to the circulation within a few hours. A healthy autologous surface of this type epidermizes in several days.

Alloplastic Bioactive Materials

Among the various bioactive materials, only penta-calcium hydroxide triphosphate, a stimulator of bone formation, is available for analysis. It can be used in otology as a powder because it is not subjected to pressure, as it is in orthopedics and oral surgery. The important factor is complete contact with the bone and with uninjured bony surfaces. In its unvitrified form as plates, adapters, cubes, etc., it cannot be used in otological surgery; firstly, because too much dead space remains where bone is never formed so that a seroma persists, and secondly, because vitrified and shaped adapters grow in a bioinert fashion but are not incorporated in the tissue. In one of our patients they had to be removed from the meatal wall two and a half years later because of pain on chewing. Plasticine is firmly molded; it serves to heal large bone defects in the superior and posterior meatal wall or in the tegmen tympani and antri in the presence of dural prolapse. It should overlap the internal and external sides of the bone edges as far as possible, so as to be able to ossify in the resulting sterile environment thanks to its large pores, high water content and normal pH. The bony walls of the cavity should be preserved as far as possible for contact with plasticine. Neighboring soft tissues have no bioactive effect on the calcium substance to induce the formation of bone.

Pharmaceutical Agents Used Before, During and After Surgery

Allergic mucosal reactions should be prevented during *local preparation* of the external and middle ears and the eustachian tube. They can cause the planned operation to be delayed. At the first consultation the patient should be asked about possible allergies; for example, to penicillin. At the same examination, the external meatus should be cleaned carefully and a specimen of pus sent for culture and sensitivity. Furthermore, the improvement in air conduction achieved by temporary cover of the perforation should be assessed. During the operation a further bacteriological specimen should be obtained from the depths of the wound; for example, from a cholesteatoma matrix, to isolate anaerobes.

Only rarely does the meatal skin require preoperative attention. If it does, antibiotic ointments should not be used, but simple disinfectants, possibly followed by baby oil. These substances must not penetrate a dry perforation with noninflamed mucosa in the middle ear, because they cause pain and secretion. Many disinfectants can penetrate the windows and endanger Corti's organ. In the pres-

ence of severe infection and secretion, prolonged local treatment does not reach the main foci of infection; for example, between the swollen folds of the epitympanum or behind a mass of cholesteatoma. Since the introduction of tympanoplasty we have learnt that the effective control of infection is only achieved by painstaking opening of all recesses of the middle ear.

Yeast infections of the meatus are frequent and must be controlled before the operation. However, they are not dangerous, since experience has shown that they resolve with thorough cleaning before, during and after the operation. The hair around the ear should not be shaved, as this damages the skin.

The addition of *antibiotics* to the gelatin sponge is advisable not only for inflamed mucosa, but also for a very thin matrix lining and even for a relatively mild inflammation of the mucosa. The following principles apply:
1. The antibiotic must be investigated to ensure that it is not toxic to the inner ear. The use of a locally very active antibacterial treatment is not damaging if the correct agent is chosen, but its omission can on occasion have serious consequences.
2. Pseudomonas, mainly aeruginosa, is the most frequent organism in chronic otorrhea, mastoiditis and cholesteatoma, followed by staphylococcus aureus and proteus. Newer penicillins are indeed active but occasionally carry the risk of allergy.
3. Anaerobes are quite common, the commonest being bacteroides fragilis. The above remarks apply to them also. Because anaerobes die very rapidly in a culture exposed to air, they are not often isolated.
4. Infection with mycoplasma organisms arising from the airways is often more serious. Mixed infection can necessitate combined treatment after operation.
5. Decongestion using a mild potassium diuretic may be advisable for very edematous swelling due to mucopolypoid and mucoperiosteal processes.

Pre- and Postoperative Treatment of the Eustachian Tube

The tubal mucosa can only be reached indirectly. The most important point, as with all mucosa of the airway, is to free it of retained secretions. The tube, its mucosal folds and the paratubal cells should be powerfully inflated a short time before the operation; any foreign material in the middle ear or the eustachian tube is sucked out. These spaces are then filled in a retrograde manner from the middle ear, and from the nasopharynx as well, with a preparation of a tested antibiotic and cortisone. The material is forced into the tube from the middle ear with light pressure on a Politzer balloon until the patient can taste it within his mouth. Air should not be blown in afterward, to ensure that the tube remains filled.

Instillation from the nasopharynx is achieved by the introduction of a catheter into the torus, under endoscopic control. The treatment should be continued for a few days only. Although prolonged treatment can eliminate infective organisms, it leads to brisk mucosal secretion and possibly to allergic reactions. The resolution of hyperplasia of the mucosal glands is achieved in an entirely physiological manner by the surgically created middle ear, especially in children with seromucinous inflammation (p. 137).

Basics of Operative Technique

Irrigation and Apiration

Drilling requires simultaneous *irrigation* of the drill head during the operation. This is much easier during dissection in a closed body cavity, in contrast to the oral cavity, for example. Continuous irrigation and aspiration may be used. For preference, simultaneous irrigation and suction are applied as required to localized areas by the surgeon, using one hand. Irrigation by an assistant, who does not have an accurate view, is unsatisfactory. Combined irrigation−aspiration was introduced for fenestration by Venker (1949) and has been repeatedly refined since.

Physiological saline solution is used for *irrigation*; in a *highly infected ear* this can be supplemented by a disinfectant; for example, 0.05% ethacrinidine lactate (Rivanol), which is completely harmless. The yellow staining of the exposed bone discolors photographs and films, so that irrigation with Rivanol solution is not used if photographs are to be taken. At the end of the operation, all the middle ear spaces are thoroughly irrigated and aspirated. This does not in any way disturb the healing of the graft. Chinolinol sulphate 0.05% is colorless.

Aspiration: contact of the sucker with mucosa or granulations stimulates bleeding. Some air should always be allowed to enter, if at all possible. If stronger suction is necessary, a compressed, highly absorbent piece of cotton wool should be interposed to prevent adhesion of clots to the mucosa; for example, in the hypotympanum. The suction is applied to this from time to time whilst resection is being carried out elsewhere.

Drilling and Polishing

Burrs of various shapes are used with long, smooth strokes under continuous irrigation to create surfaces and to sculpt. Diamond burrs polish and sculpt at the same time. Pointed conical diamonds (0.4−0.5 mm at the point) can also cut in every shape of curve. Drills, on the other hand, bore holes and do not sculpt.

Burrs may be conical, cylindrical or round in shape; the latter are often mistakenly referred to by the old term "rose head burr." Those with the finest cutting surfaces are called "Finierer." Lempert (1941) and others used them for fenestration of the lateral semicircular canal. Diamond burrs were introduced into bone surgery by H. L. Wullstein in 1950.

The blades of all round burrs are oblique so that they cut only when turning clockwise, whereas the blades are vertical on a cylindrical drill. The latter cut sharply and without vibration if the cutting surfaces are cross-cut, because the grooves are then less likely to fill with bone dust. These burrs are particularly suitable for rapid superficial removal of bone (for example, from the temporal squama), without producing powerful bone conduction noise and marked vibration.

Three or four sizes of burrs and diamonds suffice. Burrs with coarse cutting edges are more dangerous when cutting, their sound is unpleasant and they sit less securely in the hand. All burr heads which can turn only to the right have the great disadvantage that they tend to jump unwanted over edges, possibly causing damage. The cutting edge of drills can catch on the surrounding soft tissue (for example, during a meatoplasty), as well as on mucosa, and tear them off.

Diamond burrs, rotating to the right or to the left, cut down to the soft tissues but do not damage them. They do not create incision surfaces which tend to heal rapidly, but glaze the surface of the spongiosa. Pressure with their point can be used to seal bleeding points in the bone.

The groove for a bone incision is made with finer and finer diamond burrs. Dissection may be less traumatic and quicker with a very small sharp-cutting round burr along the inner cortex of the temporal squama before the pointed conical diamond burr is brought into use.

As dissection approaches the cochlear capsule, the use of the drill must be brief and precise because of sound trauma. This is also true of aspiration; very sharp noise, especially close to the subiculum around the round window, easily evokes the stapedius reflex.

The burr or the diamond are used to create the desired shape along the longest circumference with long, even strokes at 40,000 to 80,000 revolutions per minute with continuous irrigation. A dry drill causes osteonecrosis, due to heat. Waving the drill about in a restless manner with the point still cutting on one surface instead of along a profile is a sign of poor training.

Operative Methods for Individual Osteoplastic Exposure of all Middle Ear Cavities

Osteoplastic epitympanotomy is technically the easiest method of tympanoplasty. It is the most reliable and thorough method: the entire pneumatic system of the temporal bone is exposed rapidly from the root of the zygoma to the occipital bone, and from the tegmen tympani and antri to the mastoid apex. Before undertaking surgery the novice should develop manual skills by studying the anatomical variations on 30 or more temporal bone preparations.

Osteoplastic epitympanotomy offers a unified surgical concept. The surgeon need not decide between antrotomy or radical mastoidectomy or between the open and closed method of tympanoplasty.

The basics laid down at the first tympanoplasty by H. L. Wullstein in 1952 still apply to the planning of any reconstructive operation on the ear: Firstly, later complications must always have priority over improvement of hearing. Secondly, improvement of hearing must only be considered when all danger has been eliminated. The type of procedure is only clear beforehand in a central perforation with completely quiescent middle ear mucosa in which the prospect of increase of hearing can be forecast by testing with a patch. Only in this type of middle ear is inspection of the epitympanum, the ossicular chain and the mastoid air spaces unnecessary. The purpose of the operation is to close the perforation with a free graft. *In all other restorative middle ear surgery the epitympanum and antrum must always be exposed for inspection.*

Osteoplastic epitympanotomy (Figs. **96–123**) leads directly to the main focus of disease in the epitympanum rather than via the retrotympanic spaces. Its purpose is:
- to expose the main focus from the tympanic tubal ostium across the mesohypotympanum and the epitympanum only as far as is necessary. Dissection might be extended to the mastoid apex, as well as the para- and sublabyrinthine cells, but is always tailored to the patient's requirements, and the minimal dissection necessary is carried out:

- to understand the embryological, anatomical and pathological basis of the disease as a basis for planning of eradication and reconstruction;
- to leave the posterior bony meatal wall intact;
- to preserve the middle ear and the external meatus with its skin sleeve;
- most important of all: to preserve the aeration pathways, especially the lower, and, if necessary, to extend the air-containing volume of the middle ear by lateral displacement of the orthotopic bony lid.

Incision

Dissection begins with drilling of the temporal squama along the temporal line down to the internal cortex of the middle cranial fossa. The roof of the bony meatus must be removed in order to reach the lateral wall of the epitympanum along the level of the tegmen tympani, to allow the lateral epitympanic wall to be excised. Anteriorly, the protympanic recess must be fully encompassed, so that the root of the zygoma is reached. Posteriorly, dissection is determined by the extent of the disease and the degree of pneumatization; at the very least, the antrum is exposed.

The skin incision begins at the level of the supratragal notch and then runs above the auricle, parallel to the helix, close to the hairline along the temporal line, and then, with a slight concave curve, posterior to the posterior meatal wall to the same level or lower than the anterior origin of the incision. The auricle is turned inferiorly; the meatal skin remains closed. In this way, the epitympanum and the aditus can be reached easily to allow creation of the bony lid.

The anatomical structures that suspend the auricle (the anterior auricular ligament, the greater helical and posterior auricular muscles) lie inferior to the skin incision and are not divided. Small bleeding points from the parietal branches of the superficial temporal artery are dealt with by bipolar coagu-

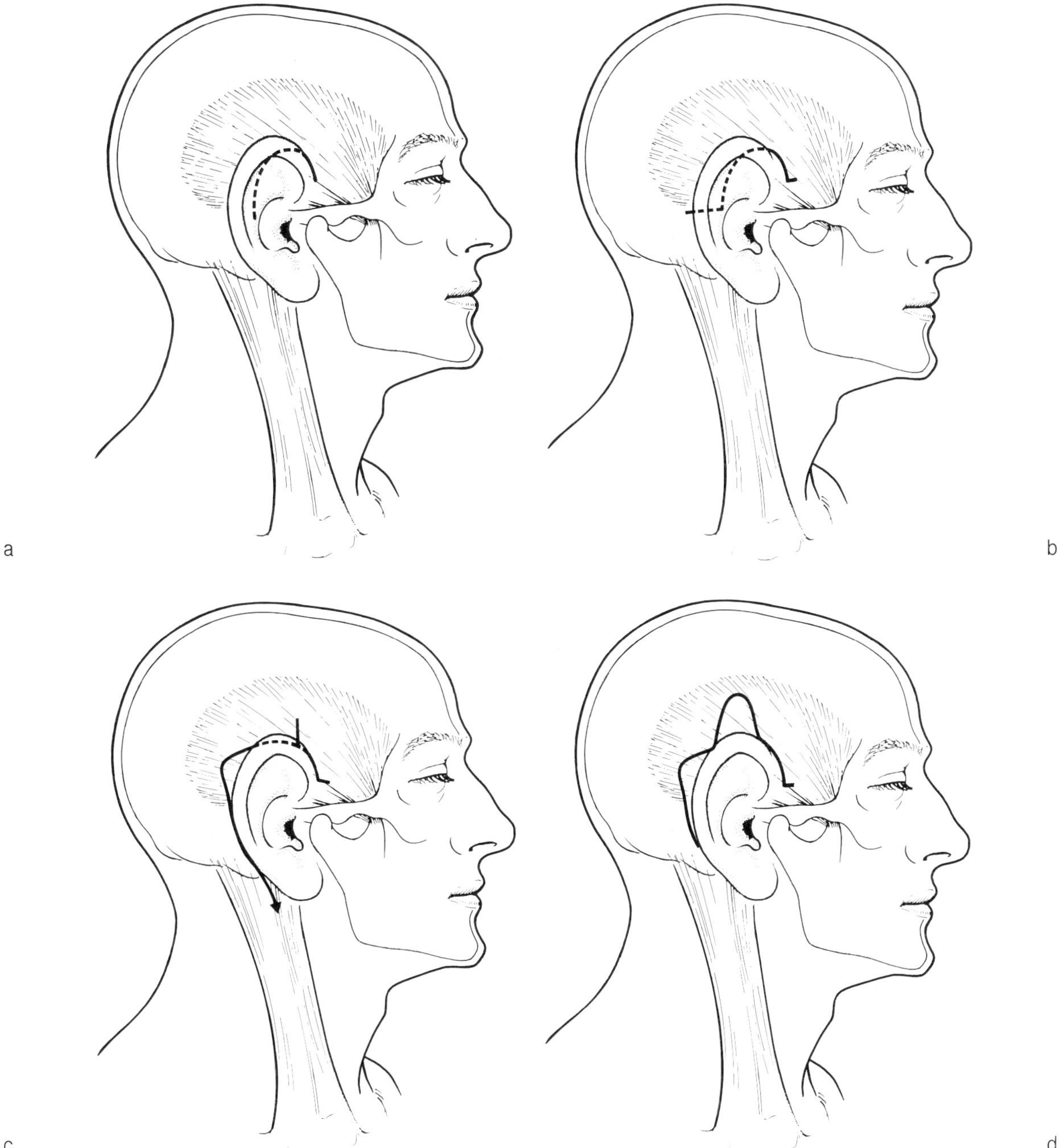

Fig. **96**   **Incisions:**

a) for almost completely absent pneumatization with a steep sinodural angle, narrow mastoid, i.e., a small base of the petrous pyramid, an anterior sinus and a low squama;

b) for a wide antrum and extensive pneumatization in the temporal bone;

c) for a wide mastoid, i.e., with a large distance from the sinus to the posterior meatal wall, and possibly extensive pneumatization extending into the occipital bone, i.e., a wide open sinodural angle and a broad-surfaced base to the petrous pyramid;

d) supplementary incision for a suppurative focus in extensive pneumatization in the temporal bone and the root of the zygoma

lation: each small persistent bleeding point requires repeated aspiration, which distorts the original pathological picture and the fine structures, whose accurate study is so important. The auricle is then divided from the temporalis fascia and turned down. Damage to the meatal skin must be avoided at all costs. The temporalis muscle is divided by a periosteal incision along the temporal line, beginning at the root of the zygoma, passing the suprameatal spine and ending at the tympanomastoid fissure. It is raised superiorly and posteriorly with a periosteal elevator. If the external meatus is very curved, the dura mater will be low and the temporal line and the squama will overhang markedly.

This incision is recommended to prevent damage to the superficial temporal artery and vein, and also to provide *the necessary access* to the petrous bone by a generous dissection of the overhanging squama in the presence of disease of the anterior and posterior paralabyrinthine danger zones, particularly for a paralabyrinthine cholesteatoma.

Radiographs using Schüller's and Stenver's (Wullstein's) steep view are valuable for the assessment of the extent of pneumatization of the temporal and mastoid bones. On these views, the occipital line lies superior and medial to the labyrinthine block.

The generous exposure of the middle ear cavity using the osteoplastic bone lid is adapted to the shape of the middle ear and to the disease. The incision must therefore be created in such a way that it can be extended to deal with changing conditions.

This incision is not suitable for glomus tumors or carcinomas of the middle ear. Orientation along the internal cortex of the middle cranial fossa is usually most advisable for atresias and middle ear anomalies. Extension of the operation to the soft tissues of the neck for phlebitis, Betzold's abscess and facial nerve lesions is possible in the usual manner.

The disease may extend from the tympanic ostium of the eustachian tube, beneath the tegmen tympani, the aditus and the antrum along the floor of the middle cranial fossa to the sinodural angle. These structures must therefore be exposed first. The space under the tegmen, which is often covered laterally in the epitympanum and aditus by the overhanging squama, should be exposed. Its removal allows direct vision of all contours of the lateral wall of the epitympanum (in the old French nomenclature, the "mur de la logette").

The embryological position of the tegmen and the anterior contour of the sigmoid sinus determine how the base of the petrous pyramid appears on the Schüller's view. A low tegmen and a steep sinus indicate (p. 25) a pointed roof angle of the petrous pyramid, i. e., a steep, narrow access to the antrum, a markedly overhanging squama and a narrow caroticobulbar angle.

During postaural antrotomy, access to the antrum is narrow and directed upwards, with particular risk to the facial nerve and the lateral semicircular canal. The entrance to the epitympanum is difficult to find and even more difficult in the small concealed antrum, especially if a Koerner's septum is present. In contrast, a wide roof angle of the petrous pyramid and a well-pneumatized mastoid process produce favorable anatomical conditions.

Signs suggesting a paralabyrinthine cholesteatoma, especially an anterior one, include intermittent weakness of the facial nerve, typical radiological findings, mild fistula signs and headaches. The skin incision is then carried upward from in front of the anterior otobasion at right angles to the concha into the muscle (Fig. **96**). The *inner cortex of the temporal bone together with the tegmen* can be divided through this incision after epitympanotomy, using the diamond burr, allowing the dura to be freed. The profile of the inner cortex can be easily reconstituted with tissue glue and plasticine, and pasted over with fascia and periosteum. Paralabyrinthine cholesteatoma, either anterior or posterior, can thus be made accessible, together with its site of origin, from lateral and above by extending the osteoplastic epitympanotomy into the floor of the middle cranial fossa.

It is advisable after making the incision and achieving hemostasis to insert only *one* robust retractor, because the insertion of several instruments can obstruct a wide view into the depth of the wound.

The removal of the squama begins with long, even strokes, using a sharp cylindrical burr so that the vault of the bony external meatus is rapidly converted into a horizontal groove which includes the temporal line. The bone dust is collected. The membranous meatus is released stepwise beyond the tympanosquamous and tympanomastoid fissures. Dissection is then continued, using finer and finer cylindrical and diamond burrs along the inner cortex of the temporal squama until a bony lid is created. The membranous meatus is seldom incised.

The tegmen is thus available in the entire length of its attachment to the inner cortex of the middle cranial fossa (possibly as far as the sinodural angle) as a plane of access for the bony lid. At the posterior tympanic spine lies the completely intact posterior meatal wall. The posterior meatal wall is largely retained on the mastoid side but can later be removed as far as necessary by an approach from above, on the tympanic side, using the diamond burr with an undercut, ensuring an unimpeded view for the thorough dissection of the sinus tympani in the presence of a steep course of the facial nerve. Replacement of the epitympanic bony lid ensures restitution of a normal meatus, and the suture of the galea restores normal contours to the auricle. Drainage of the mastoid process from its tip may be necessary for a few days.

During osteoplastic epitympanotomy, the surgeon should not sit lateral to the operated ear and especially should not face the patient's feet, but should sit closer to the patient's skull, almost in the same position as for a transtemporal extradural access to the internal meatus. In 1973 Goodhill proposed changing the position of the microscope during the operation, using circumferential access to extend the mobility of the operative procedure and to improve the view of the tympanic sinus (Fig. **97**).

The surgeon develops the operation from the tegmen to the hypotympanum, and, if necessary, posterior to the posterior meatal wall into the mastoid apex, thus achieving a wide, uninterrupted view of the operative field. The pars tensa, if it has not been destroyed, is completely preserved by this operation, facilitating repair of the tympanic membrane.

The meatal skin adheres tightly to the annulus at the tympanic fissure. The connective tissue fibers and the auricular branch of the vagus nerve in the tympanomastoid fissure must be divided with a round or sickle knife. Appreciable bleeding does not occur at this point and is first to be expected close to the annulus fibrosus, where the branches of the deep auricular artery run transverse to the axis of the meatus or close to the bony origin of the tympanosquamous fissure. At that point the preauricular branches of the superficial temporal artery are easily damaged during mobilization of the relatively thick connective tissue strands. This bleeding can be brought rapidly under control with bipolar diathermy or by waiting for a brief period. The meatal skin becomes thinner and thinner as the tympanic membrane is approached.

The delicate epidermis of the pars tensa can be easily elevated over the bony annulus and from the posterior, rather robust, part of the para flaccida with a round or sickle knife. It tears easily at its anterior, very delicate, epithelial attachment. If an epitympanic defect is present at this site, its edges must be excised very carefully to prevent inversion when they are repositioned, causing an iatrogenic transplant cholesteatoma. Interposition of fascia between the collagenous fiber layer and the epider-

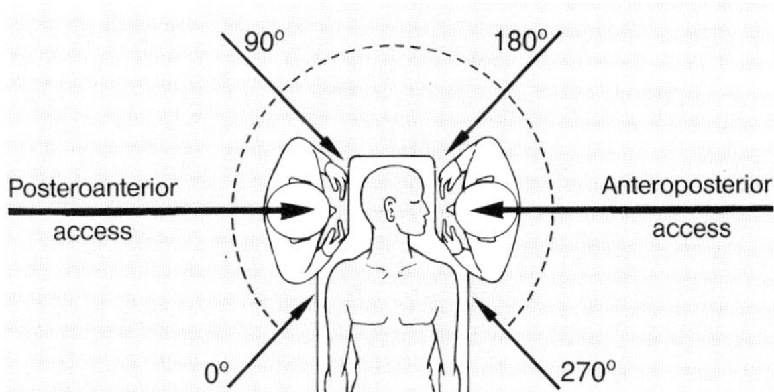

Fig. **97 Goodhill's access** (Goodhill 1973)

mis without an incision in the meatal skin is the preferred technique for reconstruction of the tympanic membrane.

The roof of the bony meatus is thinned using a fast-cutting, pear-shaped burr. Dissection continues beyond the suprameatal spine, far anteriorly into the root of the zygoma, and at that point, into the internal cortex of the floor of the middle cranial fossa.

The internal cortex can be recognized by the lightly discolored bone with small blood vessels and bleeding points. Development and thinning of the bony lid is determined by the individual circumstances; for example, a low dura, the height of the epitympanum, and the extent of pneumatization superiorly and anteriorly into the lateral epitympanic wall. The bony lid must be as thick as possible, but the dura must not be exposed or damaged.

At the zygoma the lateral wall of the epitympanum lies further medial than it does over the antrum. It is therefore necessary to cut the thick bone more deeply toward the anterior tympanic spine than over the aditus. Also, the bony projection of the tympanic bone at the tympanosquamous fissure and at the start of the tympanic annulus should be generously bevelled to expose the floor of the inferior aeration pathway and the protympanic recess widely. A thin layer of cells in the lateral epitympanic wall and the temporal squama along the middle cranial fossa with swollen mucosa may give the mistaken impression that the limit of the tegmen tympani has already been reached. It becomes clear from the radiographs and from the cortical bone exposed with the burr and diamonds that this groove medial to the deepest curvature of the middle cranial fossa must lie higher toward the arcuate eminence.

The bony groove leads directly along the anterior wall of the epitympanum upward as far as the tegmen tympani. There it bends at a right angle posteriorly and follows the outline of the middle cranial fossa along the tegmen tympani over the adi-

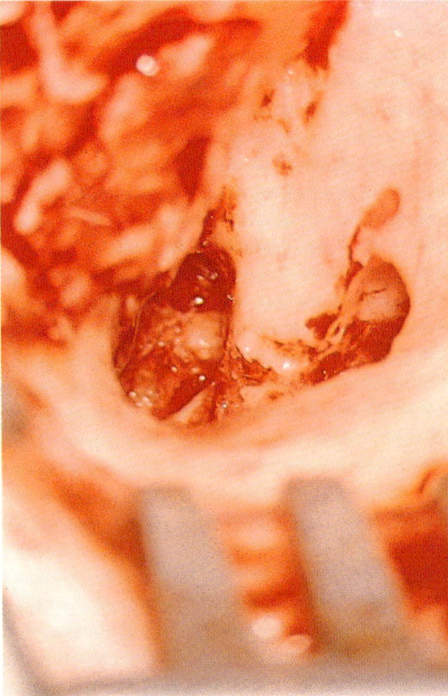

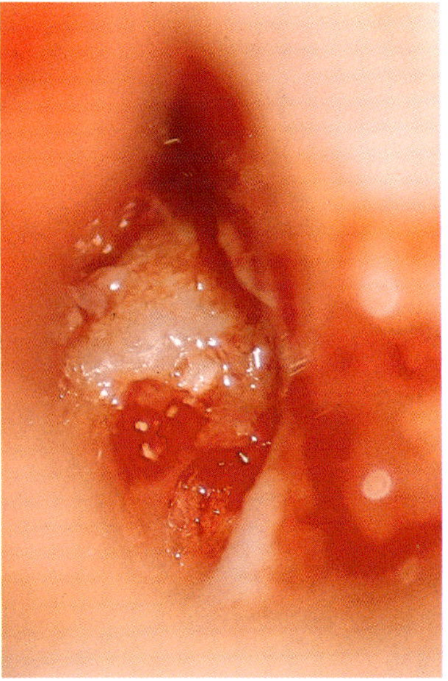

Fig. **98 Osteoplastic epitympa-notomy after removal of the bony lid.** Left ear. Using the supra-auricular access. The surgeon sits at the head of the patient and looks from above downward into the depth of the mesohypotympanum. At the right of the picture is the opened antrum. Above that lies the broad, undisturbed posterior bony meatal wall between the mesohypotympanum and the mastoid

Fig. **99 Osteoplastic epitympa-notomy** showing the same position as in Fig. **98** under higher magnification for better assessment of the oval window niche, the stapes and the sinus tympani. On the right-hand side of the picture lies the posterior stapedial crus, and on the left, the anterior. The long process of the incus is absent

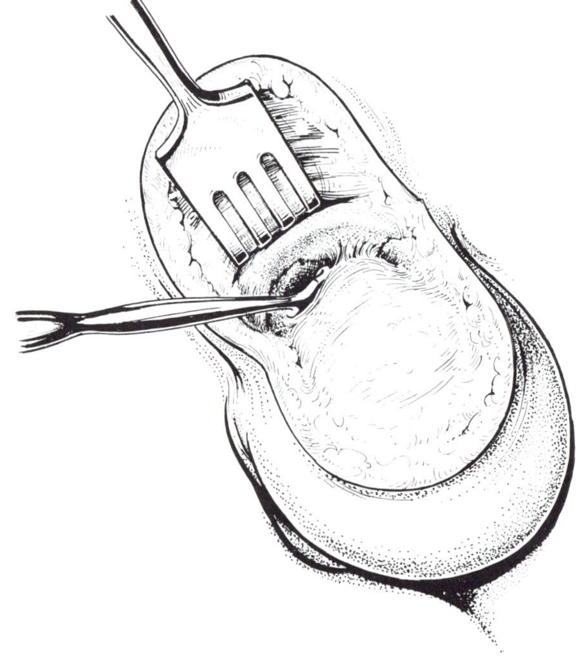

Fig. **100 Osteoplastic epitympanotomy.** The periosteal incision around the superior half of the meatal entrance is followed by release of the closed meatal tube with the raspatory beyond the tympanosquamous and tympanomastoid fissures

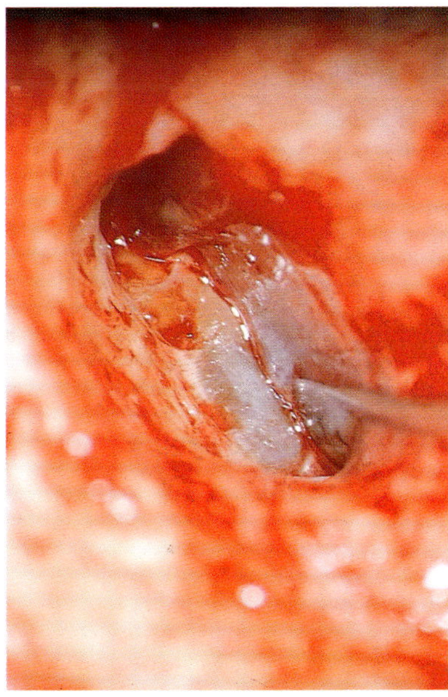

Fig. **101 Osteoplastic epitympanotomy.** Before the upper control window is created, the epidermis of the pars tensa is elevated for interposition of the fascial graft (in this case, to strengthen a very atrophic postero-superior quadrant)

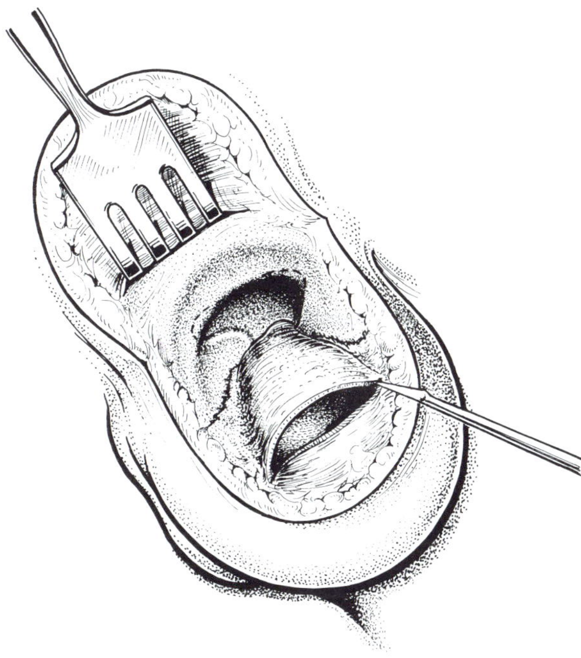

Fig. **102 Osteoplastic epitympanotomy.** The formation of the meatal skin flap is continued to the middle of the anterior meatal wall as far as the fibrous annulus. The skin tube can be opened at the entrance of the bony meatus with a vertical incision

tus to the start of the tegmen antri. The tegmen sinks slightly toward the aditus and then rises again steeply over the antrum and often only reaches its highest point in the sinodural angle.

An upper control window must be made by releasing the pars flaccida and, as far as necessary, the neighboring pars tensa, in order to permit early inspection of the incudostapedial joint and the upper mesotympanum. To achieve this the anterior and posterior folds of von Tröltsch must be divided. The perforation is often encountered in this area. In order to obtain a view of the superior and inferior aeration pathways, the tympanotubal ostium, the entire anterior hypotympanum, and the pars tensa must be released from the anterior tympanic spine, the bony annulus, and the posterior tympanic spine, to allow evaluation of the round window niche and the tympanic sinus as far as the posterior hypotympanum. If possible, the chorda tympani is dissected free from the fold, but if it is covered by the matrix of the cholesteatoma, it is immediately sacrificed.

At this point it is useful to evaluate the tympanic diaphragm and sinus, using straight endoscopes 2.7 and 4 mm in diameter, with angles of 0° and 30°, a 70° telescope 2.7 mm in diameter, and a 30°, 4-mm,

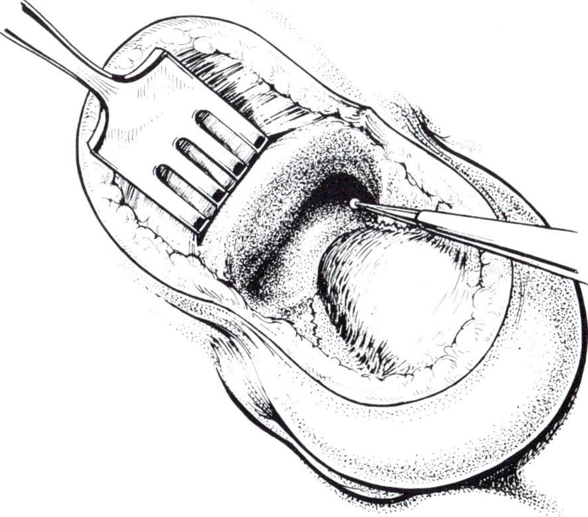

Fig. **103 Osteoplastic epitympanotomy.** When the temporal squama has been drilled down, the shaping of the bony lid begins, using smaller and smaller drills and diamond burrs (H. S., S. R. Wullstein 1976)

wide-angled telescope. The findings can determine whether an osteoplastic epitympanotomy is necessary or whether a simple myringoplasty is justifiable because of the benign nature of the disease.

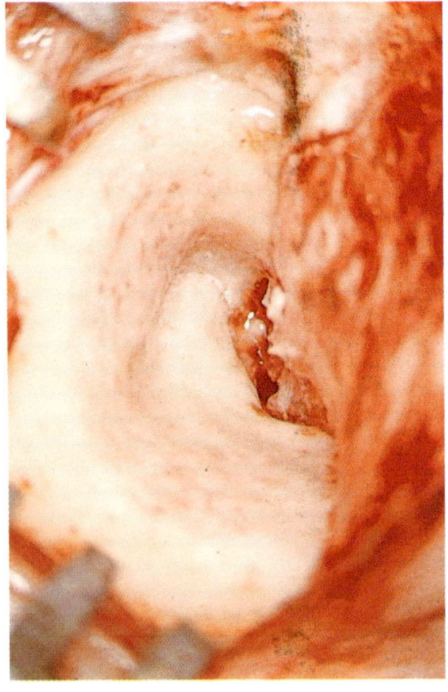

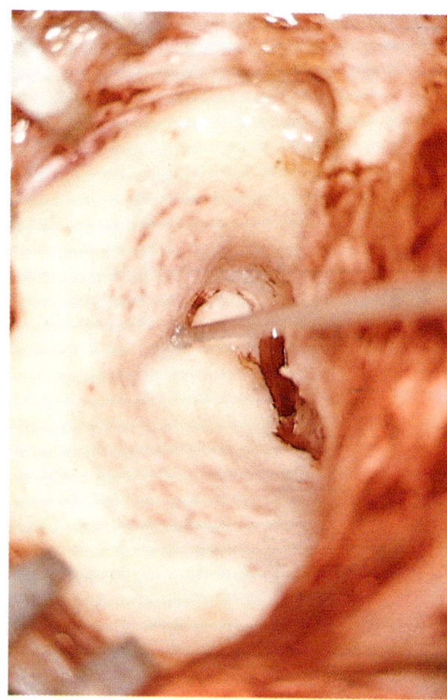

104   **105**

Fig. **104   Osteoplastic epitympanotomy.** The temporal squama has been drilled down and the site for the actual trephine has been prepared. The mesohypotympanum can be assessed through the superior inspection window and posterior to the closed meatal skin. Elevation of the epidermis of the pars tensa from the collagenous fiber layer of the tympanic membrane is continued

Fig. **105   Osteoplastic epitympanotomy.** The bone gutter is formed along the tegmen with smaller and smaller diamond burrs until the blue line can be recognized.

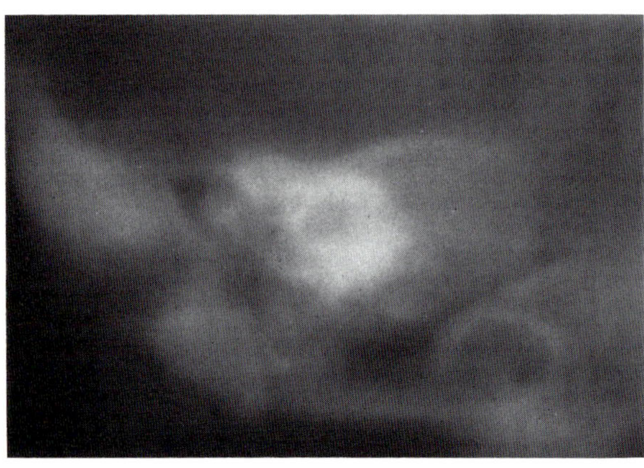

Fig. **106   A preoperative sagittal tomogram** to demonstrate the lateral epitympanic wall, which is trephined at epitympanotomy

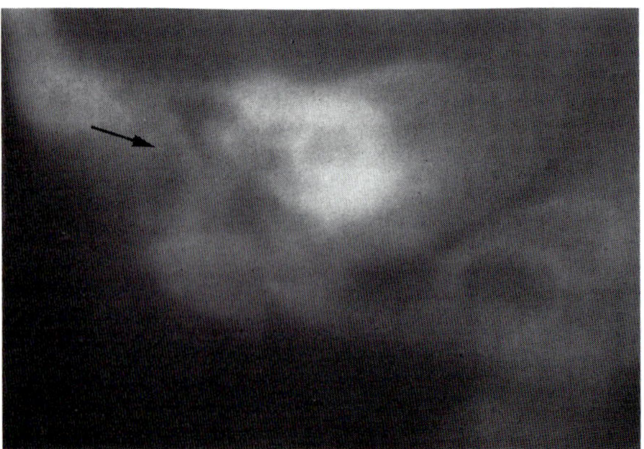

Fig. **107   The postoperative polytomogram of the same ear as shown in Fig. 106, eight days after the replacement of the bony lid at its original site.** The arrow indicates the line of trephine. The unchanged wide air space between the internal surface of the bony lid and the lateral surface of the ossicles should be observed

At the start of creation of the epitympanic bony lid, the facial wall of the protympanic recess anterior to the long process of the malleus is palpated with a slender 90° needle to determine its limits. The groove for the bone incision is started with a small diamond burr at this point, which lies as far forwad as possible.

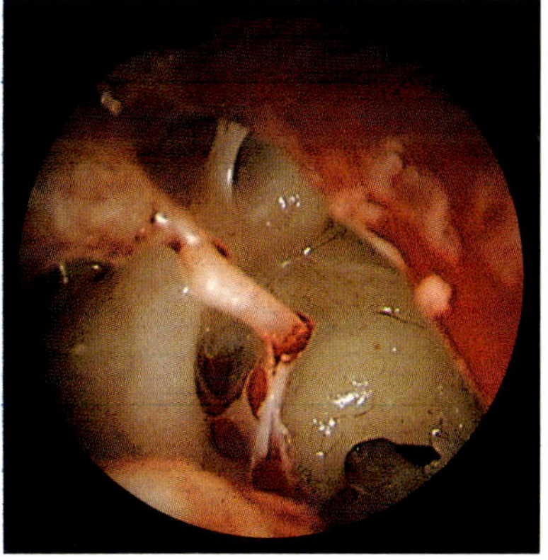

Fig. **108** **The same middle ear as in Fig. 104**. The region of the tympanic diaphragm, the oval window niche with the stapes, the cochlearform process with the tensor tendon and the round window niche are visible from the same site, using the wide-angled endoscope (0°, 4 mm) passed through the upper control window into the lumen of the middle ear cavity

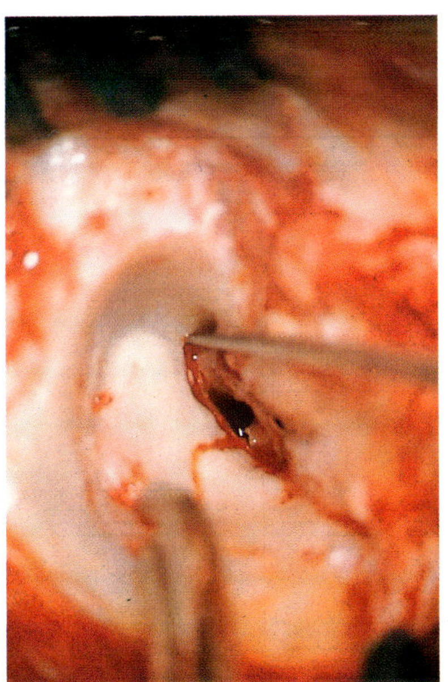

Fig. **109** **Osteoplastic epitympanotomy.** Palpation of the anterior wall of the epitympanum

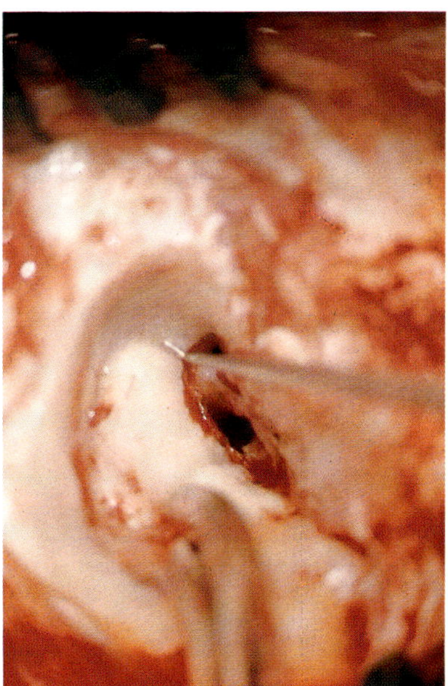

Fig. **110** **Osteoplastic epitympanotomy.** The 90° needle palpates the anterior wall of the epitympanum from outside at the point where trephine of the bony lid begins

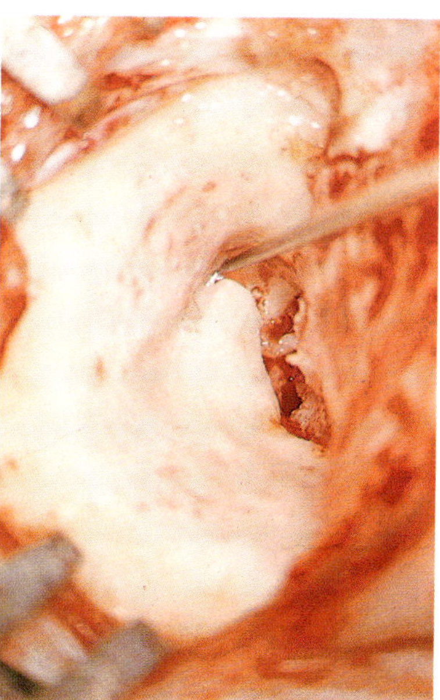

Fig. **111** **Osteoplastic epitympanotomy.** The same 90° needle as in Figs. **109** and **110** shows where the upper limit of the bony lid impinges on the roof of the epitympanum and the trephine is continued almost at right angles along the profile line of the tegmen

Trephining of the Orthotopic Bony Lid

The bony lid corresponds in size exactly to the lateral wall of the epitympanum and the aditus, but it can be extended over the entire antrum and the mastoid as far as the sinodural angle. The edge of the bony lid runs back to the facial spine in a broad arch over the aditus or beyond the antrum, depending on the radiological findings. The posterior limit of the bony lid in the incudal fossa lateral to the incus is palpated with a 90° needle immediately above the exit of the chorda tympani. At this point over the facial spine, a groove is made externally with a diamond burr to form the fulcrum, where the bone lid will later be fractured rather than cut through, to protect the facial nerve.

The groove for the fulcrum must run over the incudal fossa exactly *at right angles* to the bone edge, i.e., perpendicular to the underlying facial nerve. *Any bevel leads not into the open incudal fossa, but into the facial canal. An incorrectly bevelled bone groove represents the only danger of injury to the facial nerve.*

A pointed conical diamond 0.3−0.4 mm thick at the point is used for the trephine. The epitympanic bone lid is cut out along the already prepared bony groove, beginning at the anterior tympanic spine. This bone incision would be too dangerous at the facial spine; therefore, it ends after the curve over the entrance to the antrum. *The transition from the deep antrum to the thick bone of the lateral semicircular canal is palpated* with the stationary pointed diamond burr. A robust round knife or a small elevator is inserted under the lid from the tegmen to break it off. The bone lid can crack along the tympanosquamous fissure; it is supported at this point with a wide elevator to prevent it breaking into two parts.

If the matrix of the cholesteatoma adheres to the internal surface of the bone lid, it is immediately dissected off delicately without tearing it. Only then is the lid lifted out with the double-cupped forceps. When it is removed it should be completely free on its surface of any inflammation. It is kept in Ringer's solution, with antibiotic added until it is replaced. The epitympanum, with its disease undisturbed, is now freely exposed to the surgeon in its entire extent, and access is created to the antrum via the open aditus (Figs. **121−123**). *Up to this point osteoplastic tympanotomy is a purely anatomical dissection which leads directly to the main focus of disease. It can be carried out more quickly with increasing experience.*

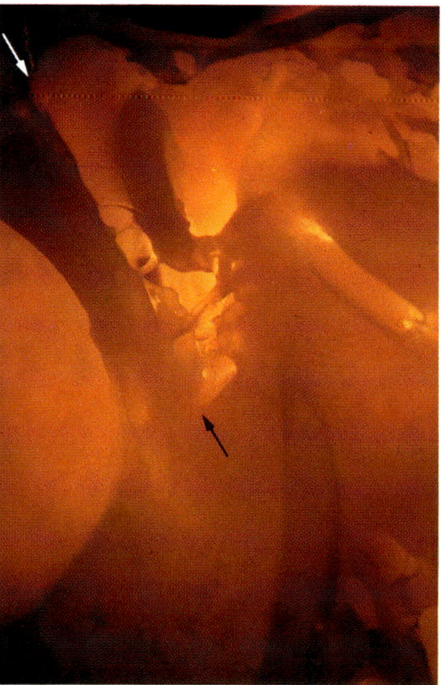

Fig. **112 Sagittal serial section of the temporal bone illuminated with a forward-looking optic (0°, 4 mm) introduced into the eustachian tube.** The lateral wall of the epitympanum which is removed during trephine of the bony lid, is indicated between the two arrows. The landmarks of the bony lid in relation to the ossicles, to the tegmen and to the lumen of the lateral and posterior semicircular canals as well as the facial nerve should be observed

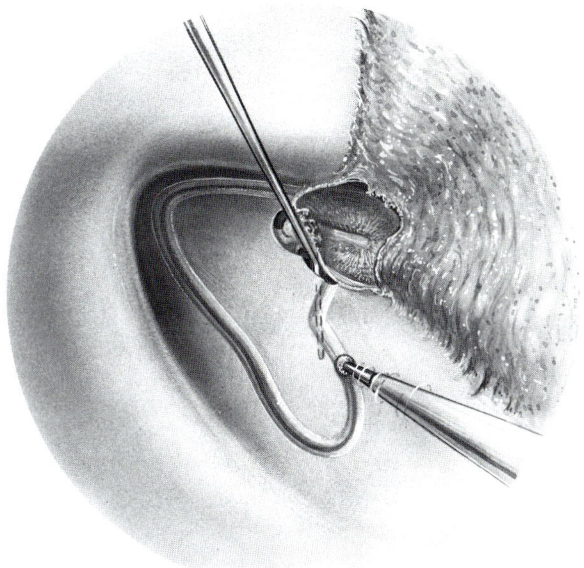

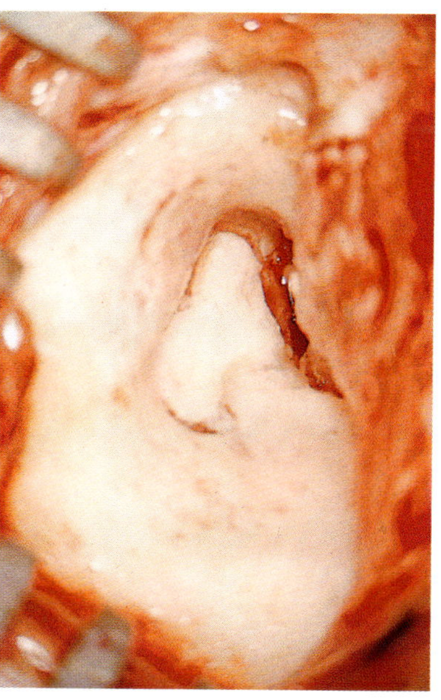

Fig. **113** **Osteoplastic epitympanotomy.** The middle length 90° needle, introduced into the epitympanum lateral to the ossicles and immediately above the chorda tympani, shows from inside at which point a bony groove must be created externally; the fulcrum indicates at which point the bone is broken at the end of trephining of the bony lid, in order to protect the facial nerve (H. L., R. S. Wullstein 1976)

Fig. **114** **Osteoplastic epitympanotomy.** The formation of the bony lid has been completed. The blue line shows its contours in which the trephine is completed, using a pointed conical diamond burr

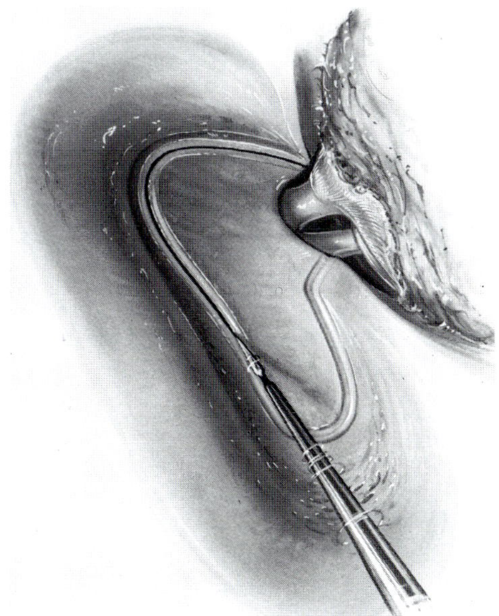

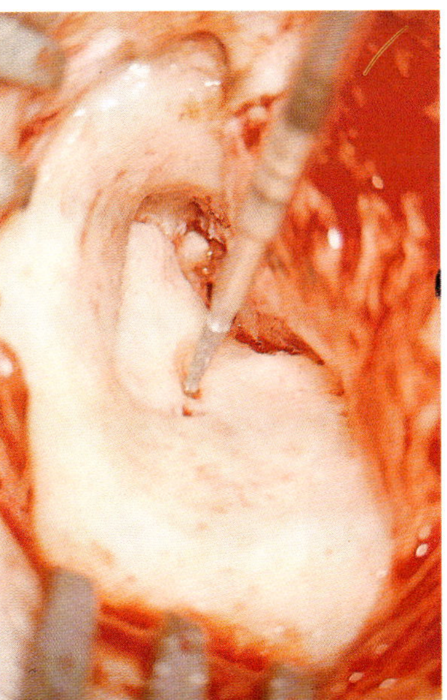

Fig. **115** **Osteoplastic epitympanotomy.** The pointed conical diamond burr cutting out the bony lid in the previously created bony groove (H. L., R. S. Wullstein 1976)

Fig. **116** **Osteoplastic epitympanotomy.** The stationary conical diamond burr is used to palpate carefully the depth of the antrum at the facial spine

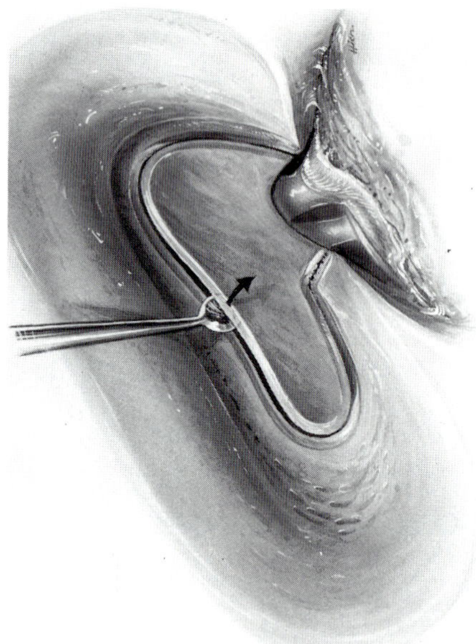

Fig. **117 Osteoplastic epitympanotomy.** A robust elevator is introduced under the bony lid at the tegmen and bends it slightly at the facial spur like a fulcrum. If the tympanomastoid fissure runs through the lid and begins to crack, the elevator must be used to elevate in front and behind it to retain continuity (H. L., R. S. Wullstein 1976)

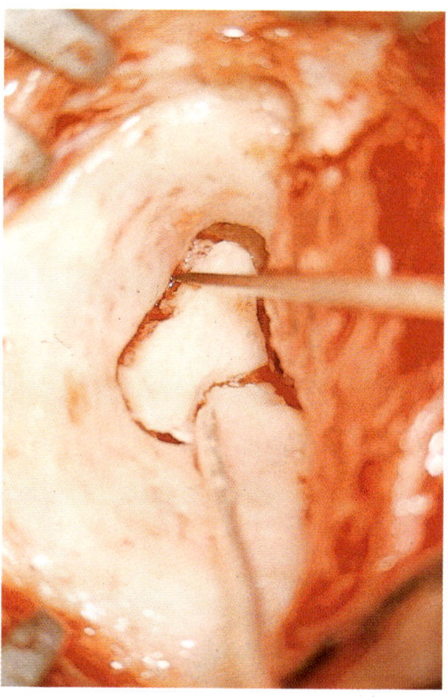

Fig. **118 Osteoplastic epitympanotomy.** When removing the bony lid, the sucker helps to provide slight contra-pressure to allow the lid to be carefully freed from the underlying pathological tissue

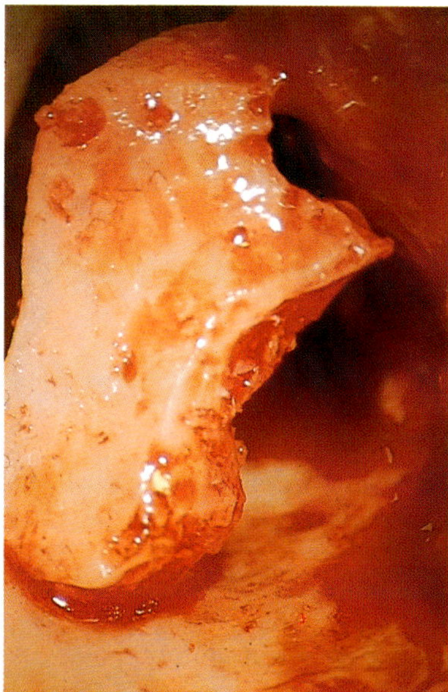

Fig. **119 Osteoplastic epitympanotomy.** The shape of the trephined bony lid corresponds exactly to the outline of the lateral wall, and the contours of the tympanic notch, the anterior tympanic wall, the tegmen tympani and antri, with an extension over the antrum and the point of breakage at the fulcrum

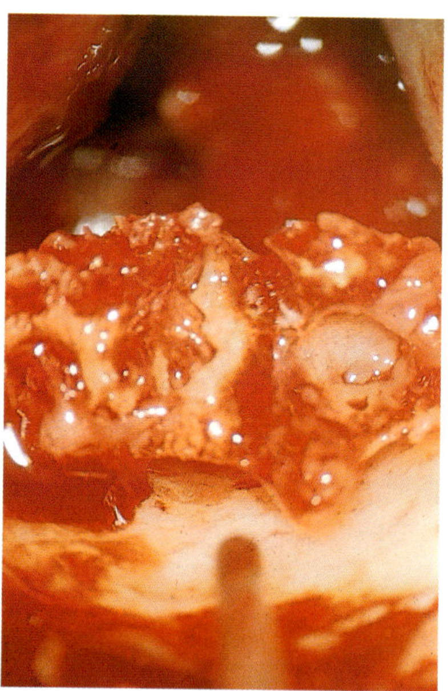

Fig. **120 Osteoplastic epitympanotomy.** The internal surface of the bony lid with the mucosal covering on which can be recognized the site of attachment of the lateral malleoincudal fold (the individual fold which cannot be retained when the epitympanum is opened)

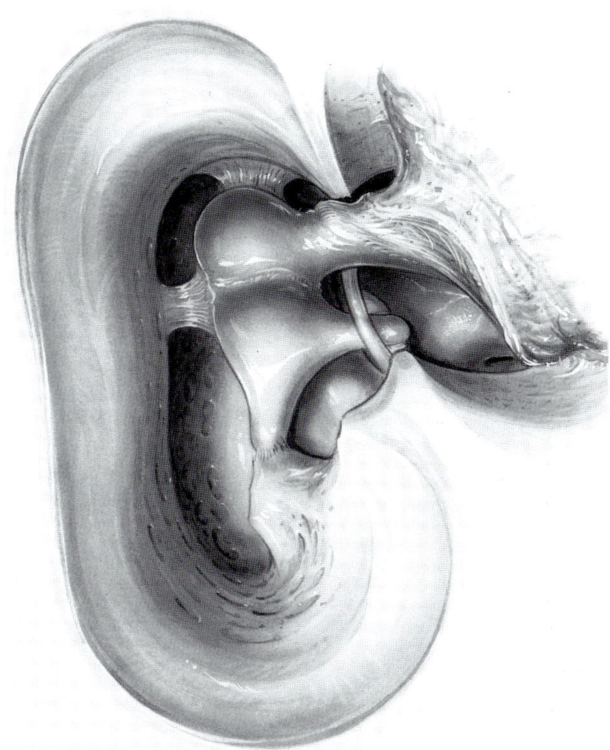

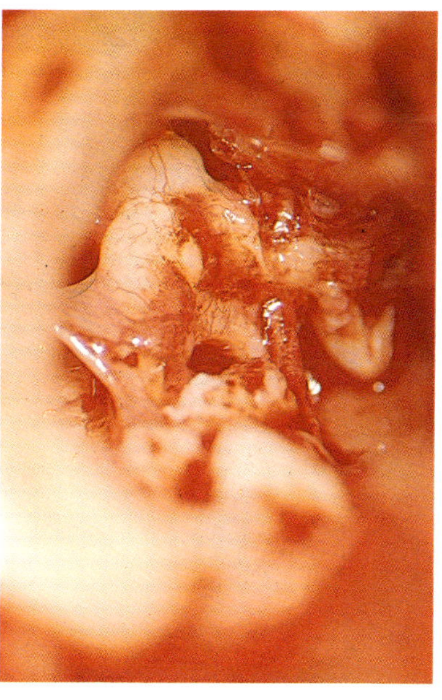

Fig. **122   Osteoplastic epitympanotomy.** Open middle ear space with intact ossicular chain. The superior malleoincudal fold runs to the tegmen and divides the epitympanic space into a medial and lateral compartment

Fig. **121   Osteoplastic epitympanotomy.** Open epitympanum with ossicles. Wide access to all segments of the middle ear (H. L., S. R. Wullstein 1976)

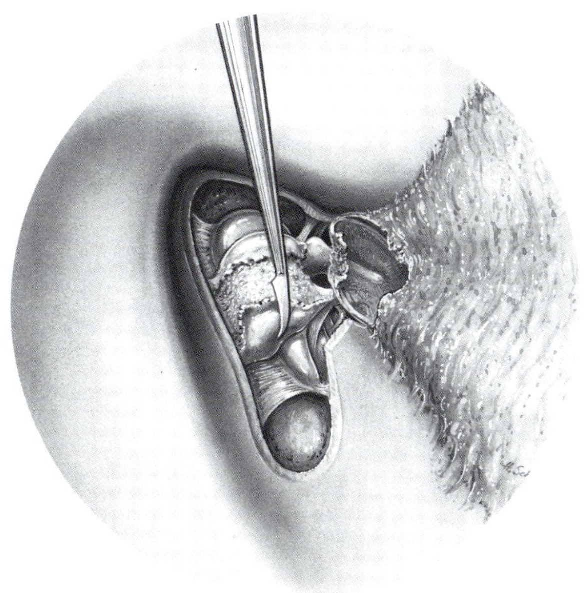

Fig. **123   Osteoplastic epitympanotomy.** After the removal of the bony lid, the cholesteatoma is carefully removed with a sickle knife

Reconstruction of the Middle Ear Space after Osteoplastic Trephine
(Figs. 124–143)

Replacement of the Orthotopic Bony Lid

Reconstruction begins with replacement of the orthotopic bone lid in its original position to allow primary healing without any restriction of the space of which it forms one wall (Fig. **124**).

The air content of the epitympanum can be increased by lateral displacement of the bone lid. The following points should be borne in mind during replacement of the bone lid:

1. The bone incision must be as fine as possible and the bone lid as thick as possible to reduce the loss of substance to a minimum. The normal contours of the external auditory meatus are thus restored to ensure correct resonance. The abundant bone dust from the temporal squama can be placed externally on the seams around the bone lid.
2. The lid must be fixed firmly in the desired position on the edges of the bone, especially anterosuperiorly and on the fulcrum.
3. The formation of adhesions is prevented by optimal positioning and the primary ingrowth of bone, especially if the ossicular chain is preserved (tympanoplasty Types I and II).

The replacement of the bony lid is very simple. It is fitted into its original position in the same way as it was removed. The narrow cleft remaining at the site of trephining is filled by bone dust and fibrin glue before adapting the overlying fascia and meatal skin. (The bone dust and glue may not be necessary.) If the loss of bone substance due to drilling is minimal and the trephine cut remains fine (which is more often the case in a sclerosed bone than in a well-pneumatized bone), then simple cover with fascia without tissue glue and bone dust is sufficient. The robust skin of the meatus together with the tympanic membrane repair always retain the bony lid in position by adhesions. Its broad, well-vascularized base on the floor of the meatus ensures smooth healing.

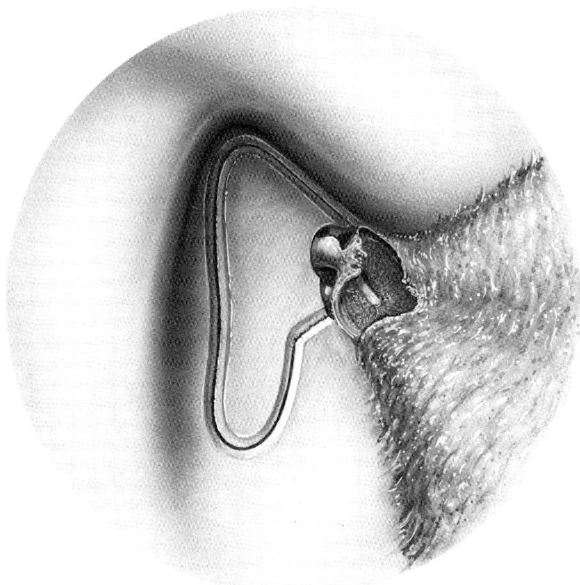

Fig. **124 Osteoplastic epitympanotomy.** The bony lid is replaced in its original place (H. L., S. R. Wullstein 1976)

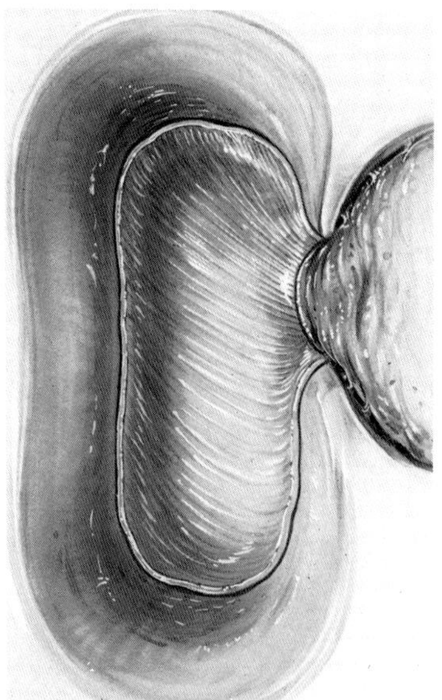

Fig. **125 Osteoplastic epitympanotomy: tympanoplasty Type I.** The fascia covers the site of the trephine and the replaced bony lid widely. The meatal sleeve is about to be replaced (H. L., S. R. Wullstein 1976)

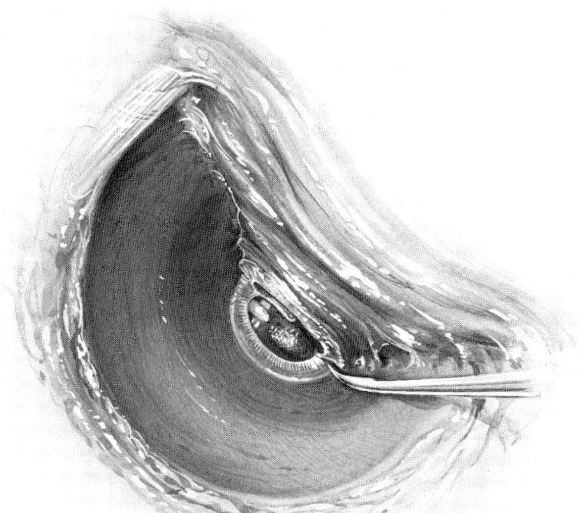

Fig. 126 Elevation of the meatal skin tube, including the epidermis of the tympanic membrane. The skin-periosteal sleeve is released superiorly and posteriorly beyond the annulus fibrosus of the tympanic membrane, as far as the edge of the tympanic membrane perforation, after a circular incision through the connective tissue at the level of the suprameatal spine, extended as far as the meatal bone (H. L. Wullstein 1968)

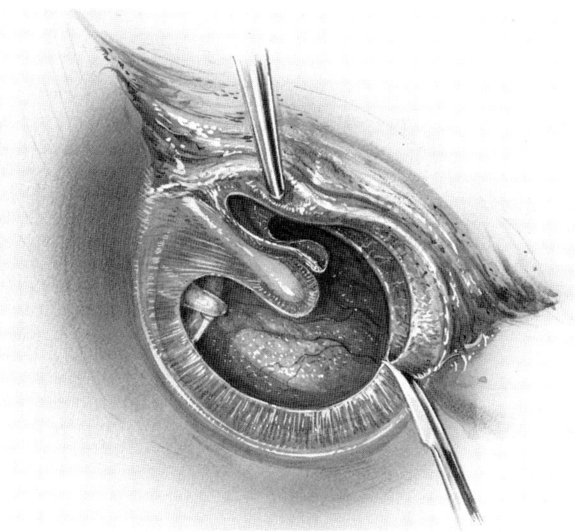

Fig. 127 Elevation of the meatal skin tube, including the epidermis of the tympanic membrane. The epidermis of the pars tensa is elevated from the fibrous annulus around the perforation continuous with the meatal sleeve, as far as the junction with the anterior meatal wall. The bony annulus is curetted thoroughly with the elevator, to remove an annulus cholesteatoma, because the epidermis is anchored to the bone with pegs at this point (H. L. Wullstein 1968)

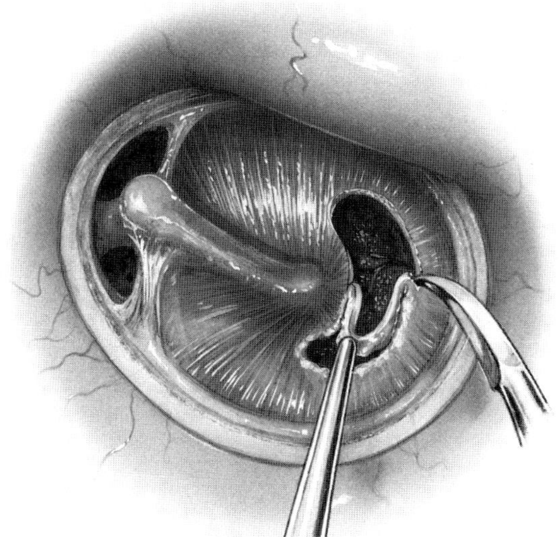

Fig. 128 Excision of the margin of the tympanic membrane perforation. After the epidermis has been elevated from the collagen fiber layer of the pars tensa, the edges of the perforation are widely incised with the point of the sickle knife so that the epidermis growing inward over the edge of the perforation is also removed (H. L. Wullstein 1968)

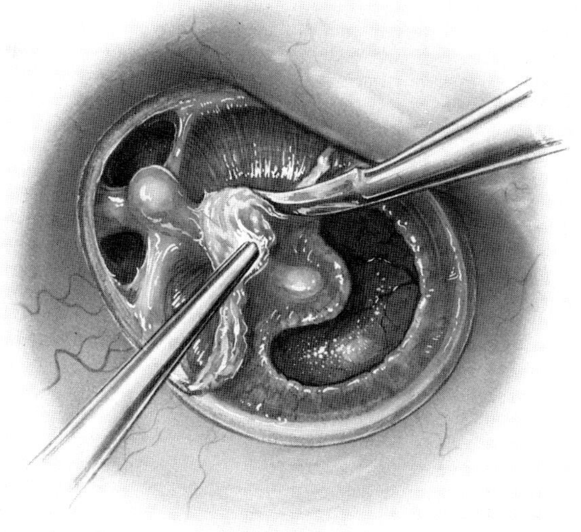

Fig. 129 De-epithelialization of the pars tensa at myringoplasty. After the meatal skin has been elevated in its entire circumference with the dissector down to the bone, directly above the fibrous annulus, the epidermis is elevated from the collagen fiber layer, using the concave side of the sickel knife. Firm adhesions are divided sharply without damaging the collagen fiber layer (H. L. Wullstein 1968)

Repair of the Tympanic Membrane

If a defect of the tympanic membrane is large and the disease in the inferior aeration pathway extensive, it is justifiable to adapt and glue the tympanic membrane graft at the start of the operation. It lies on the floor of the meatus and is not in the way, irrespective of whether the graft is used as an underlay, as an overlay or is interposed between the layers of the remnant of the pars tensa. One piece of the fascial graft is used to repair the tympanic membrane, and a larger piece is used to cover the bony lid and the line of the trephine. When the latter is being fitted from above, loose adaptation of the graft in the tympanic notch can be achieved by dividing the fascia in two to prevent tension and the formation of scar tissue. The surgeon must strive to create a new flexible pars flaccida and under it, a wide Prussak's space.

Variations in Shape of the Bony Lid

Variations of the size, breadth and thickness of the bony lid should be planned individually before the operation. Osteoplastic closure is still possible if exposure must be extended beyond the antrum.

Lateral displacement of the bone lid, to extend the tympanic diaphragm and the space lateral to the ossicles, is the most frequent supplement of the osteoplastic procedure; it causes no loss of bone substance. Furthermore, the increase in air capacity of this region, especially if the ossicles are retained, ensures a more reliable coupling of the epitympanum and the mastoid to the ventilation and to the mucociliary clearance of the mesohypotympanum running to the eustachian tube.

If a large bone lid was planned (for example, because an extensive cholesteatoma was suspected), the surgeon can be surprised. Two examples follow:

1. A long-standing middle ear inflammation with cholesteatoma. The interruption of the aeration at the boundary between the anterior and the posterior segments led to indrawing of the atrophic pars tensa in the posterosuperior quadrant and to the genesis of an invagination cholesteatoma with consequent disruption of the ossicular chain, due to erosion of the long process of the incus and of the stapes (Figs. **130–132**). After exposure, cholesteatoma was found lying only in the incudal fossa. A "macroantrum" in Schüller's view simulated advanced bone destruction.

2. A nearly normal Schüller's view can almost completely conceal an occult medial cholesteatoma in the presence of extensive pneumatization (Figs. **133–134**).

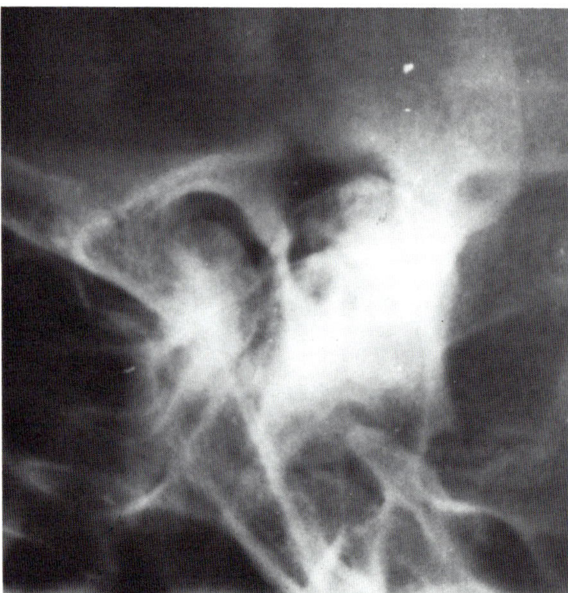

Fig. **130 Preoperative Schüller's view of poor pneumatization and a large clear area in the antrum.** The posterosuperior quadrant of the tympanic membrane showed a defect filled with flakes of cholesteatoma. An audiogram showed a conductive hearing loss of 40–50 dB. The patient was suspected of having an extensive cholesteatoma

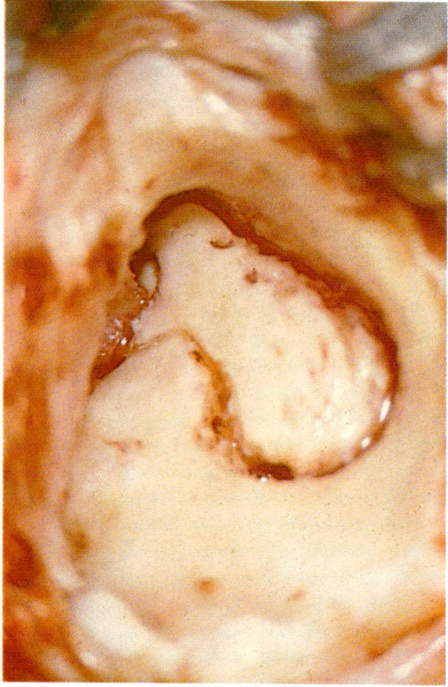

Fig. **131 Osteoplastic epitympanotomy, showing the same ear as in Fig. 130.** A very large bony lid was created because of the suspicion of an extensive cholesteatoma

A bone lid of ample size over the antrum is always better than one which is too small, even if no cholesteatoma is suspected. Supra-auricular access posterior to the closed meatal skin tube offers complete freedom of movement.

As a rule, the meatal packing is removed on the third postoperative day, and the replacement dressing is left in place for more than two weeks. Thereafter, progressive epidermization of the tympanic membrane is noted through the almost normal meatus, and the supra-auricular incision can scarcely be seen.

If exposure of the retrotympanic spaces, with complete clearance of even the smallest cell, is necessary as far as the thick bone of the labyrinth, the sigmoid sinus, the bony facial canal and the cortical bone of the posterior cranial fossa, it is still possible to achieve osteoplastic closure of the middle ear space with coupling of the posterior segment to the function of the anterior segment. Two different methods can be chosen, as the following examples show:

1. After removal of the bone lid, drilling of the temporal squama is continued directly along the tegmen antri toward the sinodural angle, always orientated by means of a Schüller's view which shows the position of the dura and the sigmoid si-

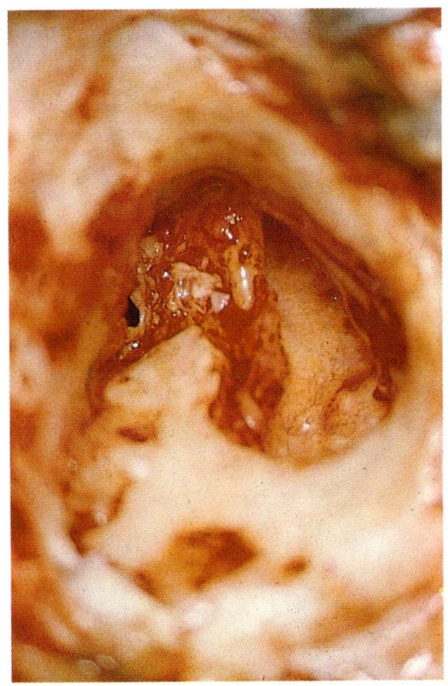

Fig. **132** The bony lid has been removed from the same ear as in Figs. **130** and **131**. The cholesteatoma extends only as far as the incudal fossa. A macroantrum had simulated an extensive cholesteatoma on the Schueller's view

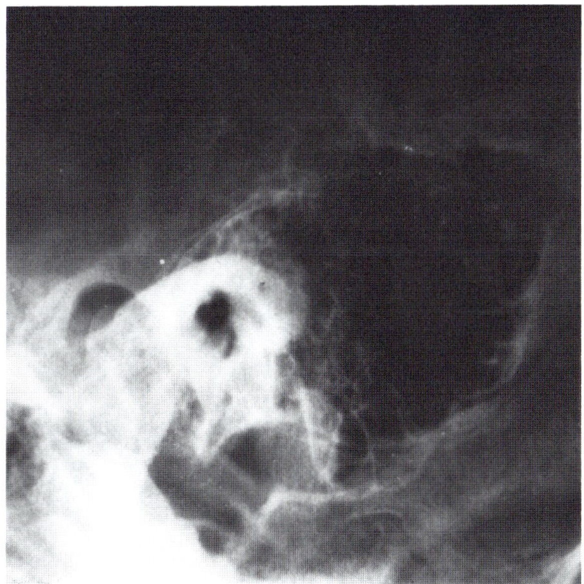

Fig. **133** **Preoperative Schüller's view, showing well-aerated pneumatization with large cells.** The anterior semicircular canal is clearly seen and, in front of it, a transparent focus in the antelabyrinthine trigone. Otoscopy showed a fine scar in the region of Shrapnell's membrane. An audiogram showed a conductive deafness of 30—40 dB

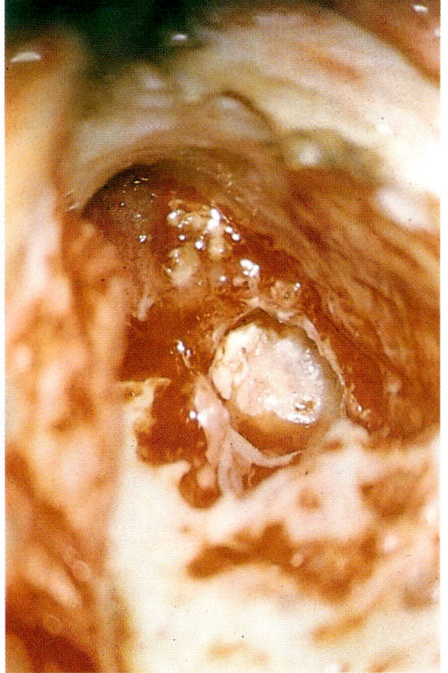

Fig. **134** **Osteoplastic epitympanotomy, showing the same ear as in Fig. 133.** Removal of the bony lid exposed a large cholesteatoma, which had extended as far as the apex of the mastoid and the sinodural angle

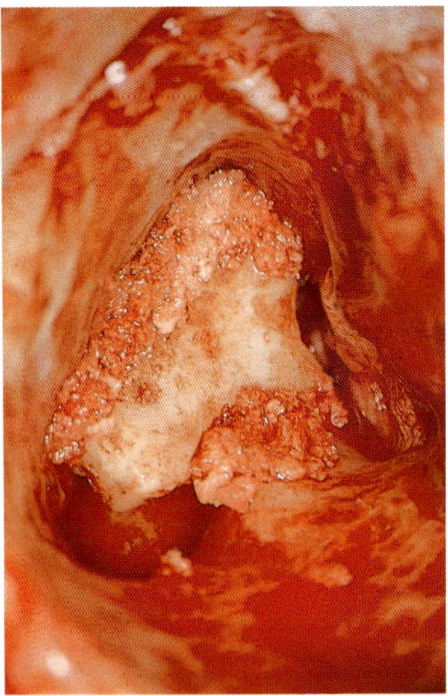

Fig. **135 Chronic otitis media with cholesteatoma arising from the pars flaccida, showing a marginal bone defect in the tympanic notch.** Osteoplastic epitympanotomy and a tympanoplasty Type III (deep) was carried out. The stapes has been built up by a sculpted allogenic incus. The defect in the tympanic membrane has been replaced with a piece of fascia underlying the remnant of the pars tensa in the mesohypotympanum and laid on the edges of the bony lid. Because of a very large cholesteatoma in the mastoid apex and the sinodural angle, it was necessary to drill down the cells further posterosuperiorly after removal of the bony lid, so that a gap was produced over the antrum leading towards the sinodural angle after replacement of the bony lid, as after a mastoidectomy. The bone defect in this case was filled with plasticine plus bone dust

nus. The lateral wall of the mastoid process is removed with a large cutting burr, initially in a posterior direction along the profile line of the middle cranial fossa as far as the sinodural angle and then directly inferiorly along the curvature of the sinus posterior to the retained posterior meatal wall. The surface of the mastoid process is exposed widely, as for a mastoidectomy, as far as the tip of the mastoid process, and is covered again at the end of the operation by suture of the galea to the untraumatized periosteum.

2. Double access for mastoidectomy and osteoplastic epitympanotomy: the mastoid cell system is opened as far as the antrum, after a generous skin incision. The entire cell system is then opened posterior to the intact meatal wall. Osteoplastic trephine of the bony lid and exposure of the epitympanum then follows from the meatus, if necessary, at a second stage. (The reverse sequence of steps is also possible.) A very large defect of the lateral wall of the mastoid process can be covered with a plasticine sheet if ample periosteum was taken, so that a surface is recreated with favorable circumstances for rapid growth of epithelium.

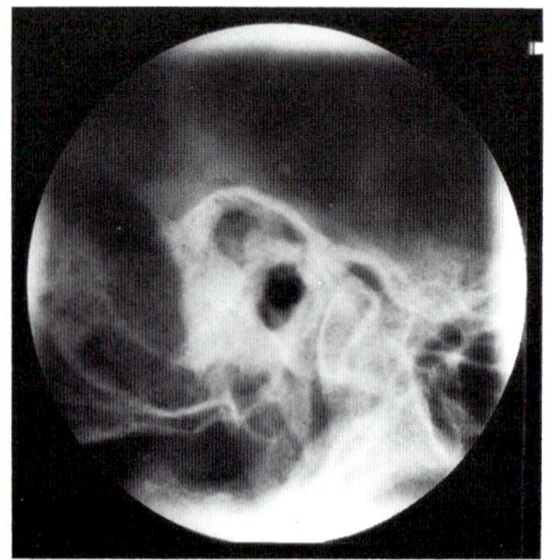

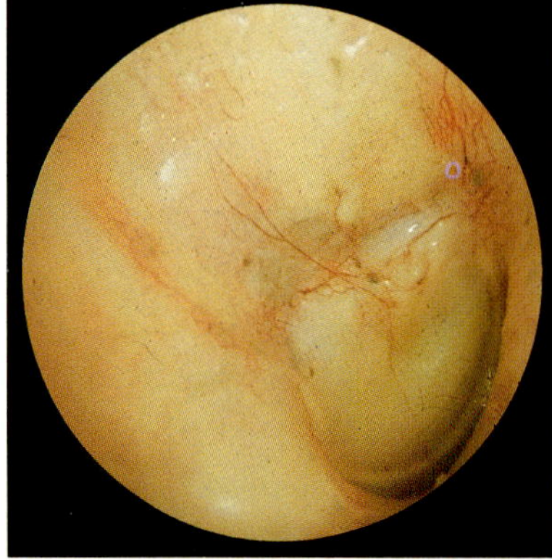

Fig. **136 Schüller's view of the same ear as in Fig. 135, six months after operation.** The lid has reunited by bone and the gap behind it has also closed by bone. The tympanum and the retrotympanic spaces contain air

Fig. **137 Endoscopic view of the same ear as in Fig. 91, six months after operation.** The contours of the meatus are normal. The plasticine and the graft have healed smoothly

136   137

Fig. 138   Combined access to the middle ear spaces with complete clearance of the mastoid cell system. An osteoplastic epitympanotomy was carried out first, followed by exposure of the retrotympanic spaces along the middle cranial fossa, as far as the sinodural angle. It was continued from that point inferiorly, posterior to the intact posterior wall, as far as the apex of the mastoid process. The posterior meatal wall was retained in its entirety (H.L., S.R. Wullstein 1976)

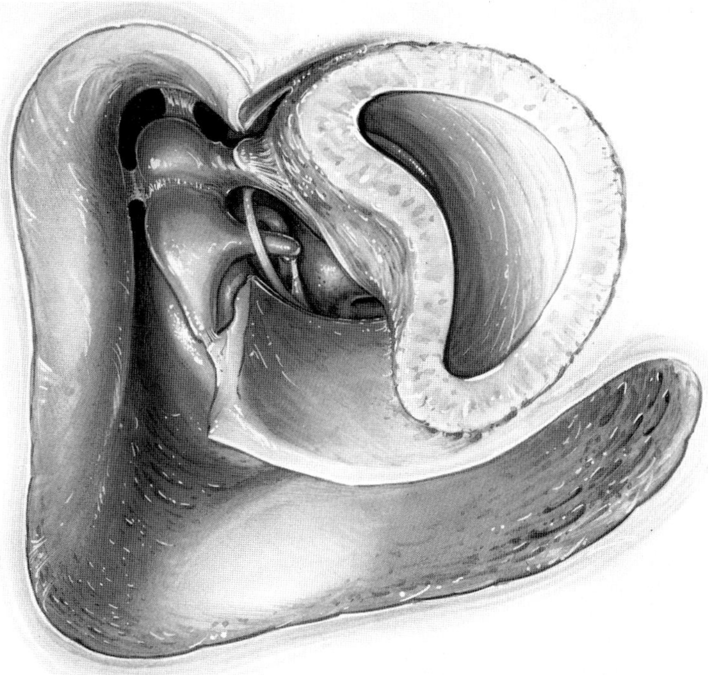

Fig. 139   Combined access showing the same view as in Fig. 138. The surgeon is looking forward from behind. The sub- and perilabyrinthine cells have been cleared, and access fo the apical cells is free. The bony lid is replaced as usual, as is the meatal skin tube. The firm layer on the posterior surface of the auricle covers the open mastoid as after an antrotomy (H. L., S. R. Wullstein 1976)

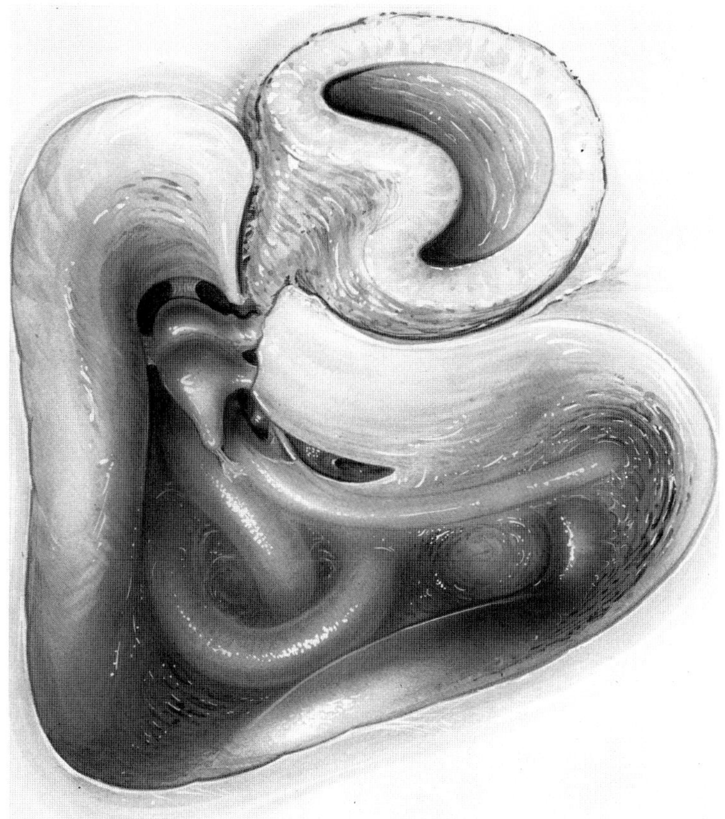

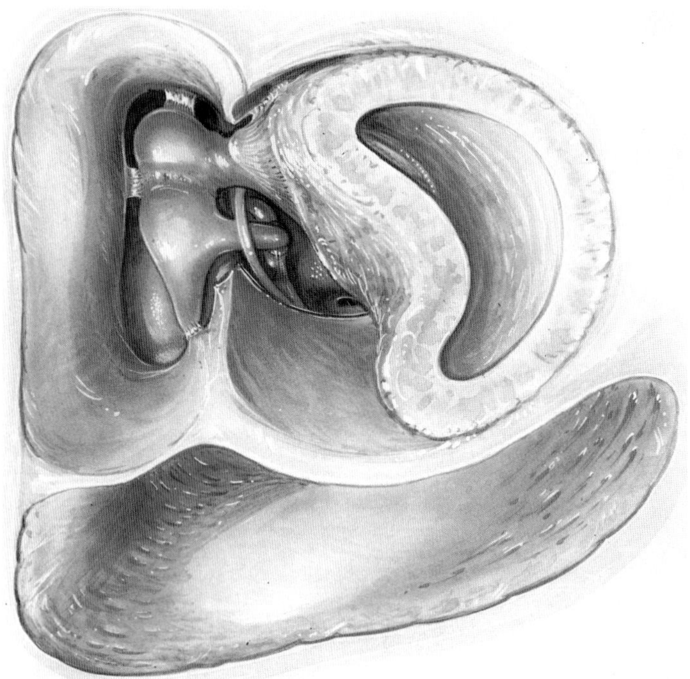

Fig. **140 Combined access.** Antro-mastoidectomy follows osteoplastic epi-tympanotomy. The direct view of the open epitympanum with the ossicular chain is shown. The bony bridge lies over the aditus and antrum
(H. L., S. R. Wullstein 1976)

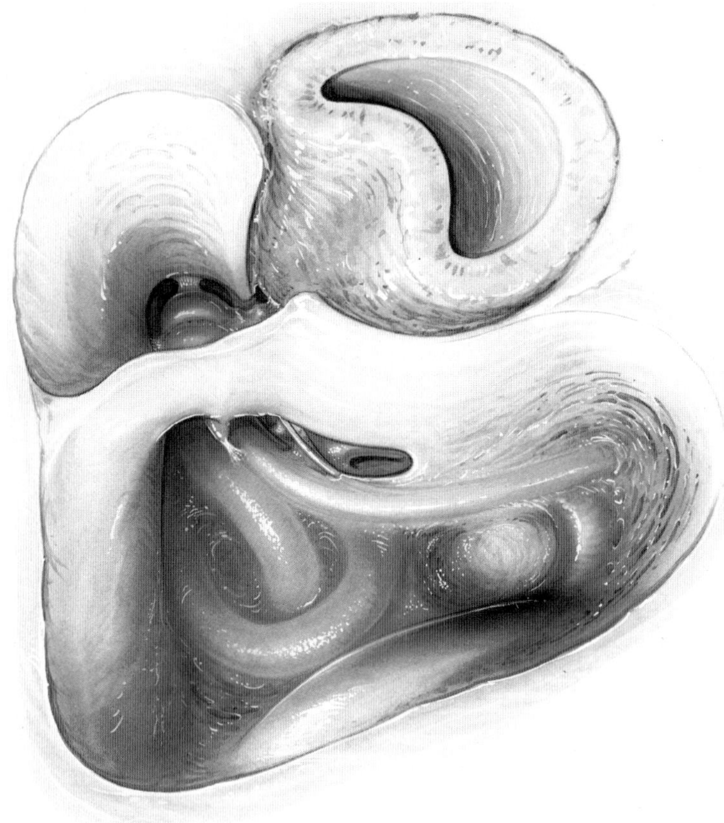

Fig. **141 Combined access (same case as Fig. 140).** View from behind looking forward, behind the intact pos-terior meatal wall and behind the bony bridge over the aditus. Reconnection of the posterior sector to the aeration and drainage of the anterior sector is achieved by replacement of the bony lid. The meatal skin tube is replaced
(H. L., S. R. Wullstein 1976)

Fig. **142 Cholesteatoma in the antelabyrinthine trigone.** If a dangerous medial cholesteatoma lies in the anterior point of danger,
possibly with a fistula into the ampulla of the
anterior semicircular canal, access to the
paralabyrinthine cells is gained by removal of
the destroyed ossicles, and the matrix is then
removed (H. L., S. R. Wullstein 1976)

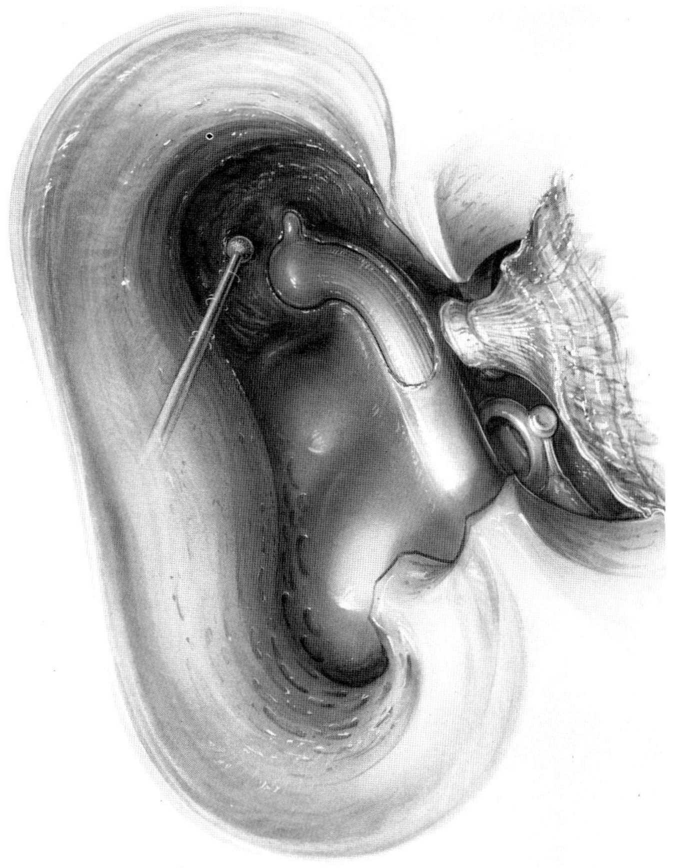

Fig. **143 The facial nerve** is decompressed
in its entire length, from the geniculate ganglion in the anterior epitympanum, as far as its
exit at the stylomastoid foramen
(H. L., S. R. Wullstein 1976)

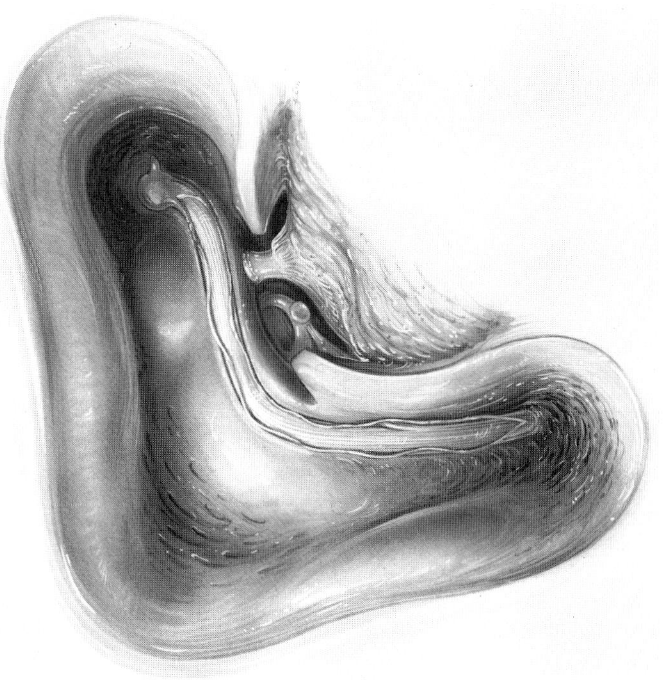

Endoscopy and Endoscopic Operations

(Figs. **144**–**153**)

Prolonged work to a precision of one-tenth to one-sixteenth of a millimeter, using the free hand, has proven itself easily possible since 1952. However, performance could not be improved further because none of the currently available microscopes permitted surgical manipulations under continuous magnification with an appropriate depth of focus.

The solution to this problem is an endoscope with a short focal length and its own illumination, which can be introduced close to the operating field. Endoscopes fulfil these criteria and can be manufactured in varying lengths and diameters. At high magnification and very short distances, from the light source to the object, the field of vision is small, and a very high degree of clarity and illumination is therefore necessary. Endoscopes are superior to operating microscopes in one important respect, in that an angled telescope provides a view in the depth behind the walls. This advance in surgical technique, however, has increased the demands on

the ability of the surgeon quite extraordinarily: it is difficult to introduce the straight endoscope directly into the middle ear, and angled endoscopes require a great deal of practice, because very vulnerable areas are examined under high magnification at close quarters.

Every assessment of the function of the middle ear must begin with investigation of the upper airway. Detailed endoscopic examination of the nose and nasal sinuses is thus one of the first steps of diagnosis. Any abnormality of aeration such as mechanical obstructions, vasomotor disorders of the nasal turbinates, and hyperplastic and atrophic mucosal lesions must be corrected before tympanoplasty.

Endoscopy of the nose and nasal passages developed by Messerklinger (1972, 1978) permits visual evaluation of all details. Circumscribed ethmoiditis lateral to the middle turbinate is often not recognized on plain radiographs, but can be picked up easily by endoscopy, using telescopes of varying an-

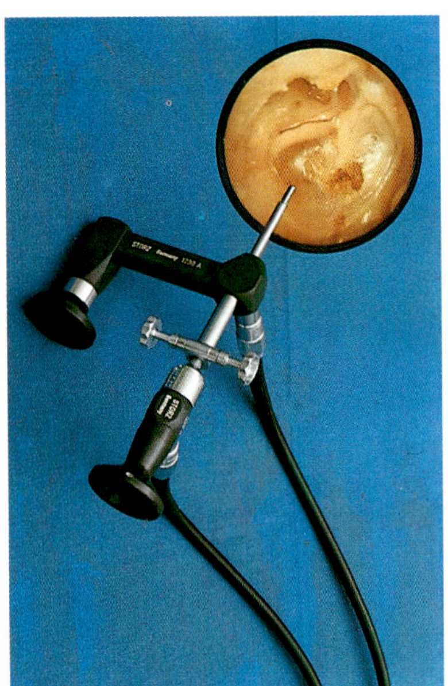
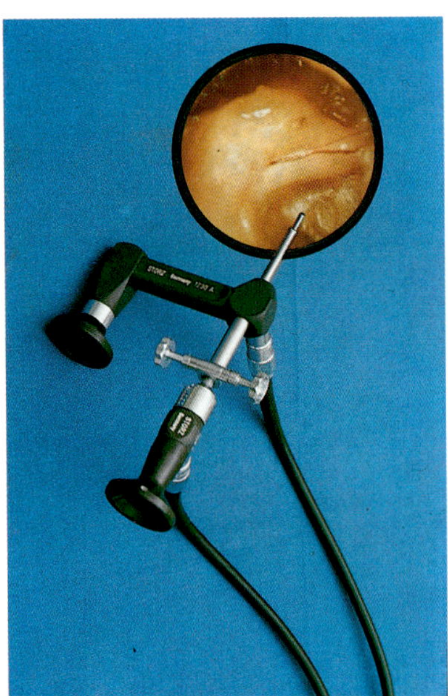

Fig. **144** **Ototympanoscope:** a large-caliber 0° endoscope with light path to allow the fine-caliber, angled endoscope (30° or 70° to be introduced without risk between the ossicles, and to allow observation and surgery through this detailed view. The practiced endoscopist can forego the large-calibre 0° endoscope

gles. All therapeutic and surgical maneuvres, both in the ethmoid and in the ear, require most careful preservation of the mucosa, to protect the cilia and the secretory flow.

Operative endoscopy is achieved transnasally and from the nasopharynx using 0°, 30°, 70°, 90° and 120° endoscopes. They slide easily over the floor of the nose and then under the middle turbinate and are then withdrawn through the middle meatus after inspection of the nasopharynx and evaluation of the torus of the eustachian tube. After evaluation of the ostium of the maxillary sinus and the infundibulum, the ethmoidal bulla and the ethmoid sinuses, the 30°, 70°, or 90° endoscope is turned to inspect the entrance to the frontal sinus and the individual ethmoid cell groups. The 0° endoscope slides into the sphenoid sinus, along the medial surface of the superior turbinate and the septum, to the superior edge of the choana and then into the ostium, which lies deeply.

The autonomic regulation of the function of the nasal mucosa is extensively assessed. However, the interaction between the middle ear and the eustachian tube, on the one hand, and the nose and ethmoid sinuses, on the other hand, is still largely unexplained, although we know from clinical experience that a reciprocal influence is present. The pathological changes of the middle ear mucosa in seromucinous inflammation are identical to those in *seromucinous ethmoiditis* (S. R. Wullstein 1985). Better aeration and drainage of the nasal sinuses improves serous otitis media in more than half of all children and adults with problems at the "bottlenecks."

In seromucinous ethmoiditis, which is so common nowadays, the entire middle and superior meati are chronically inflamed, red and swollen. Access to the posterior ethmoid and to the olfactory cleft is impeded, if not closed completely, by scar tissue. Adhesions form across the posterior part of the nasal septum, obstructing aeration and drainage of the sphenoid.

Operative endoscopy of the middle ear. Various endoscopes (0°, 30° and 70°) of different diameters (2.7, 4 or 6 mm) are used for endoscopic preoperative investigation of the middle ear. The ototympanoscope can also be used; it is a combination of two different endoscopes. The first straight endoscope (0°, 4 mm) carries the second angled endoscope (30° or 70°) into the depth. The actual diagnostic procedure is then carried out with this angled endoscope. During this procedure one hand is used for guiding the endoscope, so that only one hand is available for surgery.

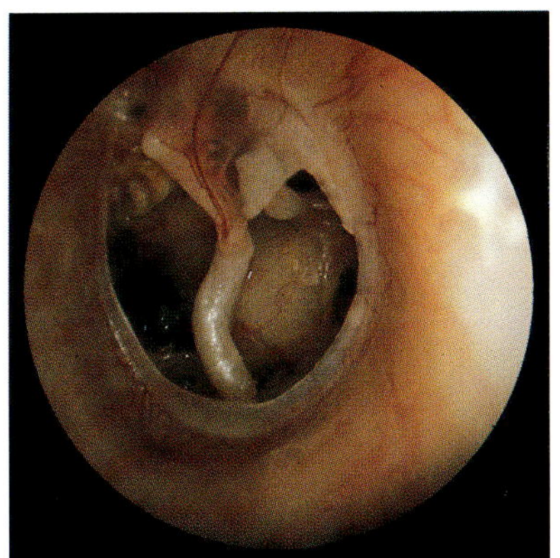

Fig. **145 Chronic middle ear inflammation.** The small cholesteatoma roots leading toward the inner ear in a dry, total perforation of the tympanic membrane disguises the fact that a more extensive cholesteatoma lies behind the tympanic diaphragm in the epitympanum and in the retrotympanic spaces

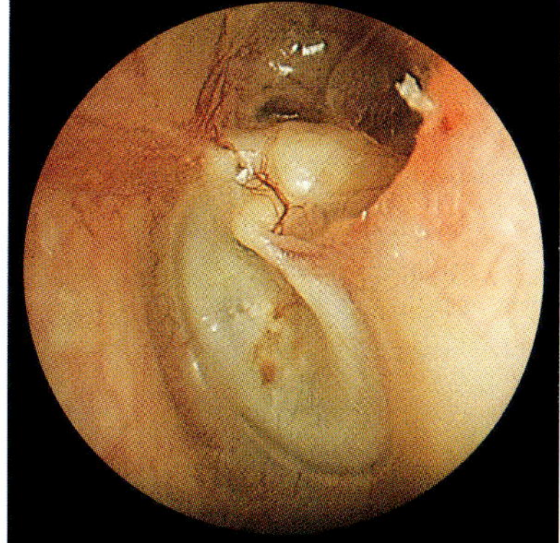

Fig. **146 Chronic middle ear inflammation** with cholesteatoma and destruction of the lateral epitympanic wall, with a retained ossicular chain and well-aerated mesohypotympanum

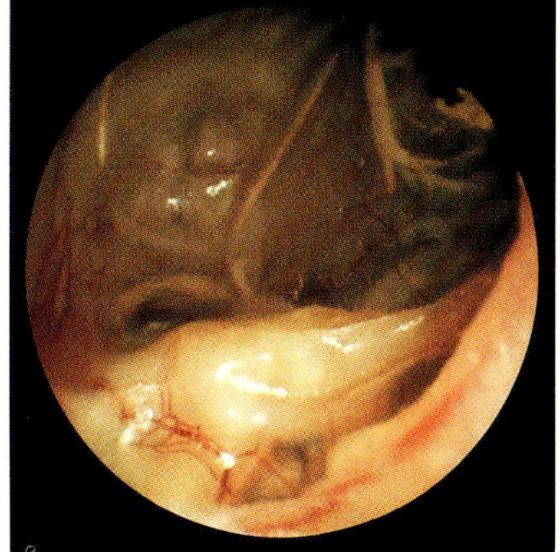

Fig. **147 Same patient as in Fig. 146.** The extension of the thin cholesteatoma matrix to the antrum can be assessed with the 30° endoscope. The cholesteatoma flakes have largely discharged spontaneously to the outside; therefore, the patient has few symptoms and relatively good hearing. The decision about the further steps of the procedure depends on the age and general condition of the patient, and the condition of the ear.

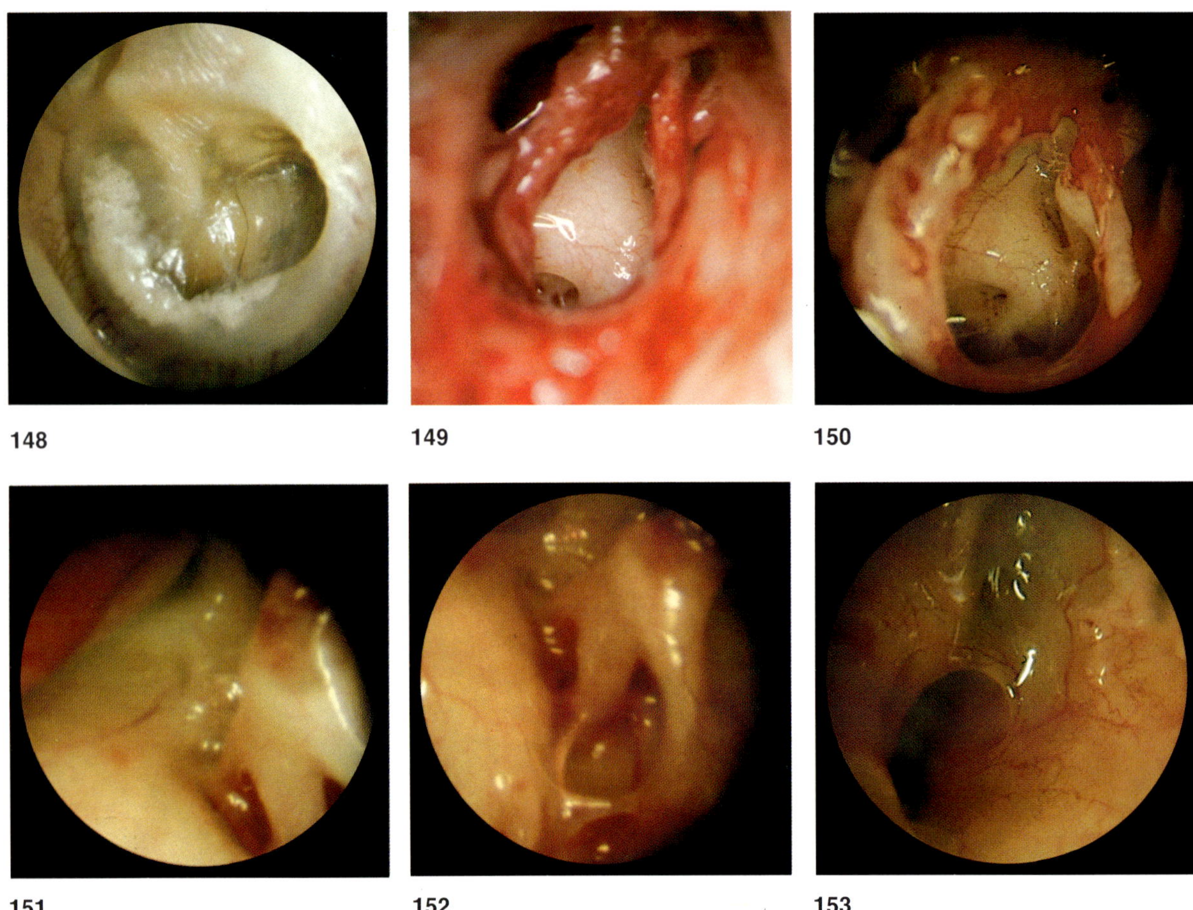

148   149   150

151   152   153

Fig. **148 Chronic recurrent seromucinous middle ear inflammation.** Preoperative endoscopy, showing retraction of the atrophic posterosuperior quadrant of the tympanic membrane, which has not bulged out after active insufflation of the tube. There is an effusion into the hypotympanum, and calcification of the pars tensa

Fig. **149 Superior inspection of the same ear through the Zeiss microscope Opmi 6.** Secretion is sucked out; the round window niche appears to be open. The middle ear mucosa is well vascularized and swollen, but capable of regeneration. It is not possible to obtain a view into the sinus tympani

Fig. **150 Intraoperative endoscopy of the same patient as in Fig. 149** with the patient's head and the surgeon in the same position. The 0° endoscope introduced through the inspection window provides information about the conditions in the sinus tympani and the oval window niche with the stapes and the chorda tympani, as well as about the condition of the entire superior aeration pathway

Fig. **151 Intraoperative endoscopy of the same ear as in Figs. 148–150.** The 30° endoscope illuminates the cochleariform process with the anterior tympanic isthmus. The opening of the eustachian tube and the

supratubal recess can be seen lying deeply on the left and above

Fig. **152 Intraoperative endoscopy of the same ear as in Fig. 148.** The 30° endoscope illuminates the posterior tympanic isthmus. An adhesion extends from the pyramidal process to the posterior crus of the stapes and to the posterior edge of the niche

Fig. **153 Intraoperative endoscopy of the same ear as in Figs. 148–152.** The tympanic diaphragm is assessed, using the 70° endoscope introduced through the aditus after antrotomy and cell clearance. The medial malleoincudal fold obstructs the free air passage through the diaphragm to the retrotympanum. The fold is severely inflamed and produces much secretion, which mixes with that produced by the remaining mucosal surface, overloading the capacity of the posterior tympanic isthmus. The air mixture delivered is inadequate compared to resorption of the reserve air in the retrotympanic spaces, causing reduced pressure in the retrotympanic isthmus. This situation of internal pressure with deficient refilling of air leads to ingrowth of the pars tensa into the posterior tympanic isthmus (see Fig. **148**), and is often the first stage of an invagination cholesteatoma

The following are assessed:
a) the fundus of the external meatus, if the tympanomeatal angle cannot be seen due to marked protrusion of the anterior wall of the meatus;
b) deep retraction pockets of the pars flaccida and pars tensa in the supratubal recess and the eustachian tube, ion the sinus tympani and, beyond that, the epitympanum and the aditus;
c) the middle ear cavity;
d) the aeration pathways through the defect in the tympanic membrane.

After freeing the closed meatal skin tube from the superior and posterior bony meatal wall, *only a circumscribed area* of the mesohypotympanum can be inspected through the middle ear using the *operating microscope* (Fig. **149**). The 0° and 30° endoscopes introduced endaurally through the upper control window give much more reliable information than does the operating microscope about the condition of the mesohypotympanum; for example, the sinus tympani, the round window or the region of the diaphragm.

There is also a set of fine instruments available to go with these 30° or 70° endoscopes, including 45° to 90° needles in various lengths, and curved fine double-cupped forceps for the removal of swellings and adhesions, fixation due to osteitis, granulations or tympanosclerotic plaques.

These endoscopes can be introduced through the mastoid process and through the antrum, posterior to the meatal wall, if the ossicular chain is preserved, to demonstrate the medial surface of the ossicles and the wall of the epitympanum as far as the protympanic recess, and inferiorly, beyond the diaphragm, even as far as the promontory. If necessary they allow microsurgical manipulations to be carried out.

This endoscopic method is of particular value through an aditus-antrum control window in recurrent seromucinous effusions, and in children from the age of four onward (see Fig. **153**).

Endoscopy of the inflated cartilaginous eustachian tube is described on p. 155.

Tympanoplasty in Chronic Inflammation of the Middle Ear

(Figs. 154–163)

The middle ear mucosa is a continuation of the mucosa of the upper respiratory tract. It forms a middle ear resistance complex based on the following anatomical and functional factors:
– the mucociliary transport system, which includes an active secretion of varying chemical composition;
– immunobiology;
– enzymes.

The mucosa almost always reacts in the same way, i.e., by reduction of ciliary activity, metaplasia of the epithelial layer, an increase in number and density of the ciliary and secretory elements, increase or reduction of secretion, hyperplasia and hypertrophy of the individual elements, disappearance of the functional elements, hyaline and fatty degeration, calcium deposits, fibrosis, and induration or atrophy of the entire mucosa. The result is the various pathological and clinical forms of chronic otitis media, which can present synchronously or sequentially. The vitality of the mucosa and the intensity and duration of the noxious influence determine the occurrence and recovery of these lesions.

In chronic or adhesive otitis media it is helpful in attempting to predict the surgical requirements to know how the early acute phase of the primary disease progressed. Much detail of the histology of the temporal bone has been known for more than a hundred years, but the surgeons' understanding has been changed by intraoperative observation of the fine structures of the epitympanum.

Tympanoplasty is nowadays almost always indicated for the results of bacterial or viral inflammations of the upper airways, due to tubal or hemotogenous spread. It is also indicated for acute injuries, congenital anomalies and tumors. In chronic inflammation, the course can be determined from the middle ear outline, its narrowings, ridges and niches as well as its spatial subdivision into segments and compartments, which are of importance to the surgeon for decisions during the procedure.

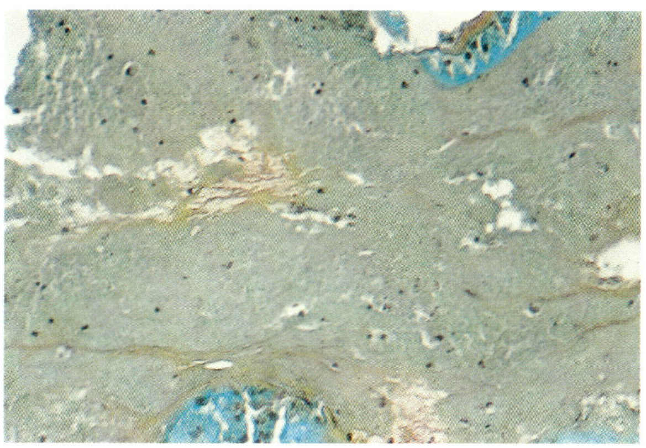

Fig. **154 Transverse section through the malleoincudal fold,** showing a fibroid subepithelial layer with edematous clefts and residual infiltrate. The epithelium is in several layers with cilia and goblet cells

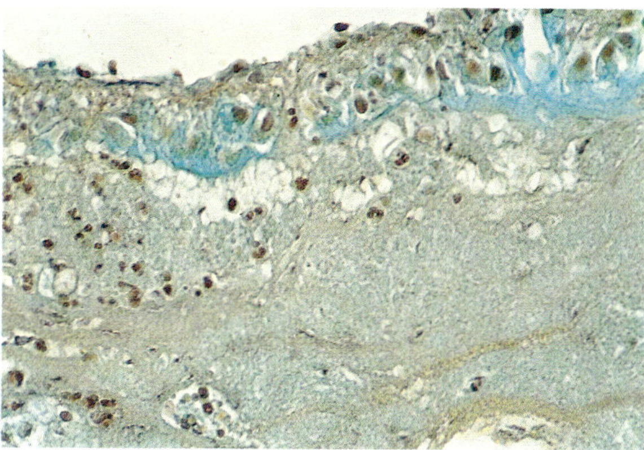

Fig. **155 Malleoincudal fold from the same specimen as Fig. 154,** showing epithelial hyperplasia, broad subepithelial edematous clefts breaking out into the epitympanic lumen, and the intercellular spaces expanded

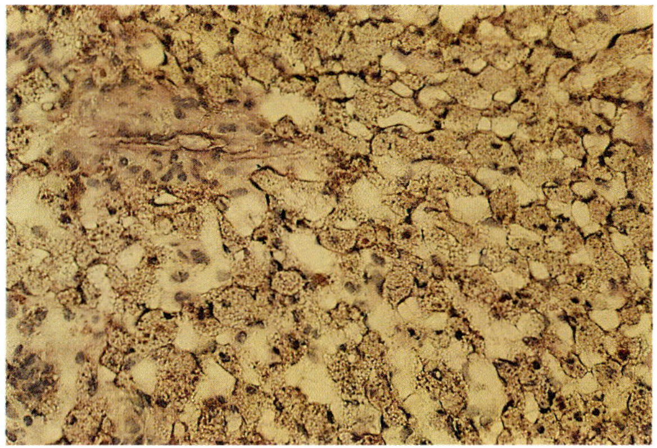

Fig. **156 Superior malleoincudal fold,** showing fatty degeneration of the subepithelial layer

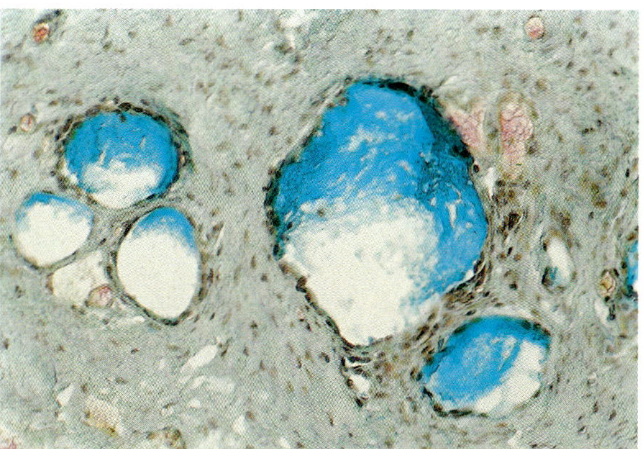

Fig. **157 Malleoincudal fold showing the same specimen as in Fig. 155,** with a subepithelial layer of conglomerate of retention cysts and transition from the active to the degenerative inactive stage of glandular epithelium

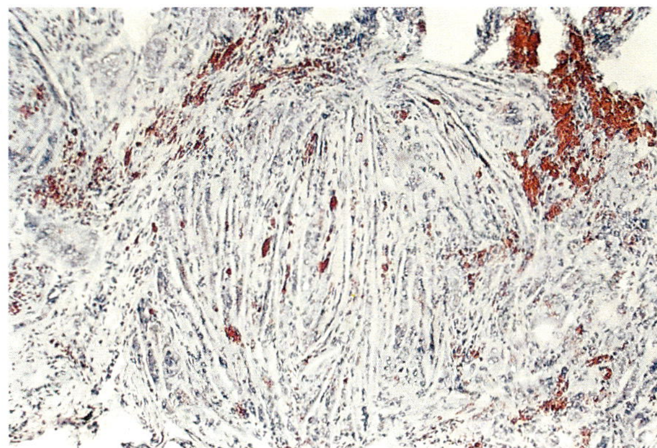

Fig. **158 Superior malleoincudal fold showing a cholesterin granuloma**

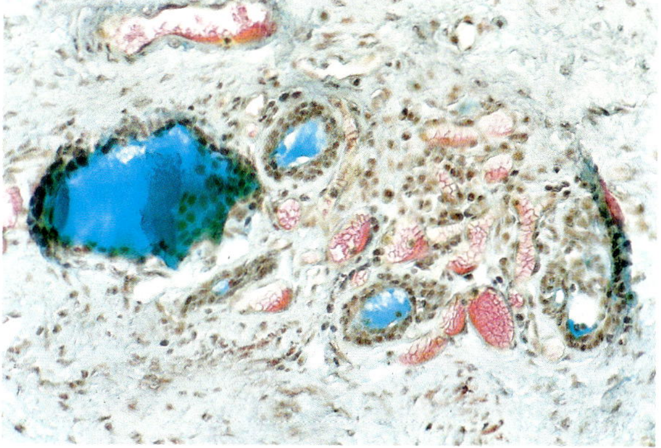

Fig. **159 Malleoincudal fold from the same specimen as Fig. 155,** showing a highly vascular submucosa with inflammatory infiltrate and cystic-glandular hyperplasia. The content of active secreting glands is rich in acid mucopolysaccarides

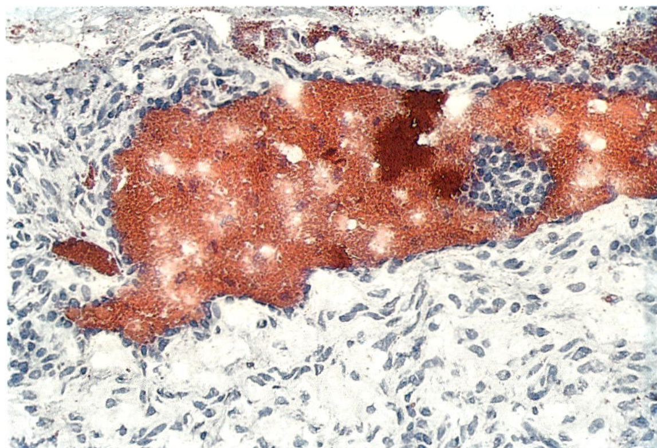

Fig. **160** **Lateral incudal fold**, showing marked adiposis of the subepithelial layer with cystic-glandular hyperplasia of the secretory elements

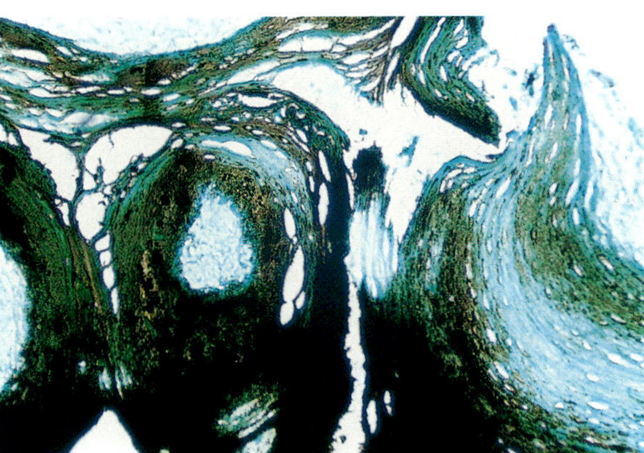

Fig. **161** **Lateral incudal fold,** showing waves and onion rings of calcified deposits in the subepithelial layer, where the hyaline degenerated primary connective tissue fibers are absent

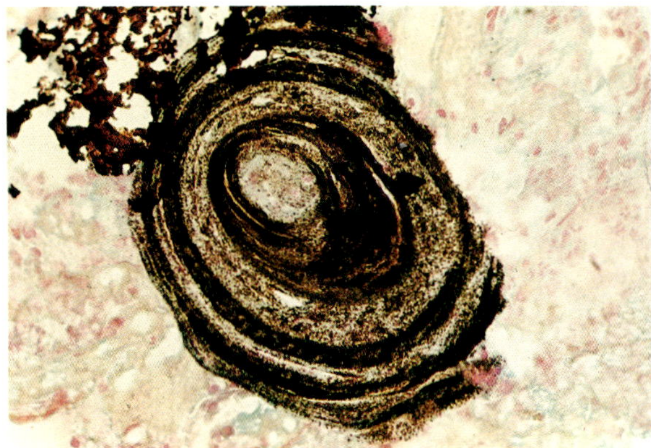

Fig. **162** **Lateral incudal fold,** showing calcified deposits of the subepithelial layer arranged amorphously in circles and which are not to be confused with pacinian corpuscles

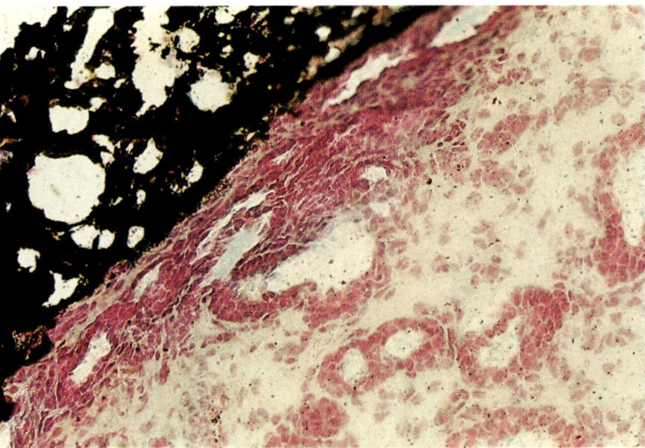

Fig. **163** **Transverse section through a lateral incudal fold,** showing calcified deposits of amorphous type close to the insertion into the body of the incus. Toward the surface, the cystic-glandular hyperplasia can be recognized throughout the entire layer of the stroma

The Mesohypotympanum

1. Chronic otitis media with perforation of the *pars tensa*, with or without *mucopolypoid* inflammation.
2. Chronic otitis media with perforation of the *pars tensa*, with or without *mucoperiosteal* inflammation.

Secondary cholesteatoma is a failed attempt at self-healing of a mesotympanic inflammation; it is discussed in the chapter on cholesteatoma (p. 101).

Chronic middle ear inflammation with a central perforation which may be marginal (for example, after scarlet fever) or central (after measles) has become much less common. The sequelae of influenza and other respiratory catarrhal diseases have also become less frequent. 80% of current infections are viral in origin, and are of many different types. With early treatment, complications are now much less frequent than previously, but seromucinous otitis media has become more common (p. 137).

If the infection and the perforation do not heal rapidly, a chronic mucopolypoid inflammation or even a deeply penetrating periosteal inflammation is set up. The foci of infection lie in the anterior segment, but mild inflammation often persists in the mucosal folds of the epitympanum, with all its pathological and functional effects on healing. Osteoplastic epitympanotomy is therefore the most advisable form of tympanoplasty to deal with this inflammation. At the very least, the aditus should be inspected with the endoscope, even if the mucosa of the promontory and the hypotympanum appears to be uninflamed on inspection with the naked eye through the perforation. If a myringoplasty alone is carried out, the inflammation of the folds does not heal with restitution of patent interossicular air spaces, because reaeration is not possible, due to adhesion of the folds.

If access is obstructed solely by a thick oedematous cushion of mucosa in the middle ear extending as far as the tubal ostium, generous scarification of the surface with the point of a sickle knife and protracted aspiration of secretions from the individual cells is advisable, using compressed surgical cotton wool as is used in ophthalmic surgery. The mucosa is thinned considerably and the outlines become clearer.

Marked polypoid and granulating mucosal disease impedes and prolongs the operation; impor-

tant landmarks are no longer recognizable. In these conditions any dissection causes bleeding which, however slight, impedes vision.

The following procedure is advisable:
Before generalized bleeding starts, the mucosa should be very delicately spread to find the incudostapedial joint. If it is still present, the head of the stapes and then the crura can be exposed by delicate dissection until the footplate comes into view. The crura must not be moved, and dissection must be carried out along the long axes of the ossicles. The continuity of the chain is thus tested. Movements of the malleus are transmitted to the oval window and are very damaging to cochlear function. Quite often the head and neck of the stapes are suspended between the lentiform process and the stapedial tendon, but the two crura are destroyed. If the ossicular chain is interrupted in this manner, the footplate is not endangered by manipulations of the malleus and incus. Dissection in the epitympanum can progress more rapidly and the surgeon can decide immediately against a Type II reconstruction and opt for a high columella (Type III deep).

The individual segments of the middle ear are opened and displayed without exposing the bone, using compressed surgical cotton wool. Aspiration is applied repeatedly to this cotton wool which absorbs edema from the mucosa of the aeration pathways, the sinus tympani and the entrance to the windows. Ultimately, all the structures of the middle ear are exposed and free of blood. The tympanic ostium of the tube and as much as possible of the bony tube are dissected and exposed carefully in this manner.

If the antral mucosa does not appear to be diseased, the mastoid remains unopened (a *tailored epitympanotomy*). The middle ear spaces are carefully irrigated with a disinfectant, which is then washed out again with Ringer's solution.

The gluing of the free graft into the perforation in the tympanic membrane can be done last, but is often better done before the dissection in the middle ear, at least before replacement and fixation of the bony lid.

The *mucoperiosteal* tympanic inflammations offer worse prospects for healing because cortical surfaces in the middle ear can be severely damaged so that new mucosa does not grow over them rapidly. The bony surface can therefore be ground down with the finest polishing burr in safe areas until delicate bleeding points appear. The surgeon must then decide whether sufficient viable mucosa is available for spontaneous regeneration, whether replacement is necessary or whether temporary cover with amnion will suffice.

Stapes and Oval Window

Assessment of the concealed conditions which can impede sound conduction in the delicate oval window may be difficult if it is angled markedly superiorly and medially under the facial canal. These circumscribed conditions include: ossification of the stapedial tendon; fixation by osteophytes; rigidity of the annular ligament due to osteitis or fibrosis; an otosclerotic focus in the anterior stapedial niche (it is possible for otosclerosis to coexist with chronic otitis media) or mild congenital anomalies of the stapes (for example, persistence of the prenatal bridging of the internal lamella of the footplate). Most of these obstructions to sound transmission can be dealt with in a one-stage procedure. Others are reserved for a second stage.

The operation is easy if marked mucosal inflammation has not extended completely into the oval window niche. Often a membrane of delicate mucosa covers a small cyst lying on the footplate. Dissection close to the footplate is then unnecessary. Achieving access to the incudostapedial joint, on the other hand, can be laborious in the presence of massive granulations, and requires persistent careful dissection, removal of granulations, and spreading of the tissue by fine strips of compressed gauze until the annular ligament of the stapes appears.

The incudostapedial joint is the weakest point in the ossicular chain. Because of its delicate structure and poor blood supply, it is the part which is most frequently interrupted. Defects of the crura are also common, although they are often hidden by dense granulations. The stapes is often extremely mobile due to laxity of the annular ligament, especially if of the incus is defective. It can therefore be very difficult to determine whether the stapes is intact or whether the head of the stapes alone remains, suspended from the lentiform process, and the crura are destroyed. The stumps of the concealed crura then often stand on the footplate, and unintended movement of them is extremely dangerous for the annular ligament. It is advisable to drill down the pyramidal process with a diamond burr to eliminate chronic foci of infection (for example, myositis of the stapedial muscle), and to open up the facial recess. The stumps of the stapedial crura can be removed with modern robust and sharp double-

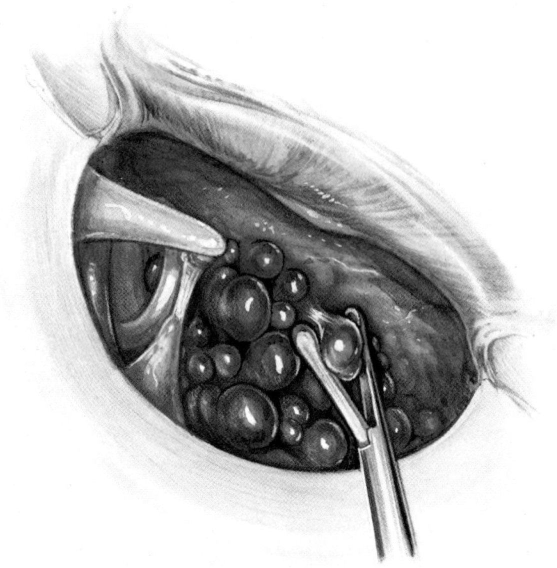

Fig. **164 Dissection of polypoid middle ear mucosa.** The mucosal polyps are removed with fine double forceps, preserving the deep tissue layers (H. L. Wullstein 1968)

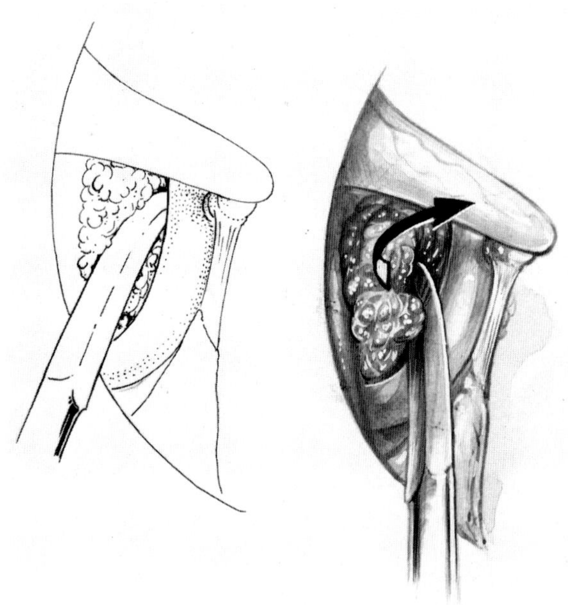

Fig. **165 Dissection of the oval niche.** Granulation tissue and mucosal adhesions or polyps in the niches and between the stapedial crura are carefully freed and removed with the point of the sickle knife, from the facial or promontory side (H. L. Wullstein 1968)

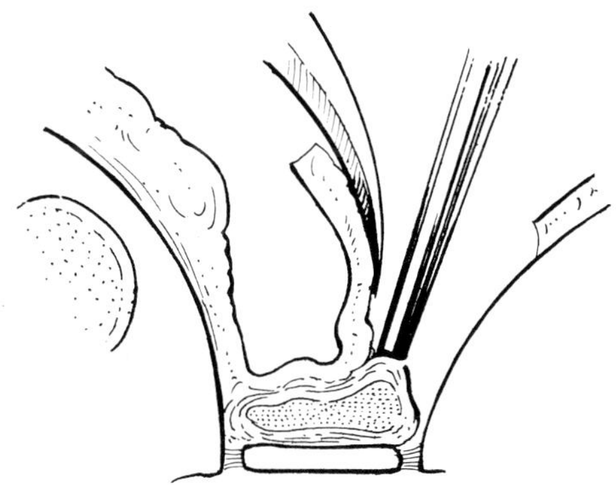

Fig. **166 Dissection of the oval niche covered with cholesteatoma matrix.** The matrix is divided on the promontorial wall of the niche and released from the bone, to allow the footplate to be inspected in order to expose and empty the mucosal cyst lying between the matrix and the footplate (H. L. Wullstein 1968)

cupped forceps or an appropriate laser. It is advisable to lay a fine antibiotic gelatin sponge on the annular ligament to avoid suction on a loose annular ligament. The bottom of the niche remains covered with this gauze during the rest of the operation. The stumps of stapedial crura can nowadays be eradicated via laser, which, however, necessitates special apparatus and operative techniques.

Facial Nerve and Oval Window Niche

A very flat but overhanging facial nerve above the oval window niche is a congenital anatomical variant which renders access to the footplate difficult. Access to the footplate is even more difficult if the oval window is relatively high and lies almost horizontally. A serious difficulty must be overcome in rebuilding a stapes which has been forced against, and attached to, the promontorial wall of the niche by granulations, so that the epithelium is almost entirely lost.

Dehiscences of the bony layer of the tympanic part of the facial canal are common. They are not to be feared during dissection, provided the instruments, particularly the sickle knife, are always used with the concave side or the point in the longitudinal direction of the nerve, and never transverse to the fibers. Drilling down the bony cover of the

nerve does not gain any space because the nerve sheath prolapses when the bone is removed. An empty niche pointing stepply upward demands a long, very narrow and angled columella (see below).

The stapes whose footplate is tilted towards the promontory should be righted very carefully; it has a tendency to spring back again. All granulations should be removed on the facial side, and all those on the promontory, as they give rise to new adhesions. The space between the denuded promontory and the stapedial crura is next filled with an epithelial graft; for example, a split-thickness graft from the lip. It is pushed in between the two like a pouch as far as the footplate, with the wall of the niche on one side and the two crura on the other. A small disk of compressed cotton wool is introduced to hold the cleft open, hold the stapes upright and firmly adapt the mucosal graft during the operation. It is removed at the end of the operation and replaced by gelfoam, to which suction is applied lightly. It forms a packing for a few days longer. A strip of silicone sheet is not used as a dividing wall because the alloplastic material is an irritant during regeneration of the mucosa.

Transposition of the facial nerve toward the promontory to gain wider access to the niche during operations (for example, for congenital anomalies or nerve grafts) achieves little because the promontory, its diseased mucosa and the wound surface of the tympanic membrane graft require all available space for aeration and healing.

Round Window and Aeration Pathways

The deep kidney-shaped hiatus anterior to the entrance to the round window niche is often completely filled with granulation tissue: it should be made accessible by introducing compressed cotton wool to which the suction is applied. This hiatus, the hypotympanic sinus (which no longer belongs to the hypotympanic cells), then opens up. It extends toward the facial nerve deeply and blindly beneath the promontory. A needle often penetrates alarmingly until its bony end is encountered. This pneumatic space must heal to allow the round window niche to recover. The bony spaces at the edge of the subiculum are palpated anteriorly, superiorly and posteriorly, and overgrowth by granulations is divided without damage to the periosteum. They are spread apart further at the introitus, and suction is then applied to the cotton wool to bring the contours of the round window niche into view. Cords of granulations are divided with a short, acutely an-

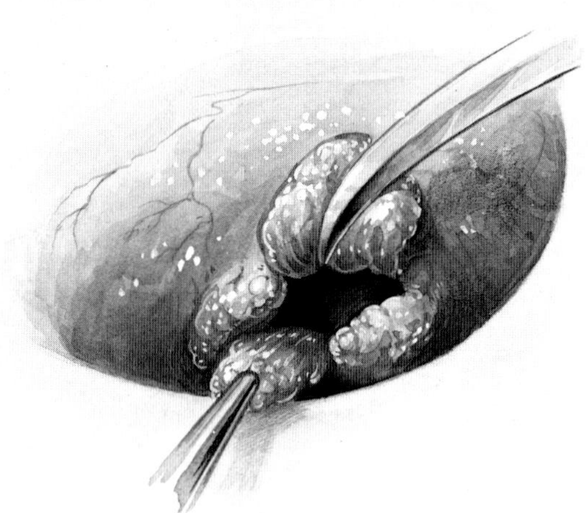

Fig. **167   Dissection of the round window niche with granulations.** Granulation tissue in the entrance to the round window niche is dissected with the sucker and the sickle knife, and small polyps and cysts are sucked away (H. L. Wullstein 1968)

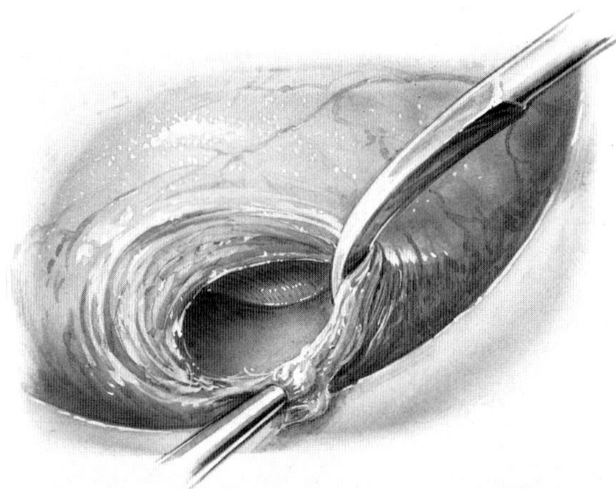

Fig. **168   Dissection of the round window niche with adhesions.** Using the point of the sickle knife directed anteroinferiorly, the adhesions are separated from the bony overhang of the subiculum; on one side, as far as the hiatus, which extends deeply under the cochlea to the hypotympanum, and on the other side, to the round window niche. Adhesions in the round window niche must be divided. To prevent connective tissue scars, the bone of the wall of the niche must not be denuded. For this reason the point of the sickle knife must never be directed anterosuperiorly in the direction of the round window membrane, and dissection must never be carried out on the bone itself. The adhesions are progressively spread apart using a 90° needle. A small compressed gauze sponge is placed between them, to press on the depths of the round window niche (H. L. Wullstein 1968)

gled needle with the anatomical flexure of the round window membrane always in view deeply. Osteophytes are occasionally found in the entrance to the round window niche in severe mucoperiostitis; they can be removed easily with a diamond burr. A view of the round window membrane is only achieved in a wide mastoid and in a wide open sinus tympani from behind and below. The restitution of the interactive pressure ("Wechseldruck" – H. L. W., 1952: indentation of the oval window resulting in a pulsing of the round window) can be easily tested in the absence of a direct view of the round window in the following ways:

1. from the *stapes*, by reflex movement of clear irrigation fluid filling the round window niche;
2. from the *round window*, using the sound produced by a fine aspirator applied anterior to the round window niche. The head of the stapes bows markedly when the stapedial tendon contracts. The sound level of the fine aspirator applied anterior to the niche is extremely high, and the test fatigues rapidly if it is repeated. Impairment of the test by a completely isolated congenital anomaly at the round window is rare.

If the round window niche is not reopened in this manner and the interactive pressure cannot be elicited, it may be necessary to take down the bony edge of the subiculum with the diamond burr as far as the *inferomedial* edge. If a burr of the correct size is used, there is no danger to the edge of the round window membrane. The wall of the subiculum should be retained *superiorly and posteriorly* to preserve its physiological function, i.e., the deflection of the aeration through the hypotympanum directly to the round window, so that the air does not flow away ineffectively into the sinus tympani. The bone should be denuded as little as possible. The round window niche including the membrane should be covered with a split graft from the lip or with amnion if only granulations are found deeply and no mucosa remains (Figs. **82** and **83**). An empty denuded niche rapidly becomes almost completely obstructed by scar tissue.

If there is any suspicion that the round window membrane is at risk due to infection, it should be reinforced by an overlay of thin fascia or amnion, or even better, by a split-thickness lip graft. There is no danger that this will affect hearing in the speech range. If the round window membrane is injured, there are two factors which endanger the function of the cochlea. The first of these is the loss of perilymph: the penetration of air leads immediately to raising of the auditory threshold (Lehnhardt et al. 1980). Is infection follows. The first step must be to

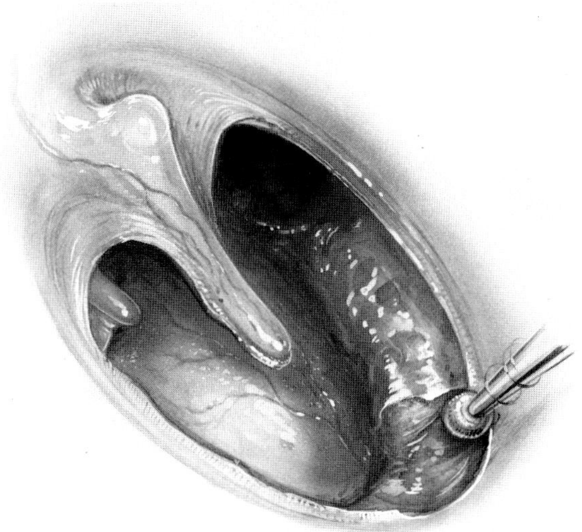

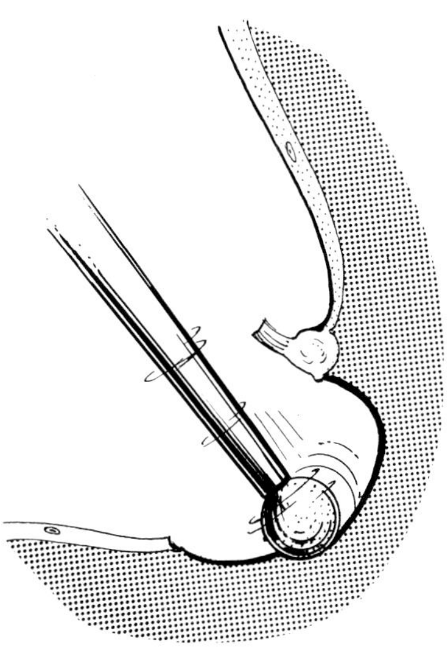

Fig. **169 Deepening of the hypotympanum.** In a shallow hypotympanum which jeopordizes the patency of the inferior aeration pathway, the bony septum of the cells of the hypotympanum and, finally, of the compact bone are drilled with a suitable diamond burr down to the jugular bulb (H. L. Wullstein 1968)

Fig. **170 Deepening of the hypotympanum.** This figure shows a section transverse to that in Fig. **169** (H. L. Wullstein 1968)

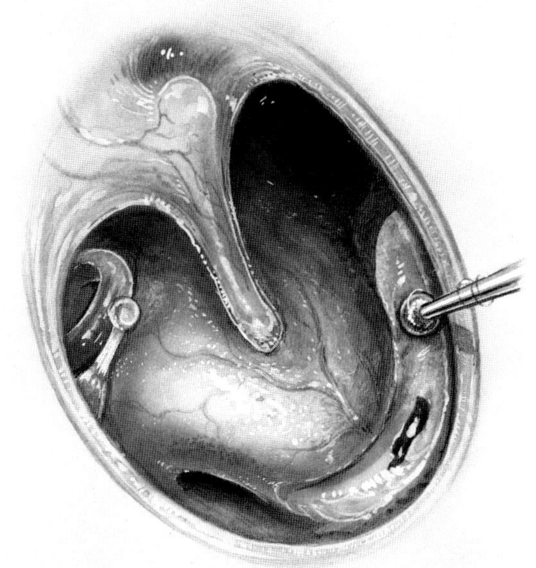

Fig. **171 Deepening of the hypotympanum.** If the jugular bulb is high, the vein wall should not be exposed, but a thin bony lamella should be left over the vein. If the hypotympanum is still not of sufficient depth, it can be extended externally in the floor of the meatus (H. L. Wullstein 1968)

fill the niche with Ringer's solution; then it is covered with a completely saturated gelatin sponge with the addition of an antibiotic which is tolerated by the inner ear. The round window membrane is closed with fascia. A previously unintended second stage is then often the most advisable course to protect the function of the cochlea.

Difficult anatomical abnormalities impede the progress of a successful tympanoplasty. They are to be sought in the course of the two aeration path-ways. The upper aeration pathway may possibly be very shallow.

Continuing granulation along the pathway from the tube to the oval window niche is probably due to *chronic myopathy of the tensor tympani muscle* if the lower aeration pathway is only a little diseased. In these cases the canal should be drilled down to the cochleariform process and curetted deeply. The tube should not need to be opened any more than necessary toward the protympanic recess, so as to

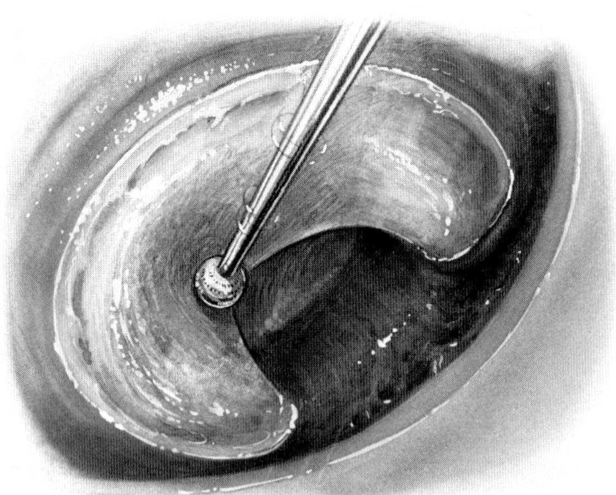

Fig. **172   Flattening of the round window niche.** The overhang of the promontory is removed with the diamond burr, as far as the insertion of the round window membrane. If the mucosa is inflamed, however, the edge of the window is often difficult to recognize

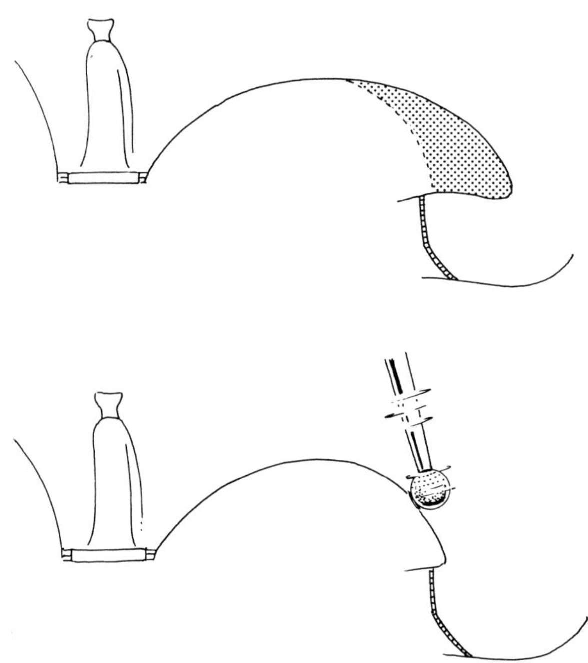

Fig. **173   Flattening of the round window niche, showing a section transverse to Fig. 172**

minimize disturbance of the balance between the superior and inferior aeration pathways.

The lower aeration pathway is often narrowed by a high jugular bulb, so that ventilation through the tympanic sinus and the posterior isthmus as far as the antrum is impeded. In extreme cases the entrance to the round window niche is almost completely obstructed. Because the mastoid process is also usually narrow, with a steep facial nerve, the sinus tympani is also often narrow. The layer of bone over the jugular bulb can be very thin or even absent, so that great care is necessary. In very rare cases the bend on the carotid artery is displaced so far posteriorly that the internal carotid artery can be accidently damaged, with the most serious sequelae. The most expensive medicolegal case in otology was due to such an accident. Schueller's and Stenver's views should act as a warning of this possibility before operation.

A well-developed hypotympanum is the best anatomical prerequisite for good hearing after all types of tympanoplasty. A shallow, underdeveloped hypotympanum is accompanied by a shallow upper aeration pathway, a flatter promontory and thus a shallow mesotympanum. A narrow tympanic sinus under a steep mastoid segment of the facial nerve can be easily blocked by granulations and is very difficult to free from a cholesteatoma matrix.

A high jugular bulb is also quite common in these circumstances. Because adhesions with the tympanic membrane graft are to be feared, it is permissible to attempt to create a new wide hypotympanum laterally in the floor of the meatus. A deep, wide groove is cut in the tympanic bone (including the bony annulus) using a diamond burr. This area must be covered with a mucosal graft.

Mucosal tuberculosis is a hematogenous infection causing small, multiple or large perforations and extensive destruction. In the exudative form it is very rare, but in the productive form it can occur in complete isolation, without pulmonary symptoms or signs. Extensive granulations should always be biopsied but the result only becomes available long after the operation is over. To our surprise, one-stage tympanoplasty has always healed well and permanently in these cases. The serious sequel of healing mucosal tuberculosis in the middle ear, the eustachian tube and the tubal torus is *persistent, extremely rigid scar tissue stenosis.* Prolonged careful aftercare lasting many months, particularly with middle ear inflation, helps to achieve a satisfactory functional result in the middle ear. Healing of tuberculosis with reconstruction of normal mucosa and aeration of the middle ear by an osteoplastic tympanotomy is shown by Figs. **174** and **175**.

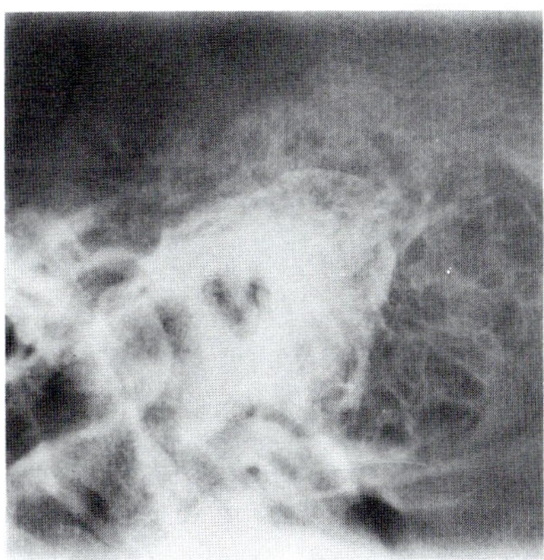

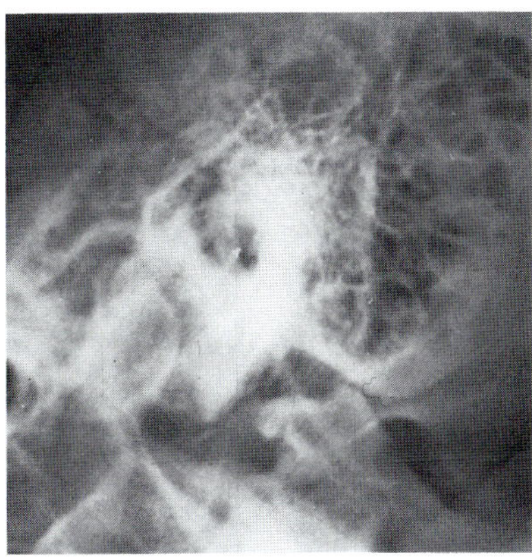

Fig. **174 Tuberculosis of the middle ear.** A Schueller's view before surgical eradication using an osteoplastic epitympanotomy

Fig. **175 Middle ear tuberculosis, showing the same patient as in Fig. 174.** Schueller's view after osteoplastic epitympanotomy. There is improved radiolucency of the entire pneumatic cell system, due to an increased air content of the middle ear

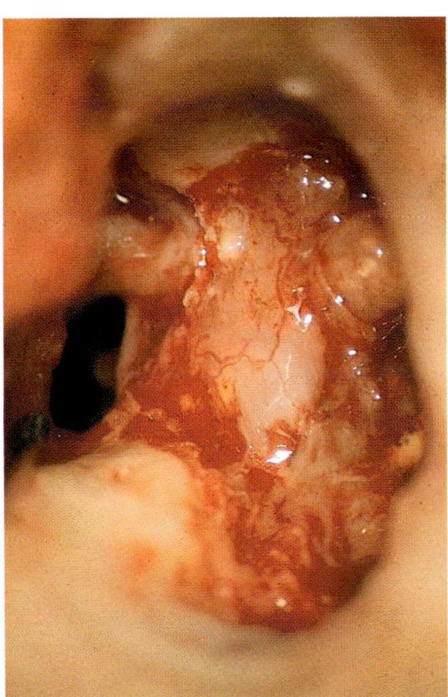

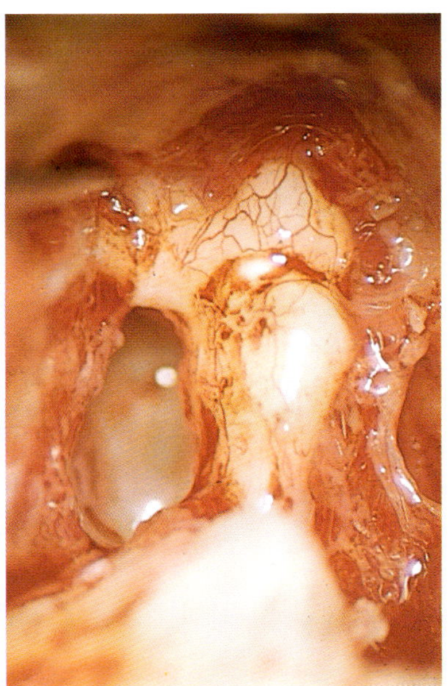

Fig. **176 Chronic middle ear inflammation with a central perforation of the tympanic membrane of moderate size,** accompanied by marked mucosal inflammation, blocking of the tympanic diaphragm and aditus. Granulations, cholesterin cysts, fibrous and fatty degeneration of the mucosal folds are present in the epitympanum. The histological picture is shown in Figs. **156** and **157**

Fig. **177 Chronic middle ear inflammation with central perforation of the tympanic membrane.** An osteoplastic epitympanotomy has been carried out, and the open epitympanum and aditus ad antrum can be seen. The ossicular chain has been interrupted, and the long process of the incus is absent. The superior malleoincudal fold is markedly inflamed and thickened, and demonstrates polypi and granulations. The histological appearances are described on p. 83

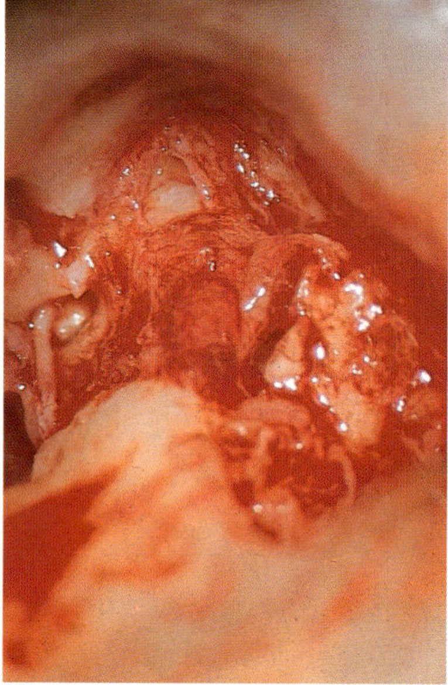

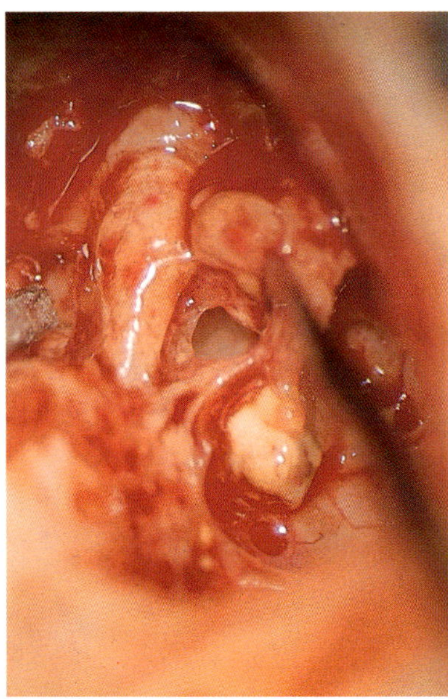

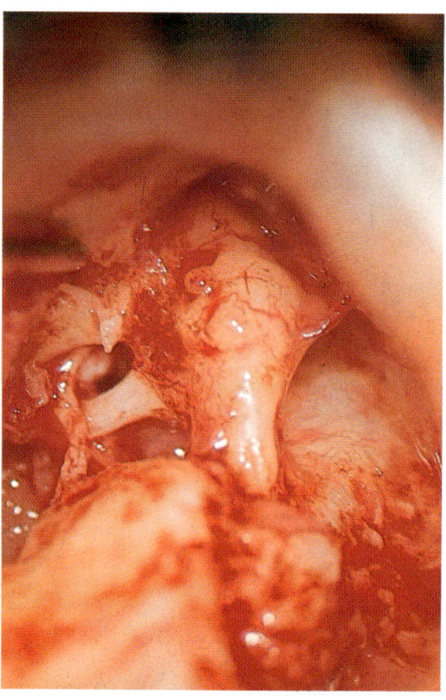

Fig. 178   Chronic mucosal suppuration. The main focus of disease is in the system of epitympanic folds. All aeration and drainage pathways are obstructed, but the ossicles remain intact

Fig. 179   Cholesterin cyst being removed from the superior incudal fold. A fatty degenerated granulation tissue polyp lies in the aditus

Fig. 180   Ossicles and chorda tympani dissected. A few small polyps have been removed from the surface of the mucosa on the body of the incus. The facial canal and labyrinthine block are covered with a thickened but well-vascularized mucosa capable of function

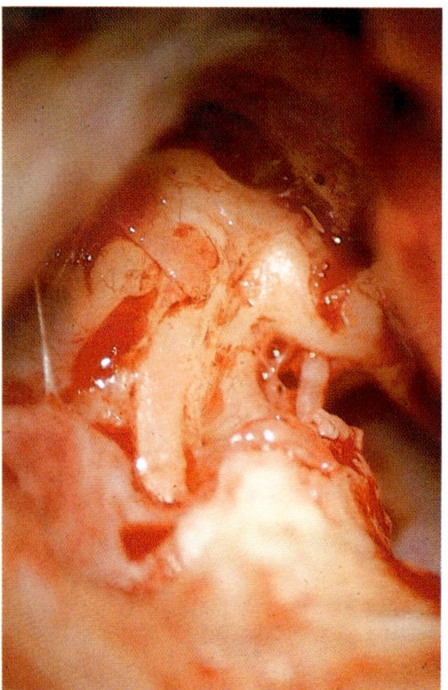

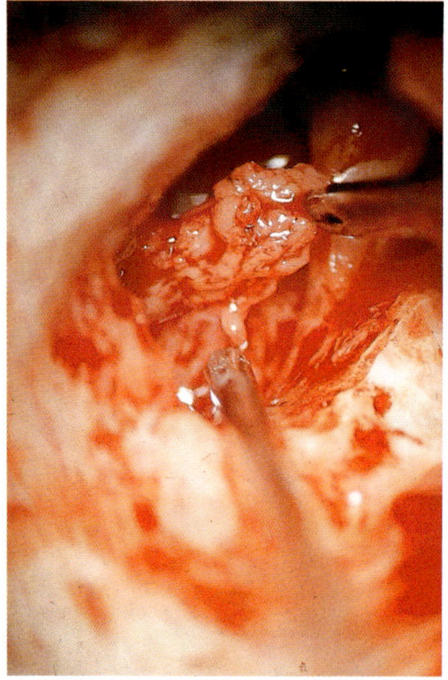

Fig. 181   Behind an otoscopically normal tympanic membrane with only a few delicate scars, a fibrous and hyaline severely degenerated calcified mucosa is hidden, with its folds in the posterior segment, which completely embed the ossicles

Fig. 182   The same location as Fig. 181. A block of thick granulation tissue has been removed from the antrum

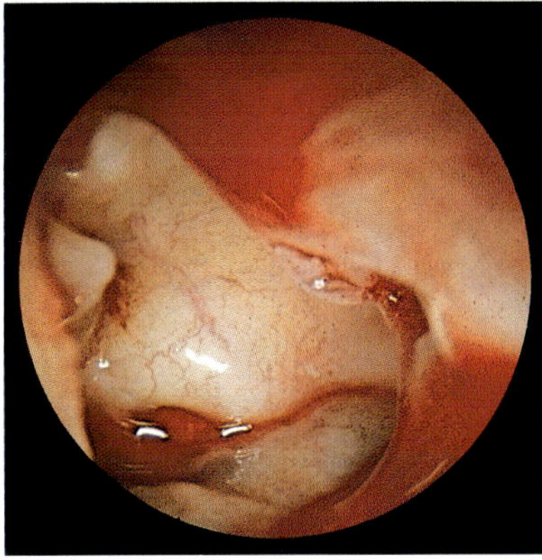

Fig. **183   Endoscopic view of the same ear as in Figs. 181** and **182.** A high jugular bulb blocks access to the round window niche. Thickened but still well-vascularized mucosa capable of regeneration lies in the mesotympanum. The eustachian tube is wide open

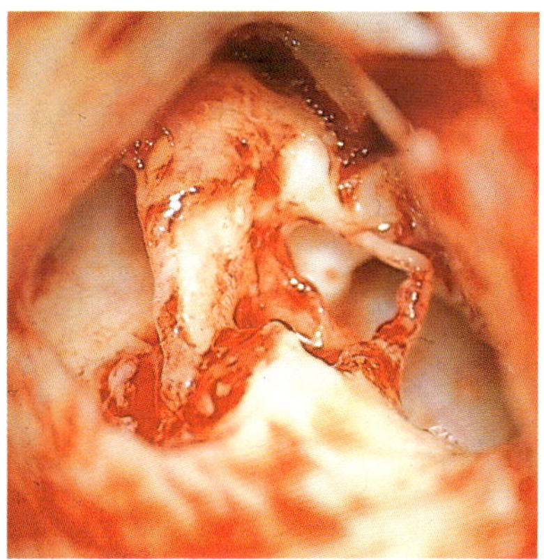

Figs. **184   The same ear as in Figs. 181−183,** showing an intact and fully mobile ossicular chain after the removal of inflammatory tissue. This is the situation shortly before the insertion of the bony lid and return of the closed meatal skin tube

Epitympanum

In the frequent tubotympanic catarrh, the infection first affects the supratubal folds and then transmits the infection into the epitympanic compartments and the protympanic recess via the anterior and superior mallear folds. An epitympanic perforation in Shrapnell's membrane anterior to the neck of the malleus without a cholesteatoma is a fairly common sequel. Tubotympanic catarrh speads along the folds of von Tröltsch and the tympanic diaphragm to the posterior isthmus, and from there to affect Prussak's space as well as the overlying folds and air cushions between the bony wall and the ossicles. A retraction of Prussak's space after healing is the most certain evidence of this (see p. 144).

The details of this previous disease cannot be clearly assessed by hearing tests and measurement of impedance. Early complete healing is an urgent necessity because of the late stages, with extensive adhesions and loss of mucosa presenting years later. Endoscopy of the epitympanum may even be indicated for the evaluation of this condition, and an osteoplastic epitympanotomy may be indicated, depending on the findings. This operation can be carried out successfully for this condition in children as

young as three or four years old. A tympanostomy tube in the anterior middle ear segment usually has no effect on the fleshy granulations which often fill the epitympanum and surround the ossicles.

These strictly localized procedures for chronic inflammation of the system of folds of the compartments can often be limited to the epitympanum if they are carried out in good time. Opening of the antrum is only indicated if healthy mucosa must be removed from its labyrinthine wall or the tegmen to fill defects of the tegmen tympani or the tympanic surface of the lid, so that new adhesions do not form around the ossicles.

Adhesions and local synechiae between the ossicles and the walls are parted easily, as described above, using needles and narrow strips of highly absorbent cotton wool. Granulations and small polyps are forced out of the protympanic recess by inflation and irrigation from the supratubal recess, to clear the anterior and medial recesses and the tubal ostium.

The folds are the site of origin of tympanosclerosis. Small plaques around the ossicles can be easily removed, but in extreme cases, all compartments are obliterated and the epitympanum is filled by a solid block consisting of tympanosclerosis and the ossicles. Removal of the masses is even then successful. Two factors are to be kept in mind:

1. Transmission of movements to the footplate endangers the cochlea, and temporary division of the incudostapedial joint is wise.
2. The absence of mucosa makes new cover of all surfaces very uncertain so that it may be advisable to sacrifice the lever system and to carry out a Type III tympanoplasty (deep). If the stapes is firmly embedded, the stapedial crura are amputated and a high columella and possibly even a two-stage stapedectomy may be indicated.

Autogenous material is used if at all possible in reconstructive procedures, but only in those with no tendency to granulate. For membranes, on the other hand, allogenic and xenogenic materials are used, the latter to avoid the medicolegal, serological and infectious problems of soft tissue. Preserved allogenic incus and malleus are available for the replacement of the ossicles. They can be easily shaped with a diamond burr to produce an oblong foot against the tympanic membrane repair, a slender shaft and a fine-forked end to interdigitate. Marquet (1981) has demonstrated that the contact surfaces of the malleus and incus are shaped differently from lateral to medial. They have a small meniscus, as was previously described by Politzer (1878); he concludes that they contribute to fine audiological tuning. He considers it more advisable to create an articulated system, using two adapted and glued autogenous ossicles, rather than a one-piece columella system.

Type II Procedures to Improve Hearing

A Type II reconstruction, i.e., with preservation of the lever system in the retained epitympanum, was previously often attempted in many different ways, most often by bridging the gap between the stapes and the handle of the malleus or the stump of the incus outside the epitympanum. It is not a satisfactory solution and good results are accidental.

The situation has been basically changed by osteoplastic epitympanotomy, so that it is now possible to decide from the appearance of the ossicles, adhesions and the degree of aeration whether repair of the ossicular chain is worthwhile. Bridging of a long process of the incus by splinting with a glued allogenic equilateral long process of the incus can be achieved through the open epitympanum (Figs. **185** and **186**). The graft may also be secured at both contact points using a small piece of adherent fascia. The defect between the lenticular pro-

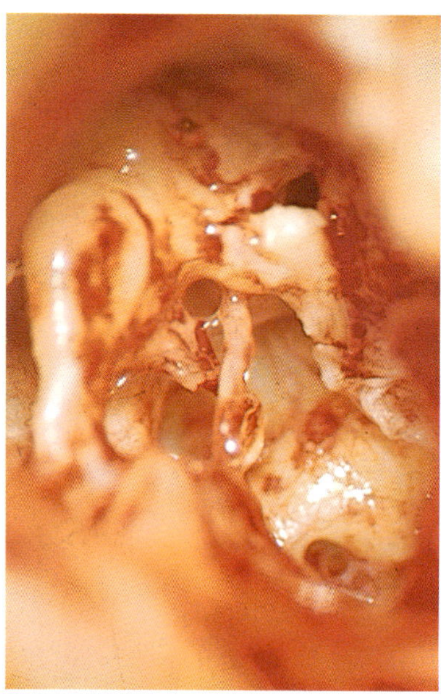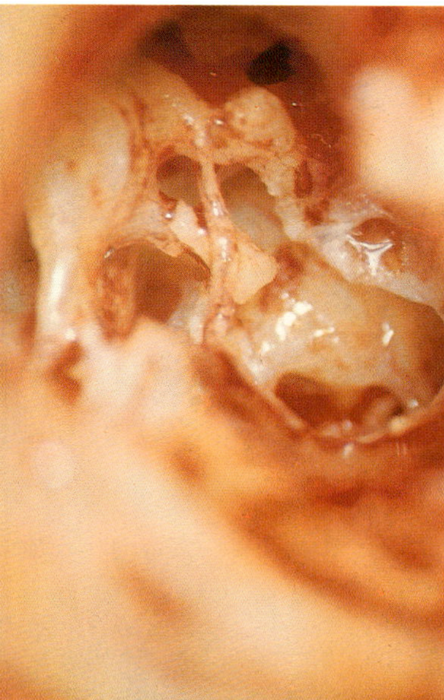

Figs. **185**–**186** **Tympanoplasty Type II.** Reconstruction of the ossicular chain with a sculpted allogenic long process of the incus from the appropriate side

185   **186**

cess and the head of the stapes can be bridged similarly.

Large anteromedial defects of the head of the malleus due to a medial focus in the protympanic recess (for example, a circumscribed anteromedial cholesteatoma, p. 108) localized at that point are not unusual. Satisfactory contact with the incus is then lost, but can often be restored by a scar tissue bridge from the neck of the malleus to the body of the incus, using a small piece of fascia.

Reconstruction of Hearing Using Type III Tympanoplasty

The Columella with a Deep Tympanic Cavity

Since replacement of the lateral wall of the epitympanum became usual, a high columella in a tympanic cavity of normal depth is the usual method, and a low columella in a shallow tympanic cavity is less frequent. Replacement materials have been extensively discussed.

A Columella in a Shallow Tympanic Cavity

A shallow tympanic cavity with a stapes and a low columella is no longer considered as an optimal audiological solution. However, this reconstruction is unavoidable in paralabyrinthine cholesteatomas because it is not possible to be certain that all remnants of the matrix have been removed. Furthermore, the subtegmental area stretching from the protympanic recess to the sinodural angle must be open to inspection through the meatus throughout the patient's life. This area is covered only by a split-thickness skin graft.

Whereas the reserve air volume of the wide antrum is retained in a Type III tympanoplasty (deep), it is absent in the shallow tympanic cavity. The mesohypotympanum must be wide open, and especially the mucosa must heal well. Shallow aeration pathways are a disadvantage. A healthy, robust, high-riding stapes reaching to the level of the facial canal is an advantage. A defect of its crura makes the choice of material for the columella difficult. Two solutions are available:

1. In the first stage of reconstruction of the mucosa of the shallow tympanic cavity without columella, one awaits complete healing. After at least three months, the tympanic membrane is elevated endaurally alongside the facial nerve, and a low columella is fitted to the new tympanic membrane.
2. Type IV procedure instead of Type III. The audiological results of Type III (shallow) tympa-

noplasty seldom approach those of effective sound pressure transformation, and a well-healed Type IV often delivers good results with sound protection. The hearing results of both solutions are thus often similar (see Chap. 12).

The Columella, its Action and its Construction

There are numerous natural examples of the audiological effect of the columella after interruption of the ossicular chain and spontaneous adherence of the tympanic membrane to the stapes (a Type III tympanoplasty with shallow tympanic cavity because the lateral epitympanic wall is absent), or after resorption of the long process of the incus (Type III with deep tympanic cavity). The collagenous layer of fibers is usually so atrophic, delicate and almost transparent that the noninflamed mucosa of the promontory can be recognized. This type of natural system can achieve the theoretical maximum sound transformation over almost the entire frequency range, although the middle ear component is absent.

Sound transmission by a columella achieves good results, as the spontaneous examples demonstrate. Many poor results are due, firstly, to unsatisfactory transmission of sound, and secondly, to ulceration at the point of contact of the columella with the tympanic membrane graft. The causes of the latter include:

1. *Unsatisfactory aeration of the middle ear.* The point of contact of the columella presents a dilemma because an attempt is made to achieve a secure tissue union. This is achieved with autogenic and allogenic ossicles, but not with any other type. Movement of the tympanic membrane on swallowing and yawning lifts the membrane from the wound surface of the graft. If epithelialization proceeds rapidly, it covers the contact points with healthy mucosa. The new tympanic membrane lies on the columella but lifts off

it easily during changes of pressure due to swallowing or yawning.

2. *Pressure ulceration of the membrane by the columella on the internal surface of the tympanic membrane repair.* In this case, chronic ulceration on the internal surface and infection at the point of contact are more frequent because neither epithelialization nor healing have been achieved. Extensive retraction and perforation of the graft are the result. Heermann (1978) therefore bridges the mesohypotympanum with fine slivers of cartilage, using his palisade technique to influence the impedance. They can be positioned in the following manner to achieve noninflammatory healing of the columella at the points of contact:

A thin, stretched, and flattened strip of fascia is prepared so that it will fit the two superior quadrants of the pars tensa and reach from the bony annulus at the anterior spine to the posterior spine. The pars tensa is thus strengthened along the anterior and posterior tympanic striae, whereas the pars flaccida is under minimal tension. The tension of the new reinforced tympanic membrane holds it away from the promontory and encourages continuous epithelialization. It thus prevents adhesions and atelectasis in the middle ear and the sinus tympani. The mucosa or granulations in the center of the footplate are carefully freshened to allow healing of a small piece of interposed fascia which prevents a perforation by the columella.

The perforation of the tympanic membrane is closed and glued in the first phases of the operation using a robust piece of fascia or, if necessary, temporal periosteum. An inert allogenic incus or head of the malleus is drilled so that it has a broad surface corresponding as closely as possible to the curvature of the tympanic membrane, and a slender shaft with a blunt end for the footplate. The columella and the fascial strip are now adjusted across the middle ear cavity, the first in height and angulation, the second in length and breadth. The pressed-out fascial strip is drawn from the apex over the columella almost to the various contact surfaces. The columella is then placed on the oval window niche, and the fascial strip fitted and glued to the two superior quadrants of the tympanic membrane. Experimental findings demonstrated on p. 42 show how these fascial strips achieve a blood circulation through the longitudinal vascular network within 48 hours. The two layers adhere, but their parallel, separate vascular supply is preserved in the long term.

Allogenic ossicles preserved in neutral cialit solution retain normal calcium phosphorus and collagen content and do not soften. They are more suitable than alloplastic materials, which are all affected by macrophages to some extent. The ceramics are the least vulnerable of the current materials, but tissue instability persists along the columella for years with all of them.

Conditions are thus created to allow epithelialization from the fascia around the shaft of the columella, whereas the sound-receiving surface between the two fascial layers is incorporated with them. Osteoplastic epitympanotomy with its wide access and deep tympanic cavity is more suitable for this type of embedding than the open technique of tympanoplasty. The closed techniques should be abandoned.

The implantation of an allogenic middle ear system as an en-bloc graft has become an acceptable operative technique only with the help of osteoplastic exposure of the middle ear spaces, because the point of anchorage of the graft to the stapes and to the annulus is widely exposed. On the contrary, when introducing the en-bloc graft through the facial-chordal angle in the closed technique, positioning of the stapes may fail, particularly in a narrow field.

Figures **187** to **192** show that an en-bloc graft of this type can heal completely, even in extremely unfavorable situations; for example, a large cholesteatoma, very diseased mucosa or narrow anatomical relationships. The maximal hearing gain is achieved, and the contours of the external meatus and the tympanic membrane are also normal. In this patient a recurrent perforation occurred due to an acute otitis media following a severe attack of influenza. A revision operation showed that the bony lid was almost completely fixed by bone, with a well-epithelialized allogenic ossicle, and *a relatively wide, delicate connective tissue bridge running from the head of the malleus and the incus to the tegmen tympani. This fold resembled the superior malleoincudal fold which suspended the ossicle.*

Prepared xenogenic membranes used to replace the tympanic membrane must be offered every aid for long-term incorporation, including the following:
– maintenance of electrolyte exchange on both surfaces;
– rapid overgrowth of both surfaces within the mesotympanum and, externally, by *autogenic rapidly vascularized* tissue, i.e., with a layer of thin fascia which overlaps the xenogenic graft on both

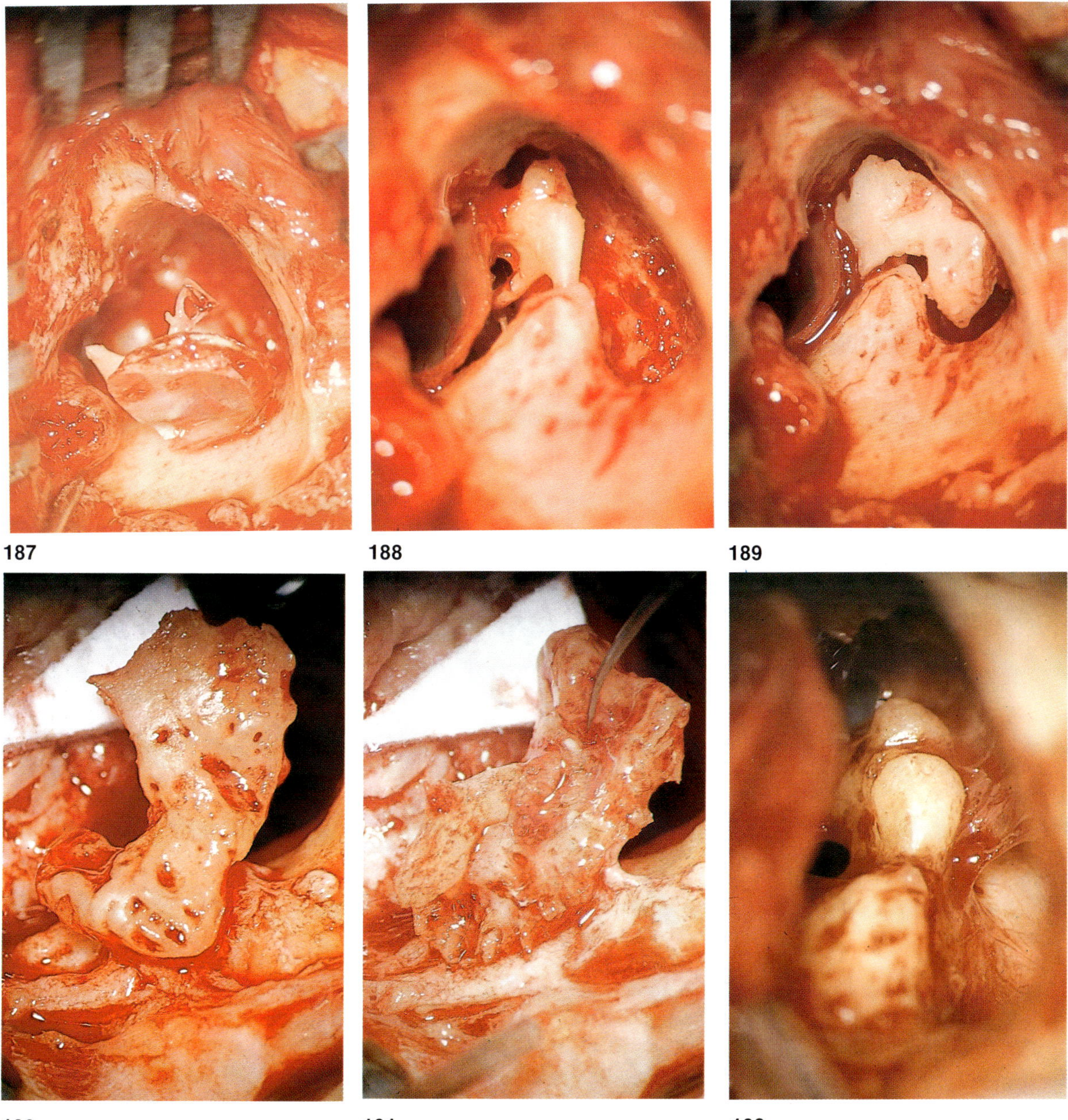

Fig. **187** **The en-bloc graft during implantation into the middle ear**

Fig. **188** After eradication of a large cholesteatoma and evaluation of all the niches, recesses, etc., the allogenic tympanic membrane, malleus, incus and the stapes, including its footplate, are inserted. The fibrous annulus allogenic tympanic membrane is carefully fitted into the autogenous bony annulus. The anterior long process of the malleus and the anterior mallear ligament are carefully adapted in the direction of the anterior tympanic spine and into the petrotympanic fissure, if possible in contact with the remnants of the autogenous anterior mallear fold. The space beneath this, leading to the cochleariform process, should remain free where the tensor tendon was previously removed, so that direct aeration of the anterior epitympanum via the supratubal and protympanic recess can be achieved. The stapedial footplate lies naturally on the autogenous foundation. A brief movement of the handle of the malleus immediately ellicits the round window reflex

Fig. **189** **The same patient as in Fig. 188.** The inserted bony lid bordering on the allogenic tympanic membrane anterior to the covering, together with the free autogenous fascial transplant. In order to secure rapid revascularization, the epitympanotomy flap is spread out over it

Fig. **190** **En-bloc graft, showing the same patient as in Fig. 188** undergoing a revision tympanoplasty three years later. It was necessary to trephine the bony lid again, using the pointed conical diamond burr in order to remove it

Fig. **191** **Bony lid removed,** showing the new mucosa capable of function on its internal surface

Fig. **192** **The same patient as in Figs. 188** and **190.** The healed en-bloc graft, three years after its implantation. Well-aerated mucosa lies in the aditus. A new mucosal fold leads from the head of the malleus and the body of the incus to the tegmen

sides to such an extent that the circumscribed longitudinal vascular sprouts invade the graft from the zone of contact with the surrounding area within a few days. Fascial grafts on the internal and external surfaces prevent adhesions with the promontory at the start of aeration of the middle ear cavity from the sixth day onward, when vascularization begins.

The healthy human pars tensa is about 0.1 mm thick, and the prepared xenogenic membrane of calf vein (Zini and Sanna 1976) is of roughly the same thickness. During healing, the membrane with its fascial layer on both sides is much thicker. If rapid overgrowth of mucosa is achieved, the mesotympanic space again becomes patent. The external fascia is also rapidly epidermized, provided that it receives its electrolyte requirements for about one week; in this case, from the saturated gelatin sponge in the meatus. In this way the new tympanic membrane is covered with robust epidermis which is not so easily injured; by manipulations, for example.

If the conditions after shaping and covering of the oval niche and construction of a columella are so unfavorable that massive obstruction of the sound transmission by the columella is likely, it is useless to preserve the epitympanum. A Type IV tympanoplasty easily achieves the desired audiological result (a 27-dB hearing threshold). Often the result is even better, with a wide tonal spectrum, probably due to concentration of the sound pressure on the stapes footplate in this deep narrow space. Provided that the patient does not have a sensorineural deafness in addition, a socially acceptable hearing threshold is achieved, as in fenestration (Lempert 1941). The construction of sound protection anterior to the round window with full-thickness skin, and covering of the oval window with split skin so that it remains wide open has already been described (see Figs. **65** and **66**).

Retrotympanic Spaces

Exposure beyond the middle ear and the antrum is carried in two directions:

1. Exposure into the mastoid cell system. After the necessary extension of the skin incision, the *osteoplastic epitympanotomy* is continued as a mastoidectomy and its extent is determined by the disease. Drilling is continued from the aditus to the tegmen antri as far as the last cell in the sinodural angle and from there, inferiorly to the bulge of the sigmoid sinus and, if necessary, as far as the bulb of the jugular vein and the mastoid tip. The cell system is eradicated with cutting burrs of suitable size as far as the level of the labyrinthine block and the posterior meatal wall. This wall must be previously bevelled; if necessary, from the *tympanic* side, so that the *sinus tympani* is widely accessible. Because the entire mastoid process lies open from the lateral side, this part of the operation is simple and rapidly carried out as a normal extended antrotomy, beginning at the site of the disease and tailored to individual needs. The lateral semicircular canal and the second facial genu remain covered with mucosa because of the risk of a fistula or exposed nerve.

Not every healthy parasinus and paralabyrinthine cell group must be eradicated, but they must be at least opened so that they can heal securely. This includes the cells in the tractus niche and those above and behind the semicircular canal as far as the crus commune. The search for the sublabyrinthine cell group must not be omitted. It often leads deeply behind a relatively compact layer of bone between the ampullary crus of the posterior semicircular canal and the jugular bulb. Unexplained bony labyrinthitis and meningitis may arise later from this point if the mastoidectomy has been inadequate. These cell groups are often poorly developed in chronic otitis media. They correspond to the posterosuperior and posteroinferior cell tracts in a well-pneumatized temporal bone. It is unnecessary to dissect healthy peripheral cell groups until firm bone is reached, provided that a large mastoid process is obliterated by a plasticine plug, and then sealed off from the antrum with fascia. From the beginning of tympanoplasty it was clear that this operative procedure and antibacterial methods allow the graft to heal smoothly, even in heavily infected ears.

The traditional principles of otological surgery demand exposure of an extradural or parasinus focus until healthy surrounding tissue is reached on all sides. This is now easier to achieve than previously, using the diamond burr and fine raspatories. If such a focus is found at mastoidectomy, drainage for several days may be valuable, preferably through a separate skin incision leading posteriorly. The inflamed sinus wall can be so swollen that there is a risk of rupture after it has been exposed. A fascial graft can be glued on in every case. However, appropriate intensive antibiotic cover is needed because a mural thrombus in the lumen of the sinus cannot be excluded; this is true as well if the dura is exposed. Firm primary closure of the wound is also advisable in the interests of healing of the epitympanic bony lid.

2. Exposure into the petrous bone. This exposure goes beyond the medial wall of the epitympanum and the labyrinthine block into the depth of the petrous bone. If necessary, dissection is continued as far as the petrous apex near the sphenoclivus angle and the greater wing of the sphenoid bone. The fine spongiosa or the two superior cell tracks lead into the pyramidal apex superior and posterior to the anterior semicircular canal. The *concealed and dangerous complications arising from the antelabyrinthine trigone were the main reason for the prolonged search for a new solution.*

If the ossicles are retained in a mucopolypoid inflammation, the space anterior and medial to the head of the malleus should be carefully dissected; the edematous mucosa is picked off and the drainage of the paralabyrinthine cells is ensured. Access to the pyramidal apex is described under cholesteatoma on p. 134.

The Empty Mastoid and Absent Mastoid Walls

A mastoid cavity is avoided by osteoplastic epitympanotomy. However, if the *subtegmental area* in front of and behind the anterior semicircular canal and in the depth of the petrous pyramid stretching from the protympanic recess to the sinodural angle must remain open for inspection because of paralabyrinthine infection, Types I, II and III reconstruction with a deep tympanic cavity are to be avoided. The operation ends with loss of the meatal roof as a Type III (shallow) or a Type IV, with a cavity open along the tegmen and the wall of the petrous pyramid above the tympanic course of the facial nerve. The mastoid cavity is filled with plasticine to the level of the facial spur, and fascia is placed over this, and the entire subtegmental surface is covered with a split-skin graft.

Several authors have attempted to extend the access at tympanoplasty to *resect and reimplant the posterior meatal wall.* In principle this is a variant of the closed form of tympanoplasty.

In the osteoplastic meato-attico-antrotomy described by Feldmann (1977), the posterior and superior meatal wall is cut out with a saw from a necessarily very extensive mastoidectomy, provided that the mastoid is not diseased. Individualized exposure and healing of the main source of the disease in the epitympanum is not possible. Because of the absent posterior meatal wall, great dificulty is encountered in the long run in holding the subtegmental region open, if this is desirable because of paralabyrinthine complications. The creation of a large permanent mastoid cavity is then unavoidable.

These cavities are then covered laterally by galea alone. As a result of the open meatal cavity, the soft tissue cover becomes easily infected, leading to a galeal phlegmon with granulations and persistent secretion. So long as the walls of the cavum are satisfactory, it is possible to fill the cavity with plasticine after thorough clearance, even if the sinus and dura have been widely exposed at a previous operation. The soft, highly infected granulations are removed carefully with a drill, if necessary, and then irrigated with a nontoxic disinfectant. The sensitivity of the bacterial flora of these heavily infected mastoid cavities is determined before the operation, to allow the correct antibiotic to be chosen as a supplement to the plasticine. With such precautionary measures even chronically inflamed walls of both cranial fossae in the mastoid cavity can be included in the filling. Antibiotic treatment must continue for about 14 days after operation. The free split skin graft which covers the plasticine on the meatal side must be carefully adapted to the surrounding skin edges so that capillary sprouts enter the free graft promptly. The result is an almost completely normal meatus.

A small defect of the posterior bony meatal wall can be closed by a plasticine wall with skin cover. If no bony meatal wall remains for filling with plasticine, the apex of the mastoid process should be amputated and the posterior edge of the bony defect is completely rounded off so that the mobilized galea of the posterior cranial fossa and the aponeurosis of the sternocleidomastoid muscle can be sutured together in the floor of the meatus, reducing the large defect to the size of a small antral cavity which is covered with full-thickness skin (H. L. Wullstein 1968).

Cholesteatoma

Classification of Cholesteatoma of the Middle Ear
(Figs. **193–195**)

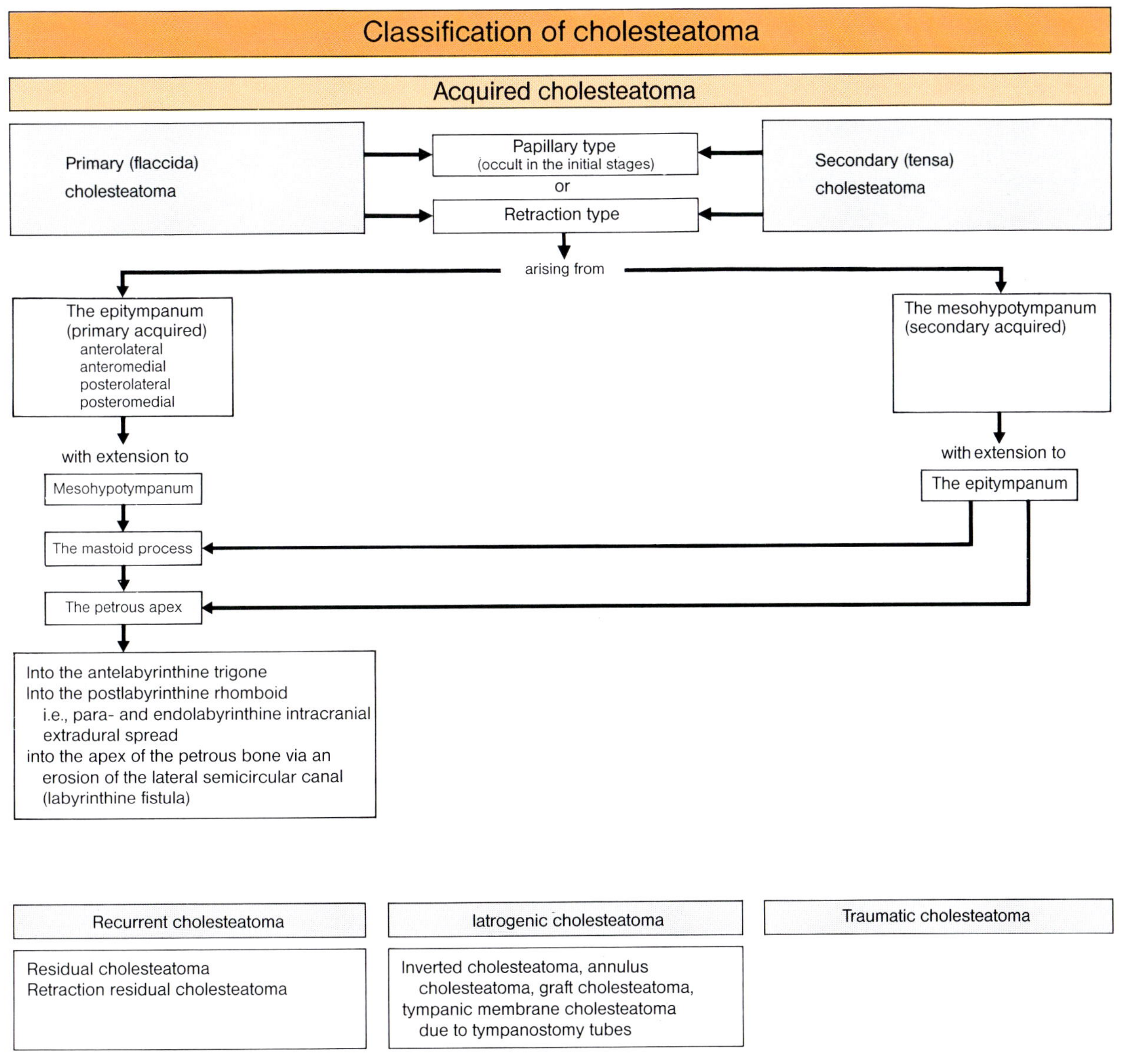

The terms primary and secondary acquired inflammatory cholesteatoma have been the subject of continuous controversy. Endless effort has been expended over many decades in the histological examination of many serial sections of the temporal bone to explain the biological and pathological course of this disease. Sadly, it was confirmed at the eighth workshop run by Shambaugh and Shea in 1984 in Chicago that there is no detailed clinical definition and classification of cholesteatoma which satisfies the otologist yet. The cause is not hard to find: numerous operative and postmortem findings of individual cases have been available for a long time, but they do not allow interpretation of the course of the disease.

Formerly there was considerable confusion about the onset, type and duration of the danger period and of the healing process of osteitis of the labyrinth. Wullstein was the first to classify osteitis of the inner ear successfully and to explain its pathological sequelae on the basis of many years of observations and radiographs (H. L. Wullstein 1948, 1968).

In a further prolonged investigation of the early stages of cholesteatoma, H. L. Wullstein (1971) established a generally valid classification of cholesteatoma based on the earliest stages in the light of the fine structures of the epitympanum, using a new anatomical and pathological method of dissection. This showed the site and manner in which the cholesteatoma matrix impinges upon the mucosal folds, and thus the direction of its further development. In old histological serial sections, the significance of the folds was not recognized because they appeared only as a line and never as a surface in the two-dimensional sections, even if they were still present.

Every inflammatory acquired cholesteatoma begins as either a *papillary type* or as a *retraction type.*

The *primary inflammatory acquired cholesteatoma* arises without exception from the pars flaccida.

The *secondary inflammatory acquired cholesteatoma* arises mainly through defects in the pars tensa.

The latter will be dealt with first because they are more easily understood.

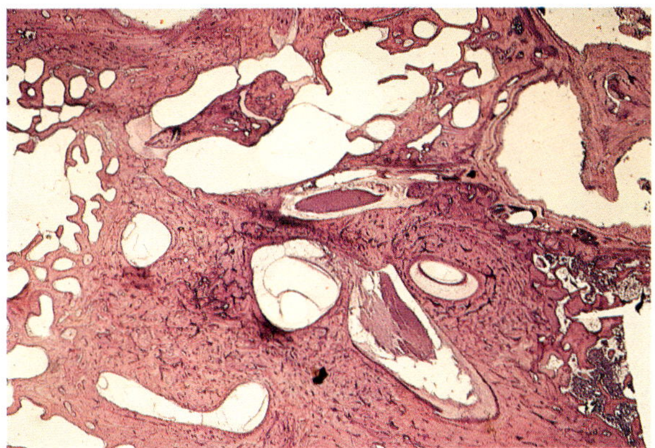

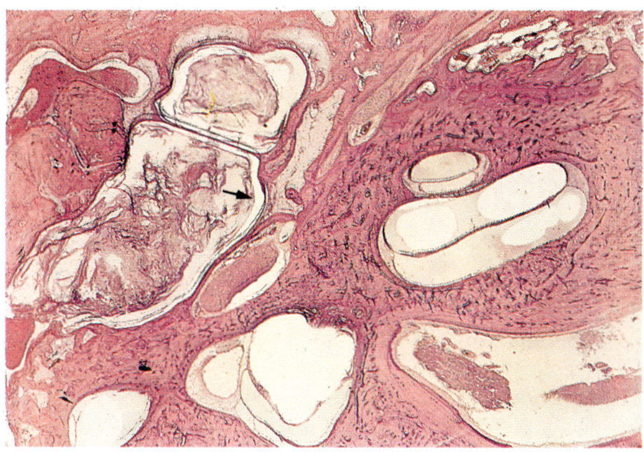

Fig. **193 Horizontal serial section through the healthy middle ear.** The mucosal fold runs from the body of the incus to the internal surface of the lateral epitympanic wall and divides this space into an anterior and posterior medial compartment. A further mucosal fold extends between the head of the malleus in a medial direction to the epitympanic wall and divides this inner space into an anterior and posterior compartment. If a medial cholesteatoma develops in this direction, it can extend further for a long time, divided into finger shapes by a medial mucosal fold of this type (Fig. **194**). If the cholesteatoma and the matrix undergo secondary infection, these fine structures are then immediately destroyed by the pressure of debris of the granulations and by the enzymatic effect of the perimatrix

Fig. **194   Horizontal serial section through the middle ear, showing chronic middle ear inflammation with a secondarily infected acquired retraction cholesteatoma.** An effusion lies lateral to the ossicles in the lateral epitympanic air cushions. Medial to the ossicles, the cholesteatoma is divided into two pouches by the medial fold. The anterior point of danger due to pressure by the cholesteatoma mass and the collagenolytic action of perimatrix in the direction of the geniculate ganglion is marked with the arrow. Compare with Figs. **193** and **195**

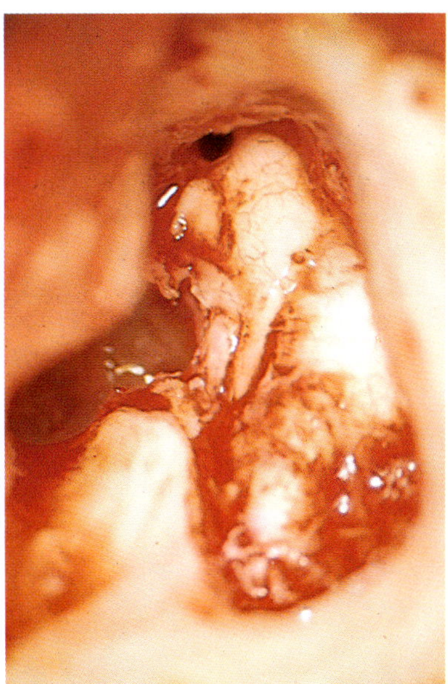

Fig. **195   Chronic middle ear inflammation with secondary inflammatory acquired cholesteatoma,** which fills the entire medial segment of the epitympanum and the antrum. The long process of the incus is absent. The intact stapes is visible in the oval window niche. These operative findings correspond to the pathological findings as described in Fig. **194**

Secondary Acquired Inflammatory Cholesteatoma

(Figs. **196–201**)

This cholesteatoma arising from the pars tensa is the result of:

1. Inflammatory irritation *of a marginal perforation* after necrotizing myringitis at the point where the flat epidermis of the pars tensa is firmly fixed by a deep papillary root at the union of the fibrous and bony annulus. It can penetrate the cavity of the middle ear at this point. Previously, this disease was particularly common after scarlet fever.
2. Mucopolypoid or mucoperiosteal inflammation with or without a *central perforation* and surrounding myringitis, with atrophy of the collagen fibers so that the lax epidermis of the tympanic membrane adheres to the walls of the mesohypotympanum.

In the absence of serious mucopolypoid inflammation in the middle ear, *the thin, flat epidermis of the pars tensa, where there are no papillae*, is the site of origin of a cholesteatoma *only where the collagenous fiber system is atrophied due to myringitis without perforation*. If this epidermis gains contact with the medial bony wall of the middle ear cavity due to retraction, it may be sucked into the epitympanum. Irritation by infected dermal debris then leads to the formation of a cholesteatoma which perforates the delicate skin close to the ossicles, and extends deeply. This matrix with no epidermal papillae does not tend to form an invasive cholesteatoma in the labyrinthine bone as does the matrix of Shrapnell's membrane. Should this not be the case, the retraction will only cause the flat epithelium to grow and cover the bony profile in the depth without causing irritation. In a central perforation of a healthy tympanic membrane the collagenous fibers are retained. The epidermis rolls around the edge of the perforation until it meets the mucosa of the internal surface, but almost never forms a cholesteatoma.

Secondary cholesteatoma due to inflammatory middle ear disease represents a failed attempt at self-healing of a defect in the pars tensa. In many countries it has become uncommon, as a result of improved living standards and immunization. It is therefore surprising that in highly developed nations, so many nonimmunized children, although surrounded by an immunized population, still suffer from this disease and its sequelae.

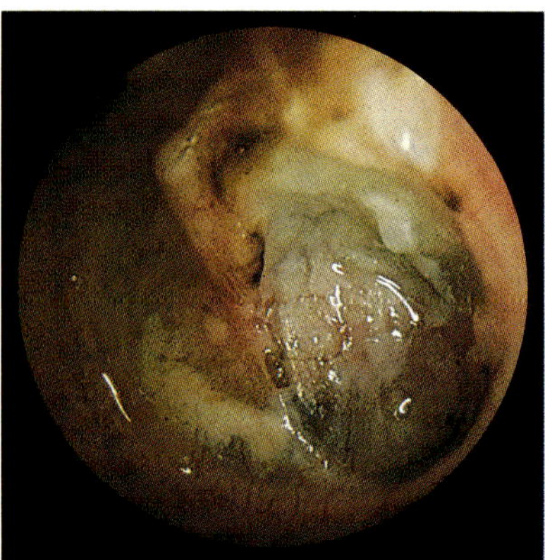

Fig. **196 Chronic middle ear inflammation with a large secondary acquired cholesteatoma.** An endoscopic view (straight endoscope, 0°, 4 mm). Deep retraction of the posterosuperior quadrant of the pars tensa with fetid purulent secretion, and flakes of cholesteatoma. The fibrous annulus is destroyed, the meatal epidermis has grown over the bony annulus and penetrated deeply into the epitympanum. The extent of the cholesteatoma can only be assessed with this view

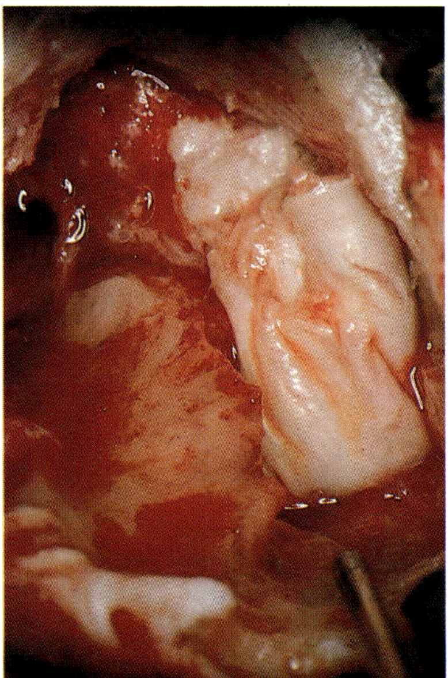

Fig. **197 Operative view of the same ear as in Fig. 196.** The cholesteatoma has been completely exposed by the removal of a large bony lid. It has already reached the sinodural angle. A sucker shows the end of the cholesteatoma, where removal of the rest of the sac begins

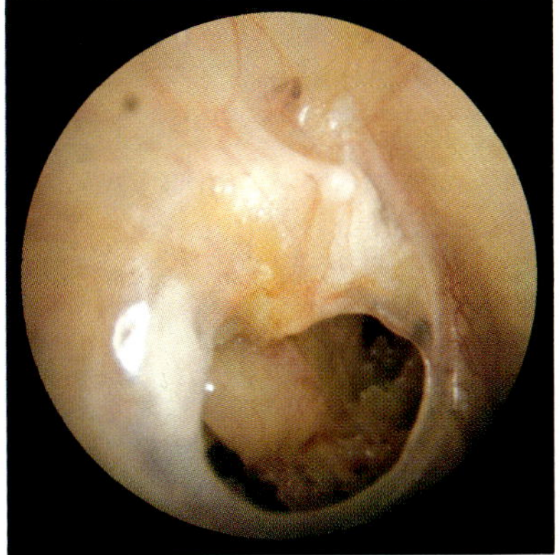

Fig. **198   Endoscopic view of a right ear (straight endoscope 0°, 4 mm).** Chronic middle ear inflammation with a dry central perforation of the tympanic membrane and concealed secondary inflammatory cholesteatoma. The non-inflamed mucosa on the promontory and in the hypotympanum can be seen through the perforation, as well as the access to the round window niche

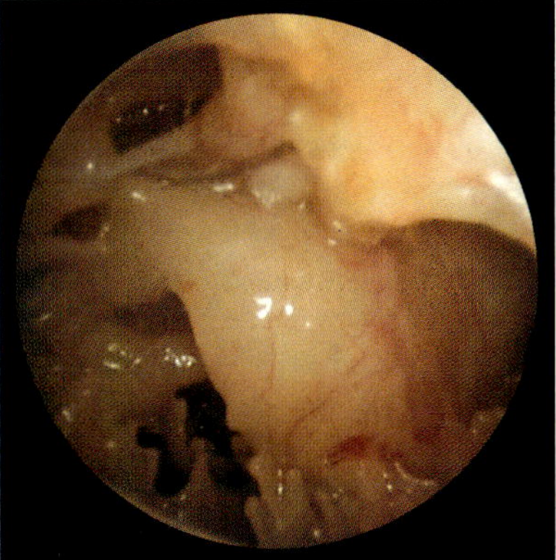

Fig. **199   Endoscopic view of the same right ear as in Fig. 198.** A view with a 2.7-mm, 30° telescope, introduced into the middle ear through the defect in the tympanic membrane. The view shows the round window niche and also the oval window niche with the stapes, the stapedial tendon and the pyramidal process. Secondary inflammatory cholesteatoma can be seen penetrating between the anterior stapedial crus and the handle of the malleus

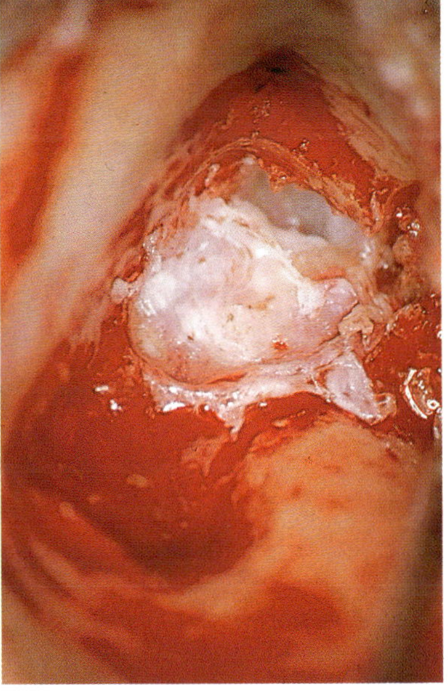

Fig. **200   Operative view of the same right ear as in Figs. 198 and 199.** After osteoplastic exposure, the large secondary medial cholesteatoma is completely exposed. The arrow shows the beginning of the development of the cholesteatoma sac, between the stapes and the handle of the malleus. The remnant of the ossicular chain is pressed against the lateral epitympanic wall and is removed because it is no longer useful

Fig. **201a   Chronic middle ear inflammation with invagination cholesteatoma arising from the pars tensa, with fixation of the head of the malleus by osteitis in the anterior epitympanum.** The cholesteatoma has developed on the medial side of the ossicles and extends up to the level of the lateral semicircular canal. The cholesteatoma is exenterated, together with the ossicles and drilling of the wall into the anterior epitympanum. A tympanoplasty Type III (deep) is created after insertion of the bony lid

Fig. **201b   After removal of the ossicles, eradication of the cholesteatoma in the epitympanum begins.** Its penetration medially and anteriorly is temporarily prevented by the tensor fold. The medial fold of the epitympanum is lined by mucosa capable of regeneration, which guarantees good mucociliary clearance

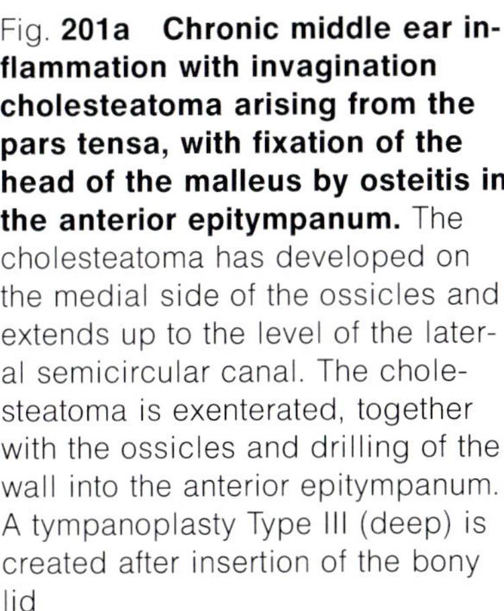

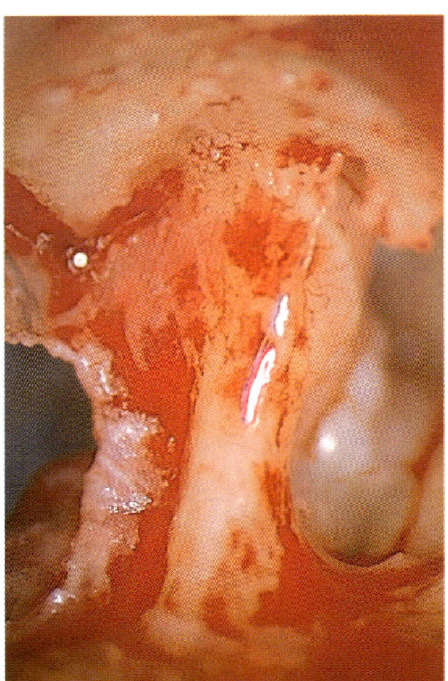

a

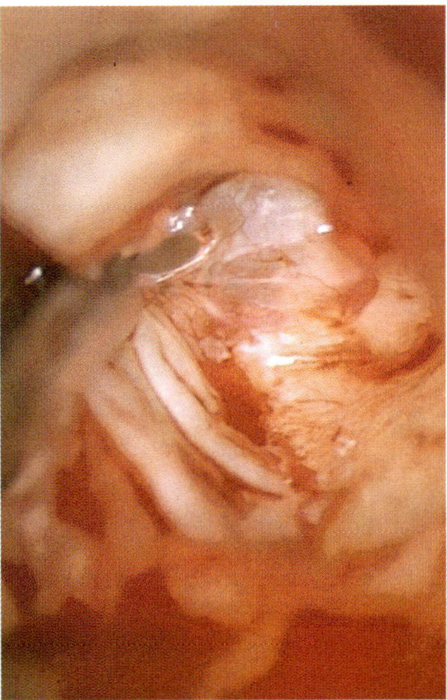

b

Primary Acquired Inflammatory Cholesteatoma

Chronic suppurative middle ear infection is becoming rarer, whereas epidermoids in Shrapnell's membrane and retraction pockets are increasing in frequency, and as a result, concealed epitympanic cholesteatoma, including occult cholesteatoma without perforation. Subacute seromucinous middle ear inflammation, the cause of these lesions, is also increasing in frequency.

The operative findings in the early stages show the principles governing the origin and development of these cholesteatomas, which may be classified as anterolateral, anteromedial, posterolateral and posteromedial (Wullstein and Wullstein 1971). *All primary epitympanic cholesteatomas must be included in this classification,* although they have two types of origin (papillary and retraction).

The term "epidermoid" is used on purely didactic grounds to emphasize the contrast with hamartomas (mesotympanic or intradural).

Papillary cholesteatomata (Rüedi 1959, Schwarz 1966) are late stages of incompletely healed, unsatisfactorily reaerated epitympanic compartments due to mild and transient tubotympanic inflammation. The loose folds with delicate stroma and active surfaces on both sides react to the slightest stimulus with marked swelling. These entirely localized tissue changes are much too slight to cause disturbance of hearing or of impedance, and cause only slight transient otalgia, which passes unnoticed. They usually arise in the early years of life at which time immunological resistance is still poorly developed. Externally, there is little more to recognize than a *slight thickening of Shrapnell's membrane*, even if the infiltration extends to the cutis at that point. A mild suppuration can occur with a temporary or permanent dry perforation. The changes may be limited to *irritation of the germinative layer*. Shrapnell's membrane is not tightly stretched, but possesses a thick stroma which is particularly lax in early childhood.

Extension of the inflammatory infiltrate from the tensor fold to the dermis causes *proliferation of its basal cell layer*. At this point the papillae sink into the stroma and lose their connection with the germinative layer completely. A pearl arises by keratinization. It forms *the origin of an occult cholesteatoma* that often lies dormant for many years, and only begins to grow after a new stimulus. *External rupture of this type of papillary pearl only occurs secondarily.* The entrance to these cholesteatomas is small. It is scarcely visible, often covered by a crust, and lies mainly in the anterior segment of Shrapnell's

membrane anterior to the neck of the malleus. This bland in flammation, especially in small children, affects the highly reactive mucosa lying close to the eustachian tube, including the obligate tensor fold, which divides the supratubal from the protympanic recess. All current operative methods are much too destructive for this type of minimal local disease that produces almost no loss of function.

Meanwhile, the cell-forming layer of the keratin pearl has gained contact with other folds and is conducted along their surfaces *either* along the lateral wall to the epitympanic air cushions as an *early anterolateral* cholesteatoma, *or* medial to the anterior mallear ligament and the tensor fold into the medial part of the protympanic recess. It then spreads further posteriorly as far as the limiting medial incudomallear fold, as an *early anteromedial cholesteatoma*. This spreading is determined by the position of the folds. The matrix adheres initially to the folds and then parts them deeply to achieve contact with the ossicles and the bony walls. Proliferation of the basal cell layer and keratinization form the nucleus of a cholesteatoma. Its late sequelae include secondary infection, destruction of the superstructure of the ossicular chain, erosions, cholesteatoma of the mastoid and petrous pyramid, labyrinthitis and intracranial complications.

Anterolateral Cholesteatoma
(Figs. **202**, **203**)

Every primary acquired inflammatory cholesteatoma arising from the pars flaccida is a lateral tympanic cholesteatoma at its onset. It remains an *anterolateral tympanic cholesteatoma* as long as the site of increased cellular proliferation, e.g., proliferation of papillae, lies in the anterior segment of Shrapnell's membrane and is directed by its migration along the anterior fold of von Tröltsch to the neck and head of the malleus and on as far as the tegmen. The stimulus is tubotympanic catarrh affecting the fold of the tensor tympani muscle between the supratubal and the epitympanic recesses and the anterior fold of von Tröltsch, together with irritation of the germinative cell layer of the neighboring Shrapnell's membrane.

Rapidly progressive liquefaction and destruction follow due to secondary infection. A persistent irritation of the inner layer of the pars flaccida arises due to the disturbance of aeration of the lateral compartment. The result is that the sprouting epi-

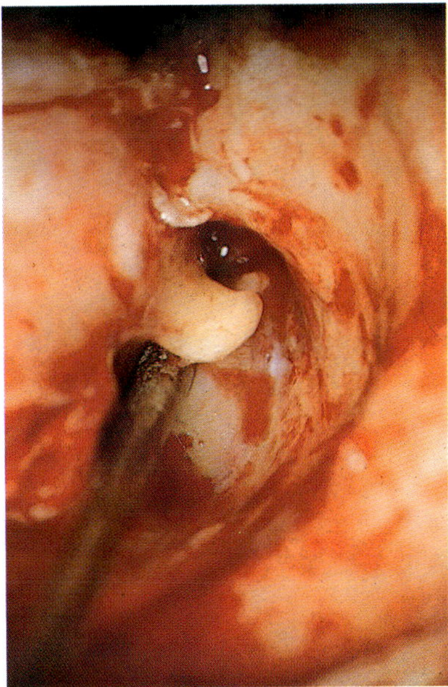

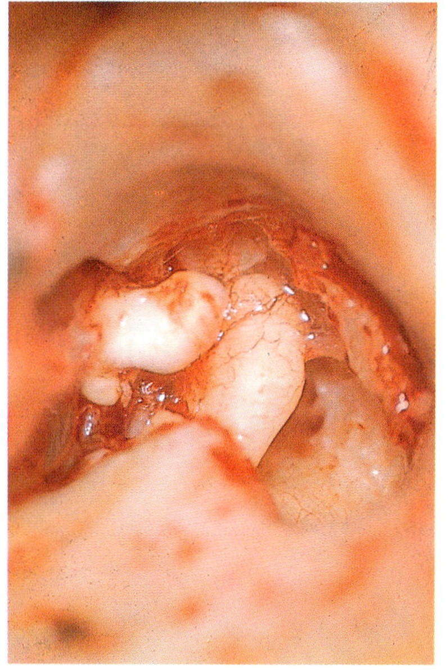

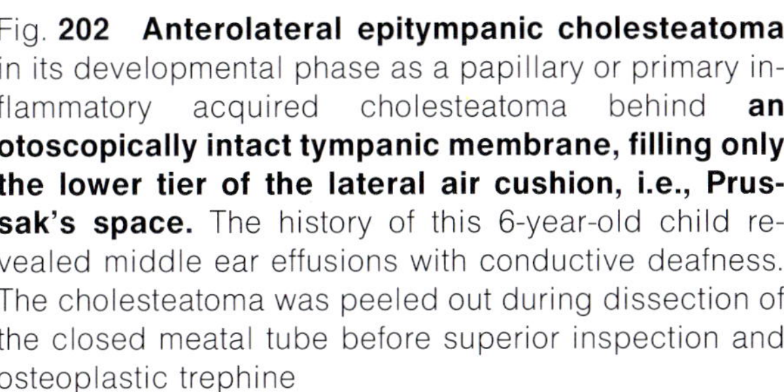

Fig. **202 Anterolateral epitympanic cholesteatoma** in its developmental phase as a papillary or primary inflammatory acquired cholesteatoma behind **an otoscopically intact tympanic membrane, filling only the lower tier of the lateral air cushion, i.e., Prussak's space.** The history of this 6-year-old child revealed middle ear effusions with conductive deafness. The cholesteatoma was peeled out during dissection of the closed meatal tube before superior inspection and osteoplastic trephine

Fig. **203 Anterolateral tympanic cholesteatoma** is one type of papillary primary inflammatory acquired cholesteatoma. It is symptomless, advanced and lies behind an **otoscopically intact tympanic membrane**, and here fills both tiers of the lateral epitympanic air cushion. The history showed a feeling of fullness and transitory deafness on landing or taking off during flying. The cholesteatoma could only be removed after osteoplastic exposure of the epitympanum

thelial papillae are directed deeply by contact guidance (Weiss 1959) in the lax stroma by the arrangement of the connective tissue fibers, although they cannot be recognized on the external surface of Shrapnell's membrane.

A perforation overlain by a dry crust anterior to the neck of the malleus, or a retraction due to the scar tissue contraction of the folds can arise without secondary infection. The direction of growth of the matrix follows the structure of the folds of the lateral epitympanic compartment between the lateral epitympanic wall and the ossicular chain.

Anteromedial Cholesteatoma
(Figs. **204, 205**)

The matrix grows medially around the neck of the malleus along the anterior fold of von Tröltsch and the anterior mallear fold. It then extends beneath the tegmen into the protympanic recess and the antelabyrinthine trigone (the anterior point of danger) lying over the geniculate ganglion and the labyrinthine segment of the facial canal anterior to the ampullary crus of the anterior semicircular canal. Destruction of the ossicular chain begins anteromedially at the head of the malleus but is entirely concealed by the remaining mass of the ossicular chain (see Fig. **204**).

Posterolateral Cholesteatoma
(Figs. **206, 207**)

These are often due to *massive retractions* of the posterior part of the pars flaccida and adhesions to the fold running from the neck of the malleus to the long process of the incus and from there to the short process of the incus and the incudal fossa or the sinus tympani. The following structures direct their growth: the posterior fold of von Tröltsch, the lateral mallear and incudal folds, the interossicular folds between the malleus and incus as well as the posterior accessory folds around the pyramidal process and the crura of the stapes. Secondary infection of the retraction pocket by keratin retention leads to external rupture. They are seldom occult.

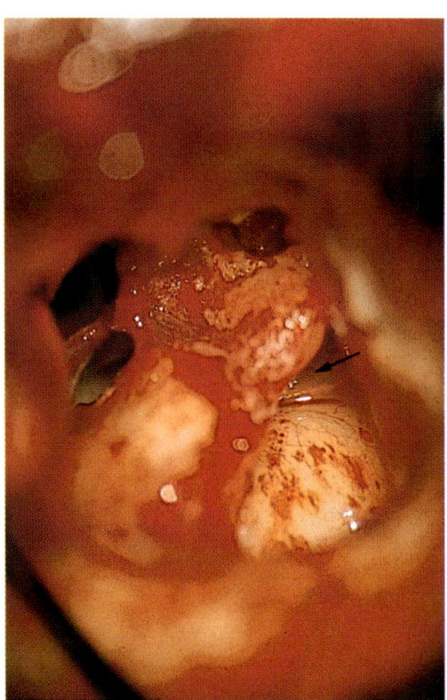

Fig. **204 Anteromedial papillary primary acquired inflammatory epitympanic cholesteatoma behind a completely intact tympanic membrane.** The history of this 22-year-old patient showed only infantile middle ear catarrh, but now an increasing conductive deafness. The head of the malleus is eroded. The medial incudal fold, shown by an arrow, initially hinders the growth of the cholesteatoma posteriorly and forces it anteriorly and medially along the tensor fold to the geniculate ganglion

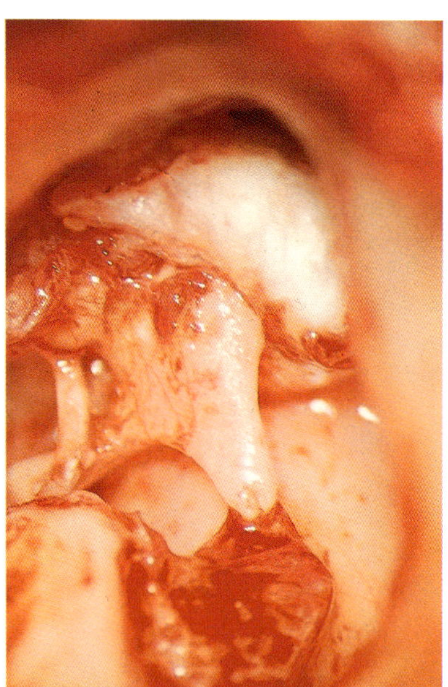

Fig. **205 Anteromedial papillary primary inflammatory epitympanic cholesteatoma** acquired in early childhood behind an **otoscopically normal tympanic membrane.** Osteoplastic exposure of this right middle ear was carried out because of conductive deafness. The ossicular chain was still intact

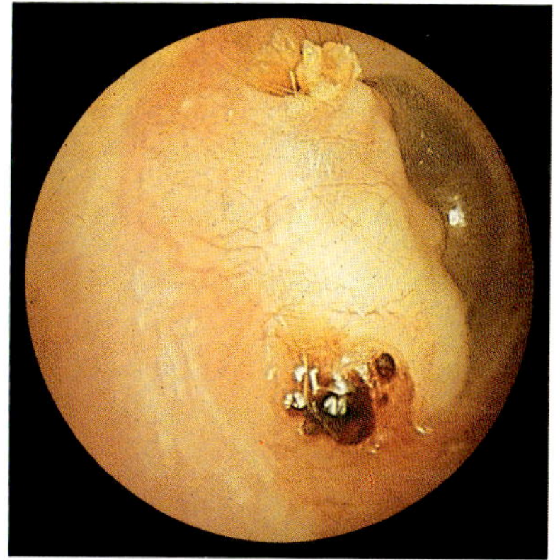

a

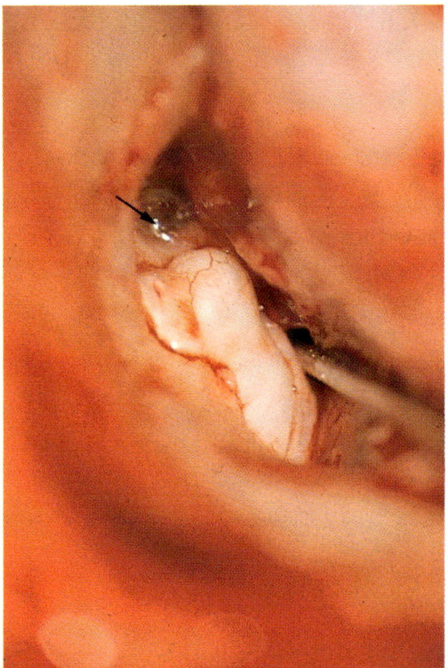

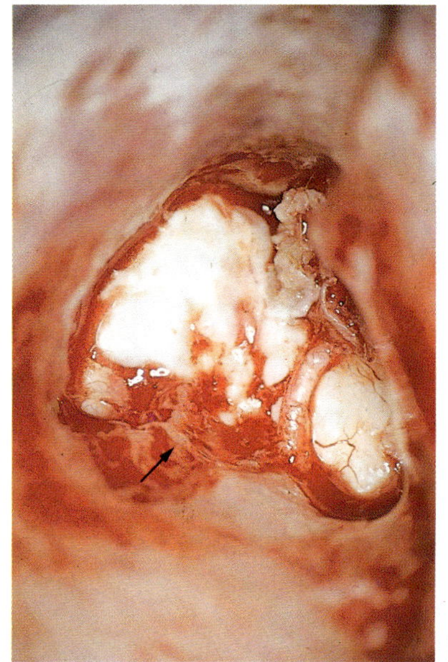

b

Fig. **206   Posterolateral primary acquired cholesteatoma** as a result of a severe seromucinous middle ear inflammation behind an inflamed, but intact, tympanic membrane. It extends as far as the sinus tympani and the aditus ad antrum. The arrow indicates the site of resection of Shrapnell's membrane with the point of origin of the cholesteatoma

Fig. **207a** and **b   Posterolateral primary inflammatory cholesteatoma** behind an intact tympanic membrane (a). Körner's septum, marked with an arrow, prevents subtegmental growth of the cholesteatoma through the aditus into the antrum (b)

Posteromedial Cholesteatoma
(Figs. **208, 209**)

This cholesteatoma arises as a result of adhesions and increasing retraction of the tympanic membrane anterior to the long process of the incus superior or inferior to the posterior fold of von Tröltsch and, particularly, the medial epitympanic fold. The matrix expands medial to the body of the incus along the labyrinthine and tegmental wall through the aditus into the antrum to the postlabyrinthine rhomboid between the two cranial fossae and the crus commune (the posterior point of danger) and finally into the mastoid.

In conclusion: a primary acquired inflammatory epitympanic cholesteatoma always begins with one of these early stages. Further directions of development are forced upon it as follows:
- mesohypotympanic;
- mastoidal;
- pyramidal, i.e., paralabyrinthine in the antelabyrinthine trigone;
- in the postlabyrinthine rhomboid;
- around the labyrinthine block, possibly with inner ear osteitis;
- endolabyrinthine, through a fistula of the semicircular canals.

The operative procedures for secondary and primary acquired inflammatory cholesteatoma are described on p. 127.

Paralabyrinthine Cholesteatoma

The earliest possible diagnosis of disease in the constriction around the labyrinthine block is decisive for the maintenance of its function. Sadly, all the *preoperative* clinical findings pointing to a paralabyrinthine cholesteatoma already indicate that the inner ear function is compromized. Therefore, a special attempt should *always* be made to determine whether the matrix extends to the points of danger or not; there, the cholesteatoma extends deeply as a narrow funnel. Direct vision must be used to ensure

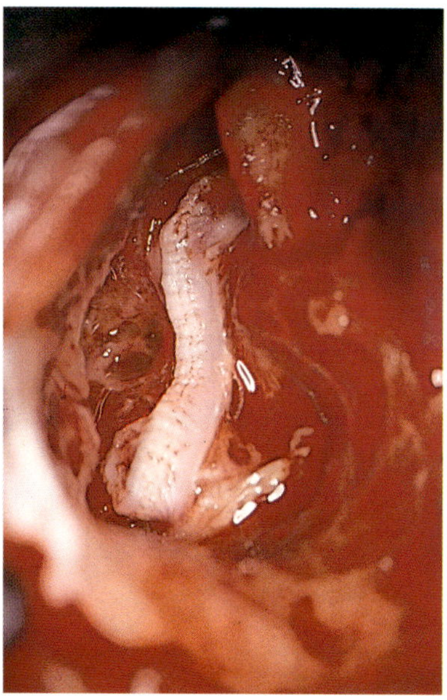

Fig. **208   Posteromedial cholesteatoma** has developed without symptoms from a retraction of the pars flaccida over many years to the sinodural angle, from where it turns and develops inferiorly to the apex of the mastoid process. This is a very unusual example: the cholesteatoma matrix has not reached the tegmen antri and is advancing only on the labyrinthine wall

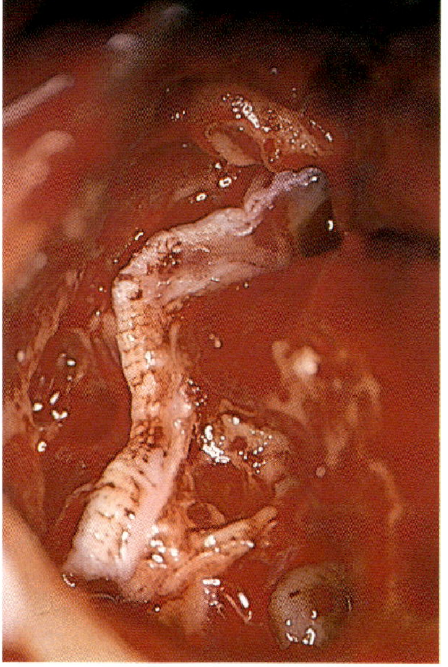

Fig. **209   Posteromedial cholesteatoma.** With the removal of the incus, the entire developmental pathway from the site of origin in Prussak's space, anterior to the handle of the malleus, to the farthest limit of its extent, in the sinodural angle, was exposed. The retraction of the pars flaccida was deflected between the neck of the malleus and the long process of the incus along the interossicular and medial incudal fold, via the incudal fossa to the antrum

that it has been removed microscopically with the diamond burr down to healthy bone.

Typically an *anterior paralabyrinthine cholesteatoma* presents with weakness of the facial nerve. The cholesteatoma penetrates the anterior triangle consisting of the nerve, the ampullary crus of the anterior semicircular canal and the dura of the middle cranial fossa. It creeps along the bony covering of the facial nerve, and erodes it. The two other sides of this triangle remain intact for a long time. An isolated *facial paralysis* can persist for many years, fluctuating in intensity due to spontaneous decompression. There may be no evidence whatever of even the smallest anterior epitympanic perforation. A peripheral facial paralysis persisting for several years may have no obvious explanation and yet it can be diagnosed in the most simple manner by a steep Stenver's view (see p. 116ff.). A round, circumscribed, radiolucent zone can be found anterior to and above the clearly visible vestibule, and above the cochlea. This space represents the cholesteatoma itself. It can expand in a tympanic direction (see Fig. **214**). A *circumscribed facial neurinoma* of the labyrinthine segment produces a similar clinical picture with similar radiological findings.

An anterior paralabyrinthine cholesteatoma later erodes the capsule of the ampulla of the semicircular canal. Because the pressure is constant, vestibular symptoms are usually absent and a fistula sign cannot be elicited. Surgical exposure shows a sharply defined defect of the capsule with healthy bony margins because secondary infection has not yet caused labyrinthitis or osteitis of the inner ear (p. 116ff.). Later still, on its way to the pyramidal apex, the cholesteatoma penetrates the cochlea from above and the fundus plate medial to the facial nerve.

A cholesteatoma of this type often penetrates the floor of the middle cranial fossa. The matrix adheres firmly to the dura from the edge of the petrous pyramid to the foramen spinosum. This type of slow superficial erosion of the dura without increased pressure does not cause headache. Occasionally only a relatively small area of the cortex of the floor of the middle cranial fossa is eroded. Matrix penetrates between the bone and the dura mater, which is elevated over a wide area. In this case the patient may be afflicted by an unexplained headache in the distribution of the meningeal branches of the maxillary or mandibular divisions of the fifth cranial nerve. The cholesteatoma is compressed between the cortex and the matrix of the dura so that spontaneous drainage is impossible. Infection of this lesion is very dangerous. Radiographs rarely produce positive findings.

A *posterior paralabyrinthine cholesteatoma* endangers both the middle and posterior cranial fossae, as well as the posterior crus of the anterior, and the superior crus of the posterior, semicircular canals.

Tension headache in the posterior cranial fossa can be the only symptom of an occult cholesteatoma for a long time if it spreads through a narrow aperture and strips the dura from the bone.

Cholesteatoma of the Petrous Apex

In exceptional cases an epitympanic cholesteatoma can surround the entire labyrinthine block during the course of many years, hollow out the spongiosa of the petrous apex and fill the entire petrous apex. It may remain noninfected. As a result, the remnants of the petrous apex and, above all, the bony labyrinthine capsule are not affected by osteitis. The facial nerve can be slowly and continuously decompressed so that paralysis does not occur or is episodic. Because of the astonishing resistance of the two inner ear functions, this extensive petrous lesion may not even be suspected, despite the clinical findings of a cholesteatoma in the middle ear. The radiological findings may indeed suggest a congenital epidermoid of the neural groove.

Cholesteatoma of the Pyramidal Apex arising from the Anteroinferior Cell Tract

It is rare that a cholesteatoma of the pyramid in chronic otitis arises from the *anteroinferior cell tract*, starting from the anterior hypotympanum, spreading through the tract, bypassing the cochlea and running along the carotid canal.

Occasionally, a relatively thick-walled group of cells lies between the tympanic ostium of the eustachian tube and the carotid artery. It is to be regarded as an unusually large paratubal cell or the connection to an anteroinferior cell tract. A purely retraction cholesteatoma arises in these cases.

Cholesteatoma of the Petrous Pyramid arising from the Posteroinferior Cell Tract

These cholesteatomas are even rarer than those arising from the anteroinferior cell tract. The posteroinferior cell tract alone can be considered as the point of origin. It lies inferior to the ampullary crus of the posterior semicircular canal above the jugular bulb, and posterior to the descending facial nerve. This cholesteatoma can penetrate slowly into the loose spongy bone of the tympanic plate without causing symptoms.

Cholesteatoma Invading the Labyrinthine Capsule

Those cholesteatomas which drive multiple roots through the perichondrial layer into the periosteal layers of the capsule are not common. It has been suggested that they take origin from the papillary skin cover of the epitympanum (see p. 115). They are to be distinguished from those which have infiltrated the small paralabyrinthine cells of the spongiosa close to the pyramidal wall of the labyrinth due to atrophy of the thinned matrix. They always lie around the anterior semicircular canal between the facial nerve and the tegmen tympani. A direct view is necessary with the microscope to recognize them in their early stages. Every root must be drilled out individually with the diamond burr, often leading close to the endosteal wall of the labyrinth.

"En-plaque" Cholesteatoma with Circumscribed Erosion of the Lateral Semicircular Canal (Labyrinthine Fistula)

The lateral semicircular canal is not entirely embedded in spongiosa like the other two semicircular canals, but lies freely to a great extent. At this point its capsule receives its blood supply externally from arterioles which arise from the stylomastoid artery in the facial canal and are a well-known cause of bleeding during fenestration for otosclerosis. If the blood supply from the arterioles of the perichondrial bone is reduced at this point due to displacement of the mucoperiosteum by matrix, the periosteal and endosteal bone are destroyed over many years.

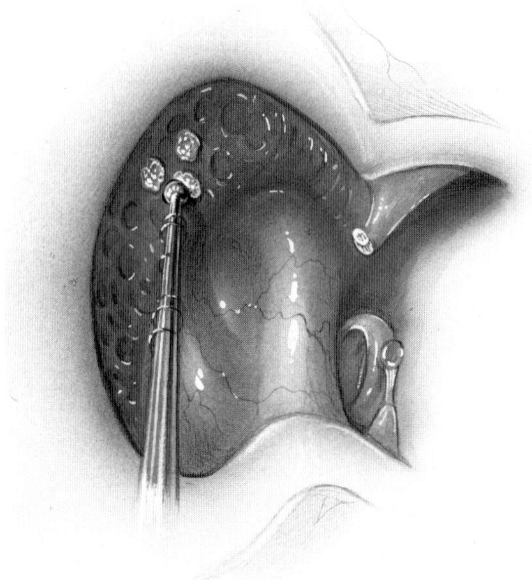

Fig. **210**   Pegs of matrix penetrating into the spongiosa or small cells of the antelabyrinthine trigone are removed with a small diamond burr

The endosteum of the semicircular canal is preserved. For that reason, the flat, noninfected matrix lies on the affected perilymphatic space and can be stripped off at the end of the operation. There is only a danger of *circumscribed osteitis* and perilabyrinthitis if the mucoperisteum is inflamed. The semicircular canal must then be removed.

Iatrogenic Cholesteatoma (Fig. 211)

Formerly, an iatrogenic cholesteatoma could arise exceptionally at the sinodural angle, i.e., in the posterior point of danger, between the two posterior vertical crura of the semicircular canals after removal of extensive *mastoid cholesteatomas* with a chisel, leaving remnants of matrix which could not discharge spontaneously. This was especially true of paralabyrinthine foci which were difficult to expose with the chisel.

The widespread ignorance of principles governing the complicated anatomy and pathology of the temporal bone, the belief in antibiotics, and the concept that many patients are willing to undergo second-look operations has led to an alarming frequency of iatrogenic cholesteatomas. Second-look operations are not carried out with such frequency in any other area of surgery, not even after life-saving operations for malignancy. H. L. Wullstein, the originator of tympanoplasty, defined the limits of the indications for tympanoplasty, and its various types, after decades of careful study of temporal bone pathology, and therefore rejected the closed technique after his preliminary attempts through the facial-chordal angle for cholesteatoma. The neglect of pathological anatomy, over-confidence due to newly available instruments and the availability of transplantation have led to iatrogenic recurrences in more than 50% of cases. Tympanoplasty of this type can scarcely be regarded as otological surgery,which was based on the principles of general surgery, which previously had at least been able to reduce fatal complications and sometimes even eliminate them.

Recurrent (iatrogenic) cholesteatomas may be divided into the following categories:

1. *Residual cholesteatoma.* The results of the closed technique (posterior tympanotomy or intact canal wall technique) show that residual cholesteatomas arise with approximately equal frequency in the epitympanum and in the sinus tympani. Originally these cholesteatomas were detected by local clinical findings or were found at revision operations to improve hearing; and later, at the second-look operation, which is considered as part of treatment.

The anatomical sites of predilection include the facial recess, the sinus tympani and the protympanic recess on the wall of the petrous pyramid. The shortest direct (i.e., vertical) view of the latter cannot be obtained from behind. In the course of time the meatal wall is resorbed if it is thinned too much from within by a recurrence.

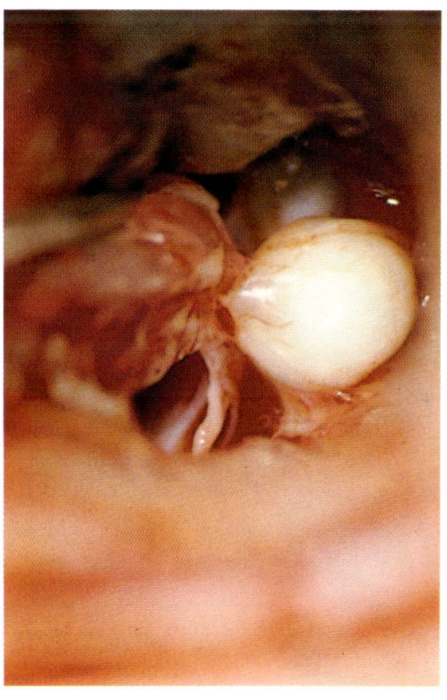

Fig. **211 Iatrogenic cholesteatoma** arising from very thin epidermis on the edge of a perforation which has inverted during repair of the tympanic membrane during underlay with a fascial graft

The recurrence which is found after a delay of 1¹/₂ to 3 years at the second-look procedure is occasionally only a circumscribed pearl of epidermis which can be removed easily if it is accessible. However, preservation of the *superior* meatal wall is usually then no longer possible. Destruction of the epitympanum indicates that the thinner *posterior* wall of the meatus also cannot be retained. As a result of the transmastoid approach, the patient has a large mastoid cavity with a defect of the *lateral mastoid wall*, which is covered by permanently infected *nonepidermized galea.* It must be reduced in size and covered with skin.

In order to prevent epitympanic recurrence with a high degree of reliability, excision and reimplantation of the epitympanic wall was developed, i.e., trephination of the *superior*, not *posterior*, wall of the meatus.

The antrum is nowadays usually opened sufficiently, so that recurrent cholesteatoma in the sinodural angle is unusual. If the matrix in the occult form has already penetrated the spongiosa between the crura of the lateral semicircular canal, this cholesteatoma progresses with resorption of the cortical bone of both cranial fossae along the surfaces of the petrous pyramid; on one side, as far as the arcuate eminence, and on the other side, through the subarcuate fossa, as far as the internal auditory meatus and the endolymphatic sac. The narrow subarcuate tract from the tractus niche through the anterior semicircular canal to the subarcuate fossa is seldom followed by the cholesteatoma, although paralabyrinthine osteitis speads by this route into the petrous pyramid.

The danger of recurrent cholesteatoma in the sinus tympani is to be sought in the shape of the inferior aeration pathway. *If the sinus tympani lies alongside a very prominent promontory, is concealed by the posterior meatal wall with a very steep course of the facial wall, and is narrow, deep and inaccessible, remnants of matrix can easily remain after removal through the meatus or through the facial-chordal angle,* even if the pyramidal process is removed. Extension of the access from the meatus by taking down the *posterior* meatal wall from the tympanic side is not possible if it was already so thinned during the approach through the facial-chordal angle that it breaks. A satisfactory result is not to be achieved under these anatomical conditions. If removal of the posterior wall cannot be avoided because of a recurrent cholesteatoma in the sinus tympani, an undesirable large mastoid cavity open to the meatus is created; the principle of the closed technique must be abandoned.

2. *Retraction (recurrent) cholesteatoma* (Fig. **212**). The cause of recurrent cholesteatoma is *retraction* of the tympanic membrane because of surgically distorted function of the essential inferior aeration pathway, even though wide access to the sinus tympani allows complete removal of the matrix. The opening into the facial-chordal angle is made so wide that increase of internal pressure caused by opening of the eustachian tube is immediately compensated for via the open posterior wall of the middle ear. The necessary reunion of the aeration pathways anterior to the tympanic diaphragm with maintainance of internal pressure is absent. Retraction occurs more easily if the collagenous fiber system of the pars tensa in the posterior quadrants of the tympanic membrane has been damaged by myringitis, or if a fascial graft without a firm fiber structure is used to form the new membrane. Invaginations of the meatal skin into the mastoid are well known to arise in this technique, leading to interruption of drainage of wound secretions, which finally become organized and cause scar tissue retraction. This retraction does not occur after facial nerve decompression through the aditus up to the

semicircular canal: wide opening of the facial-chordal angle is unnecessary, because the nerve is decompressed in its mastoid course along the posterior surface of the meatus. Furthermore, the healthy fiber structure of the pars tensa is still present. The countours of the sinus tympani are left in their original condition in this case.

To prevent this escape of internal pressure from the lower aeration pathway into the mastoid and thus to secure ventilation and drainage, attempts have been made for a long time to obstruct the surgical opening by a silicone or cartilaginous plate, but unfortunately these were unsuccessful.

The consequence of these various difficulties for the choice of surgical access is as follows: a narrow, poorly accessible sinus tympani is made fully accessible from the meatal side by undercutting with a diamond burr along the facial nerve during osteoplastic epitympanotomy. The continuity of the pars tensa, the annulus and the meatal skin is preserved, and no incision is made in the closed tube of meatal skin. *For this reason the posterior meatal wall is breached neither in the external meatus nor in the middle ear cavity at osteoplastic epitympanotomy, as it is in the radical operation or at operations through the facial-chordal angle.* A deep tympanic cavity connected to the antrum is created by the reimplantation of the bony lid, making aeration more effective than by a simple Type III tympanoplasty, which produces a shallow mesohypotympanum.

3. *Iatrogenic cholesteatoma arising from the tympanic membrane* includes inverted cholesteatoma, annulus cholesteatoma, cholesteatoma of a free skin graft, and a tympanic membrane cholesteatoma originated by ventilation tubes.

The *inverted tensa cholesteatoma* is a result of inappropriate interposition of a fascial graft between the collagen fiber system and the epidermis of the pars tensa. As already explained, the epidermis can almost always be elevated easily from the underlying layers, beginning at the tympanic striae, with a closed meatal tube. Epidermization of the fascial overlay proceeds rapidly from the edge of the perforation, in some cases within days. Whilst the fascia is being adapted, the delicate epidermal edge can sometimes roll inward, giving origin to an epidermoid which can penetrate under the edge of the fascia into the middle ear lumen. However, it usually develops externally and is then easy to enucleate under the microscope with the sickle knife.

This type of iatrogenic cholesteatoma can be prevented by introducing a small piece of gelatin foam into the perforation before the fascia is interposed.

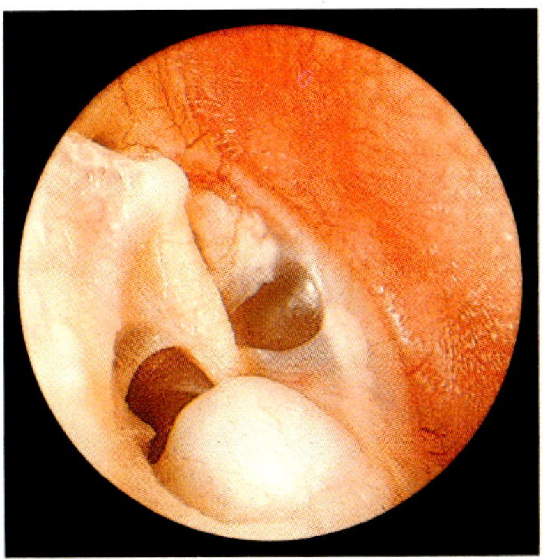

Fig. **212**   **Recurrent cholesteatoma** arising from a repair of the tympanic membrane due to inadequate eradication of epidermal pegs at the bony annulus during overlay of the fascial graft

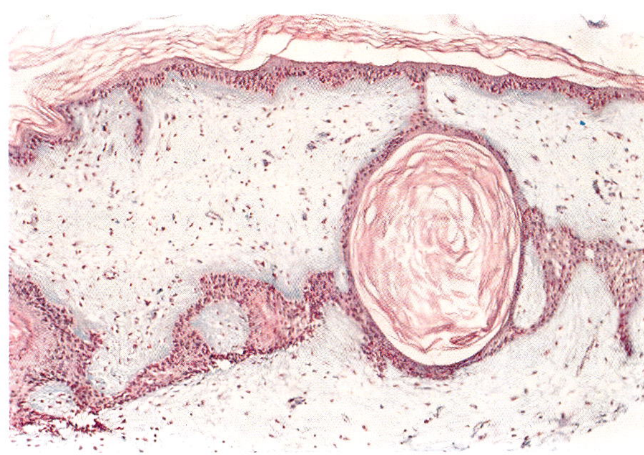

Fig. **213**   **Graft cholesteatoma** due to disordered metabolism in the early healing phase of a full-thickness skin graft

It remains there until the collagen layer of the meatal skin tube has been replaced, and is then removed. The very thin layer of the tensa epidermis is thus rolled outward effectively.

The epidermis on the tympanic membrane is thin and free of papillae, but it is anchored by deep pegs at the annulus. Beneath it small harmless *annulus cholesteatomas* can develop, covered by the graft. Before fitting an *overlay* graft at the annulus, the bony groove should be curetted with an angled round cutting knife to remove the epidermal pegs.

Graft cholesteatomas of the free skin graft are due to irritation of the basal cell layer of the epidermis in the early healing phase. Their histological picture includes cell proliferation and formation of papillae, and resembles that of papillary cholesteatoma of Shrapnell's membrane. This type of graft may experience a disturbance at circumscribed points during the healing phase, which may be so slight that it cannot be observed during the first and second weeks of the healing of the graft. Nonetheless, a subclinical but prolonged irritation is caused in the subcutis. This is characterized by an infiltration of small cells, which persists for many years, an increase of papillary formation in the depth, growth of the germinative cell layer and central keratinization (Fig. **213**).

Graft cholesteatomas in full-thickness skin grafts were previously more common. They were due to *inadequate thinning, leaving the skin appendages.* Skin is a very demanding organ compared to fascia, periosteum, etc. Despite that, it is very suitable for covering large cavities, and it reduces the size of the cavity because of its thickness. Is has proved valu-

able for covering an extensive pneumatic system in addition to the semicircular canals and aditus, for which a Lempert flap is too small (Fig. **66**). If the epidermal papillae are cut off too shallowly to allow the skin to be fitted more easily, the inner wound surface heals far beyond the middle ear with keratinized epidermis. This iatrogenic cholesteatoma is prevented if the full-thickness skin is cut transversely and is not thinned in the marginal area down to the skin adnexae.

Iatrogenic tympanic membrane cholesteatoma is caused by prolonged retention of the *ventilation tube of the middle ear.* Epidermis grows over the edge of the site of the myringotomy to the inner surface of the tympanic membrane. Unfortunately, the pars tensa must be largely sacrificed in order to eliminate this cholesteatoma. Hearing results can be disappointing, especially if an adhesive process or tympanosclerosis later sets in.

Traumatic Cholesteatoma

(see p. 157)

Congenital Cholesteatoma: Mesohypotympanic and Intradural Hamartoma (p. 164)

Clinical Features of Paralabyrinthine and Endolabyrinthine Cholesteatoma Contrasted to Osteitis of the Inner Ear

All forms of osteitis of the inner ear lead *either to spontaneous healing or to intracranial complications. The latter is usually a basal leptomeningitis* due to spread via the internal meatus or by extension of a pachymeningitis on one or both surfaces of the petrous pyramid. This occurs both in acute total osteitis and also chronic circumscribed osteitis with sequestration (see below). Acute total osteitis of the inner ear never causes a diffuse osteomyelitis of the spongiosa of the petrous pyramid, and vice versa. *The only exceptions are paralabyrinthine and endolabyrinthine cholesteatomata, which have not the slightest prospect of self healing.*

These deep-lying, concealed cholesteatomas develop slowly because they are initially almost noninfected. If the mass becomes acutely infected, then all the routes for the development of leptomeningitis are indeed open, via both cranial fossae and the internal auditory meatus.

The hearing and balance are maintained for many years even in a large para- or endolabyrinthine cholesteatoma, until a secondary infection spreads from the middle ear. The noninfected paralabyrinthine cholesteatoma causes loss of function only in the area of a progressive circumscribed pathological lesion. This progresses so slowly and slightly that it is not noticed by the patient. Since the very inception of tympanoplasty, the recognition and elimination of a *cholesteatoma endangering the labyrinth* (H. L. Wullstein 1948) has been one of the indications of early operation, irrespective of whether it is one or two stages.

Radiography of Paralabyrinthine and Endolabyrinthine Cholesteatoma

Because of the paucity of the clinical symptoms of this cholesteatoma, the typical radiological findings are the basis of diagnosis. It is therefore essential to demonstrate them by examples compared with those of other osteitic inner ear diseases (Figs. **223–230**).

The views to be considered are plain films, CT and MRI scans, the first usually in the long axis of the petrous pyramid. They thus correspond to the preferred direction of histopathological sections of the temporal bone. In plain films, superimposition of bone including the zygoma, the floor of the middle cranial fossa and the occipital line, in front, behind and below must be taken into account. The immediate relation of the middle ear and the inner ear block is the subject of investigation: the typical Stenver's view is slightly foreshortened, therefore, and the pyramid is elevated as far as possible above the bony base of the skull by marked tilting of the head (Wullstein's view for classification of inner ear osteitis, later called Chausée III view).

CT scans, either axial or coronal, demonstrate both ears on one view in sharp detail, but without the smooth transition which arises from the deep osteitic effect, particularly at the inner ear nucleus. Furthermore, only the detailed views mentioned allow the temporal bone to be rotated free of the bony base of the skull so that the cortex of both cranial fossae, the contour of the inner ear and the paralabyrinthine structures can be assessed in isolation, if the bone is well-pneumatized at the point where the four cell tracts lead through the bottleneck to the retrolabyrinthine space. These tracts are too foreshortened on the bilateral views as a result of the almost diagonal position of the petrous pyramid in the base of the skull.

The cortical bone of the *posterior* surface of the petrous pyramid presents a regular grey color on Stenver's views of whatever type, whereas the cortical bone of the *middle* cranial fossa presents dark contour lines due to the bone edges. The labyrinth, the internal auditory meatus and the carotid canal are shown against this background of the surface of the petrous pyramid. Progressive defects of the cortical bone in paralabyrinthine cholesteatoma do not obliterate this background and the edges of the upper surface of the petrous pyramid. Assessment of the paralabyrinthine density, especially in differential diagnostic serial views during acute total osteitis, is better achieved by plain films than by a CT scan. Also, relatively small paralabyrinthine cholesteatomas require years before they produce circumscribed destruction of the semicircular canal system.

The early posterior paralabyrinthine cholesteatoma stands out clearly against the cortical bone of the posterior and middle cranial fossae. Anterior cholesteatomas are submerged in the interior of the petrous pyramid and, for a long time, produce no defect in the cortical bone.

This type of obliteration by posterior paralabyrinthine cholesteatoma resembles that of early *acute total* osteitis, which always takes origin at the nucleus of the semicircular canals. However, after about 8 weeks, total acute osteitis begins to form bone apposition, with an increase of regular density without labyrinthine structures. In contrast, destruction of bone continues throughout life in a paralabyrinthine cholesteatoma (Figs. **214–222**).

The vestibular and cochlear functions fail rapidly in total acute osteitis, but only gradually over many years in a para-endolabyrinthine cholesteatoma. *Acute total osteitis has a very limited period of extreme danger after which it heals and enters a purely endosteitic chronic phase if the middle ear infection resolves. In contrast, the danger of intracranial spread is ever present in para- and endolabyrinthine cholesteatoma, in addition to the gradual loss of inner ear function.*

In the acute stage of osteitis, plain films taken every two weeks for ten to twelve weeks until bony healing is achieved are sufficient to monitor the course of the disease. After operations on the paralabyrinthine area, a plain film is needed as a base line for comparison with the postoperative paralabyrinthine and labyrinthine status years later. The evidence provided by serial radiological observations is critical if paralabyrinthine cholesteatoma threatens to progress to an acute total osteitis due to secondary infection. They are indispensible during the subclinical phase of *labyrinthitis, during and*

after the loss of the functions of the labyrinth (for example, during the transition from a circumscribed to a total membranous labyrinthitis) to allow an osteitis to be detected before infection spreads to the CSF.

The course of purely *membranous labyrinthitis* has been explained on postmortem findings, by transverse histological sections. The disease heals rapidly by scar tissue *provided that* the causative middle ear inflammation also resolves. The various forms of osteitis heal independently of the membranous labyrinthitis, either within a specific interval (after acute total osteitis, in about 12 weeks) or only after many years. In cholesteatoma, the inner ear never heals, even if the function is maintained. The necessary long-term follow-up of chronic circumscribed inflammation until secure healing is complete can only be achieved with radiological follow-up.

Because the paralabyrinthine area forms the immediate relation at every tympanoplasty, the decisive phases of these diseases are given in table form (Table **1**) in comparison with the radiological findings.

Table **1** Synopsis of the Interdependence of Membranous Labyrinthis and Osteitis of the Bony Inner Ear.
Inner Ear Cholesteatoma Compared with Inner Ear Osteitis

Soft Tissue Labyrinthitis on the Basis of Histological Findings Based on Zange's Monograph (1919)	Bone-Destroying Labyrinthitis (H. L. Wullstein 1948)
Acute membranous labyrinthitis Acute diffuse serotoxic labyrinthitis, which can heal with maintainance of function, acute diffuse purulent or hemorrhagic-purulent labyrinthitis, acute diffuse granulating proliferating labyrinthitis, acute diffuse necrotic labyrinthitis, acute traumatic labyrinthitis, including iatrogenic forms. *Chronic circumscribed and diffuse membranous labyrinthitis due to persisting chronic otitis media, granulating-proliferative.*	Acute osteitis of the bony inner ear, para- and endolabyrinthine. *Acute total osteitis:* primary granulating *in acute and chronic otitis media is always the same in time and space* and is exclusively determined from the moment of the loss of the two inner ear functions, caused by interruption of the last vascular supply via the internal meatus in addition to the two paralabyrinthine vessels from the stylomastoid artery and from the subarcuate fossa and the arcuate tract. *Acute osteitis of the bony inner ear affecting only the endosteum because the blood supply from the paralabyrinthine vessels is maintained (see above):* primary granulating, i. e., with blurred inner contours, primary necrotic with necrotizing membranous labyrinthitis (i. e., initially sharp inner contours), posttraumatic forms, including iatrogenic forms. *Chronic, purely circumscribed osteitis* with persisting chronic otitis media, including fistula of the lateral semicircular canal. *Chronic diffuse endosteal osteitis* with persisting chronic otitis media − chronic partial. *Necrotizing osteitis* i. e., true partial or total sequestration of the inner ear. *Paralabyrinthine cholesteatoma:* anterior, lying in the antelabyrinthine trigone; posterior, in the postlabyrinthine rhomboid. *Papillary invasive cholesteatoma with roots penetrating the anterior semicircular canal.* *Pure endolabyrinthine cholesteatoma* arising from a *labyrinthine fistula.*

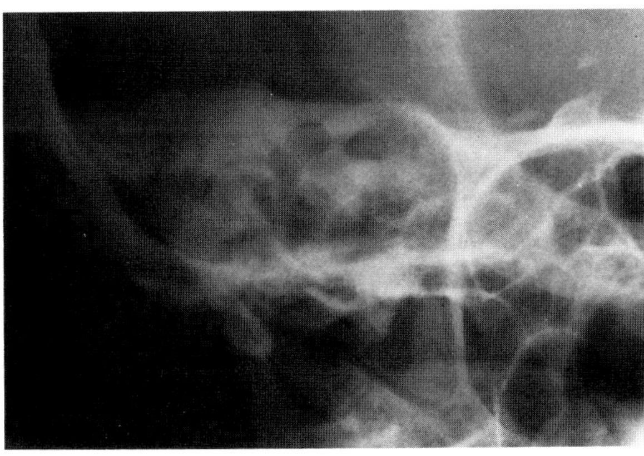

Fig. **214 Example I: paralabyrinthine cholesteatoma** arising from the antelabyrinthine trigone lying on the facial nerve anterior to the ampullary crus of the anterior semicircular canal and beneath the cortical bone of the middle cranial fossa, producing a circular defect superior and medial to the vestibule and lateral to the fundus of the internal auditory meatus

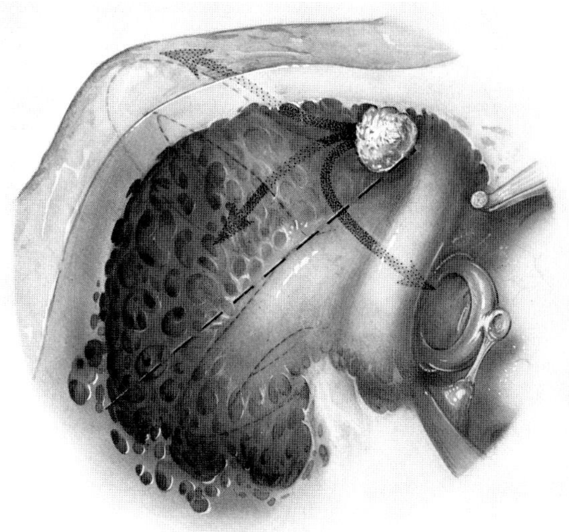

Fig. **215 Developmental pathway of the antero-medial cholesteatoma.** Penetration of the cholesteatoma from the anterior epitympanum into the spongiosa of the pyramid, anterior to the ampulla of the anterior semicircular canal and superior to the facial nerve. This cholesteatoma tends to extend in the spongiosa in the direction of the arrows, i.e., to the middle cranial fossa close to the arcuate eminence, to the posterior cranial fossa, and from above into the vestibule, medial to the ampullary crus of the lateral semicircular canal behind the facial nerve. The facial canal has been previously eroded (H. L. Wullstein 1968)

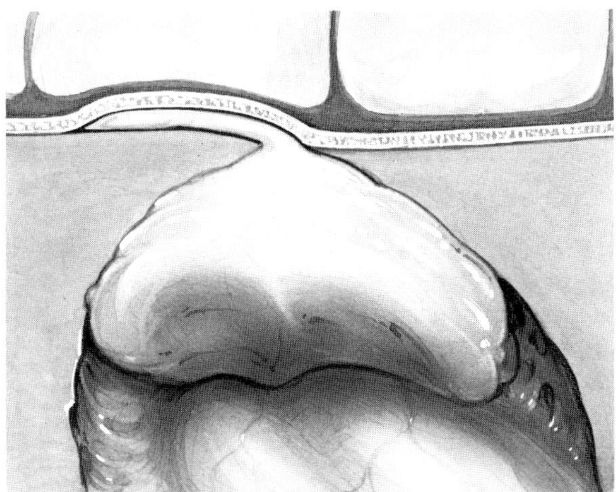

Fig. **216a Example 7: Widespread erosion of the cortex of the floor of the middle cranial fossa in the tegmen tympani,** arising from the antelabyrinthine trigone, with superficial extension of a cholesteatoma pocket between the cortex and the dura. The lesion was scarcely visible in a radiograph, in contrast to Example 6 (H. L. Wullstein 1968)

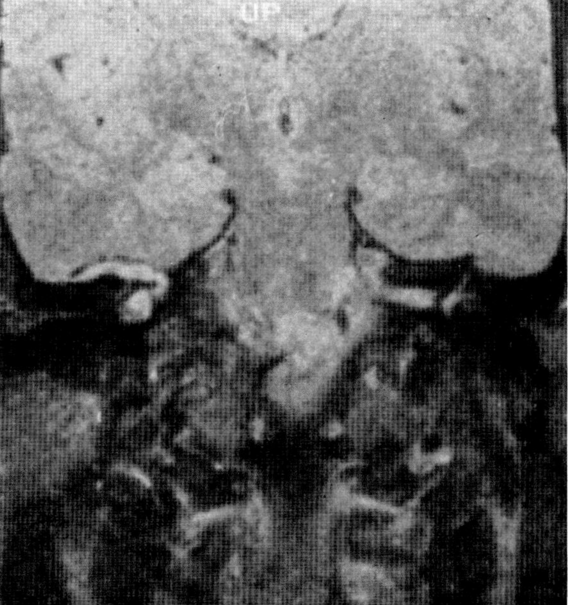

Fig. **216b MRI, frontal section. Paralabyrinthine cholesteatoma** developing from the anterior point of danger, causing erosion of the inner ear and the tegmen tympani. Intracranial, subdural spread presenting "cholesteatoma en plaques" (courtesy of Dr. Vignaud and Dr. A. Hasso)

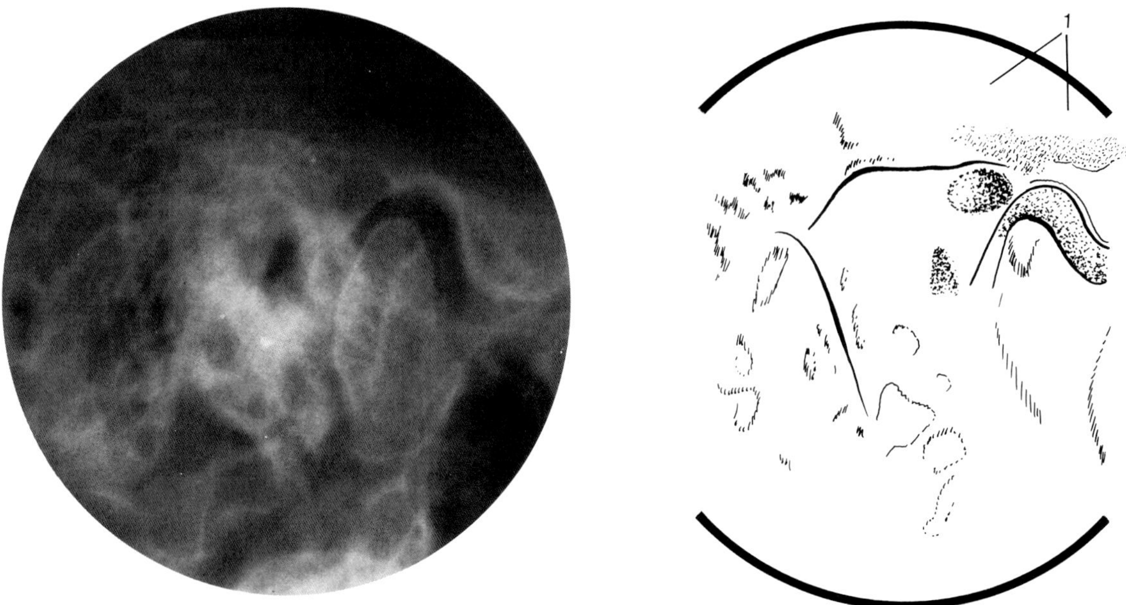

Fig. **217** **Anterolateral cholesteatoma.** 1. Erosion of the cell system with localized breakthrough into the socket of the temperomandibular joint and into the middle cranial fossa

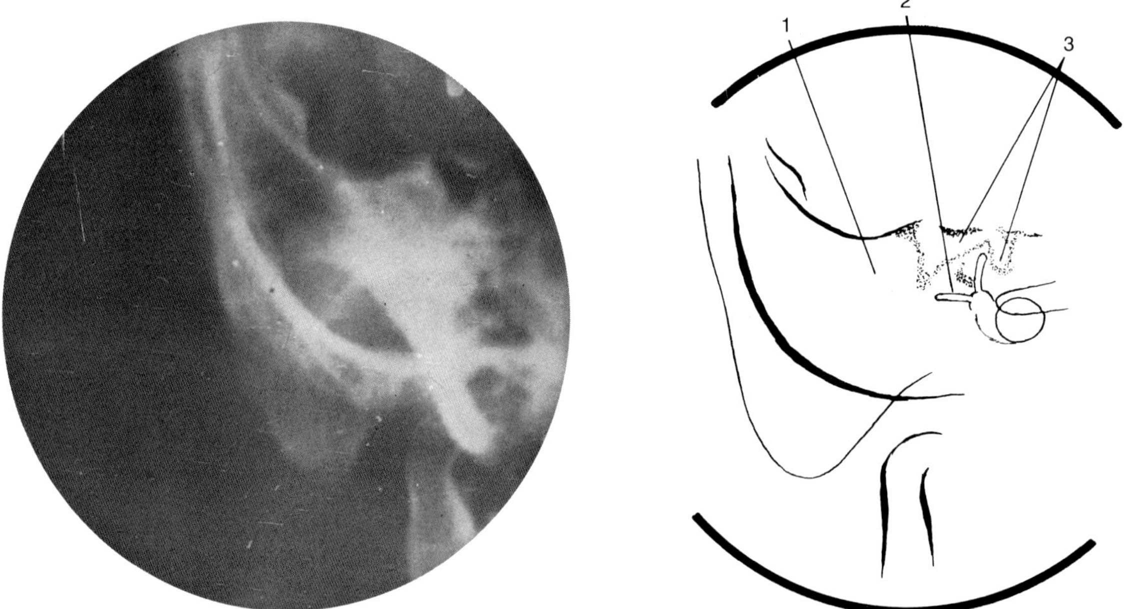

Fig. **218** **Posterior paralabyrinthine occult cholesteatoma with a normal tympanic membrane arising from the postlabyrinthine rhomboid.**
1. Sclerosed mastoid, 2. Lateral semicircular canal, vestibule and basal turn of the cochlea, 3. Erosion of the cortex of the middle and posterior cranial fossa lateral and medial to the posterior crus of the anterior semicircular canal

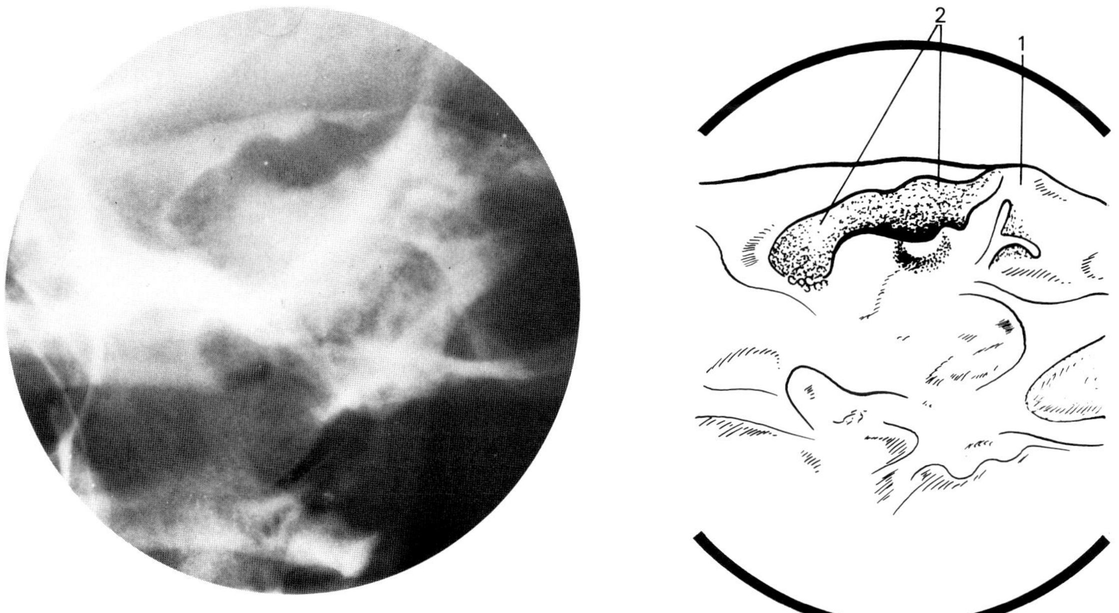

Fig. 219   Anteromedial cholesteatoma extending from the antelabyrinthine trigone around the labyrinth into the petrous apex. Anterior to the arcuate emminence is a small erosion of the cortex of the middle cranial fossa with a flat, extensive cholesteatoma between the floor of the middle cranial fossa and the dura. The patient had a facial nerve paralysis, but both inner ear functions were retained. There was no osteitis.
1. The dome of the anterior semicircular canal, 2. A cholesteatoma cavity medial to the inner ear

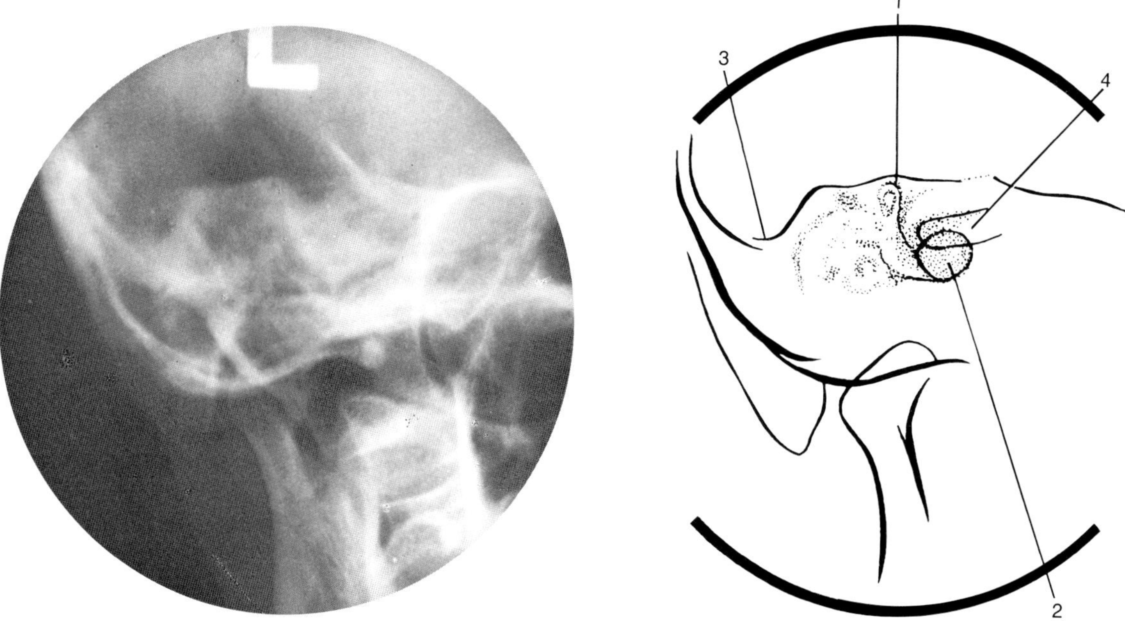

Fig. 220   Small anteromedial cholesteatoma. Symptomless erosion of the inner ear over three decades, with minimal facial weakness. The patient died within two days of convexity meningitis due to a fundus abscess in the internal meatus.
1. Remains of the dome of the anterior semicircular canal at the arcuate eminence, 2. Remnant of the cochlear eminence, 3. Low middle cranial fossa dura; elevation of the petrous pyramid edge between parts 1 and 3 due to periostitis, 4. Clouding of the internal meatus in its fundus. Operation showed a small cholesteatoma of the epitympanum and cholesteatoma roots leading to the semicircular canal and the cochlea. There was no osteitis

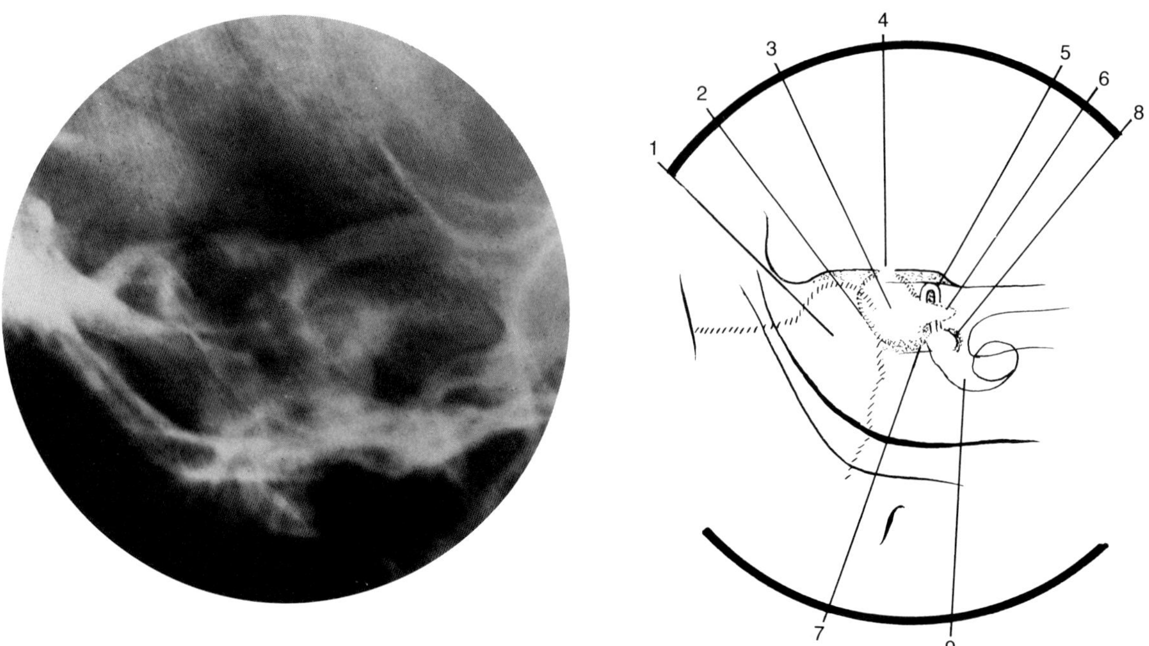

Fig. **221 Recurrent (residual) cholesteatoma behind a radical mastoid cavity.** 1. Radical mastoid cavity, 2. Partial bony wall anterior to the cholesteatoma cavity, 3. Extensive erosion of the cortex of the posterior surface of the pyramid, 4. Erosion of the cortex of middle cranial fossa. 5. Remnant of the anterior semicircular canal, 6. Cholesteatoma roots leading through the subarcuate tract, 7. Defect of the lateral semicircular canal, 8. Vestibule, 9. Cochlear with basal turn. **There is no osteitis.** Vestibular and cochlear function are retained

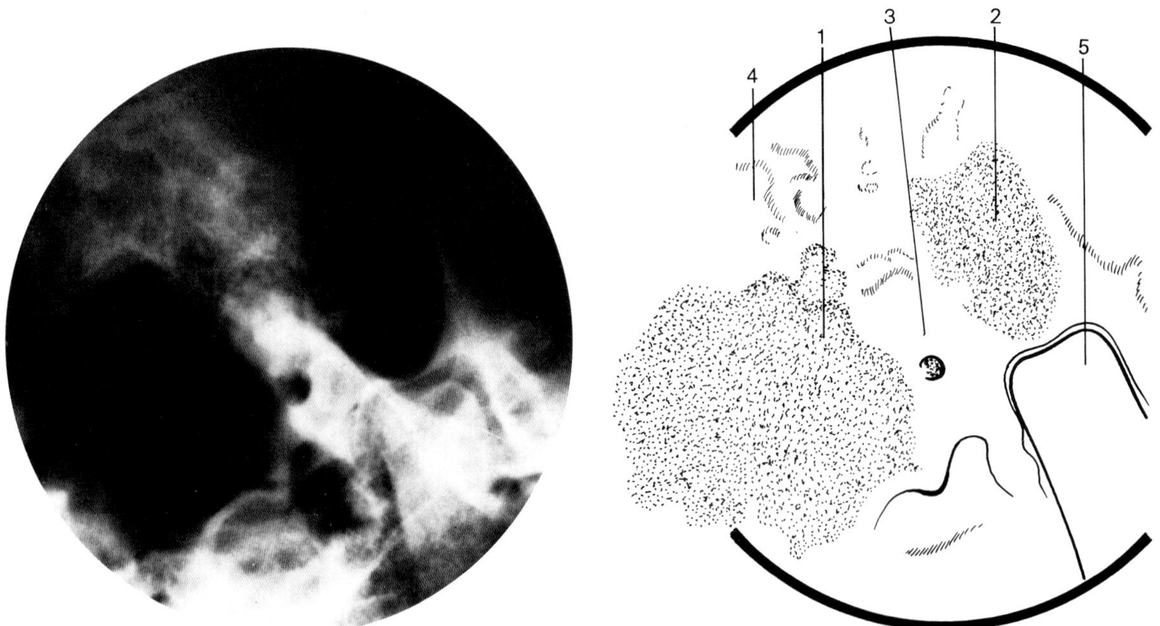

Fig. **222 Extreme example of middle ear cholesteatoma invading the entire pyramid.** 1. Destruction lateral to the nuclear area of the pyramid, 2. Medial to this point, 3. Remnants of the massive central nuclear region of the pyramid, 4. Sinodural angle, 5. Temporomandibular joint

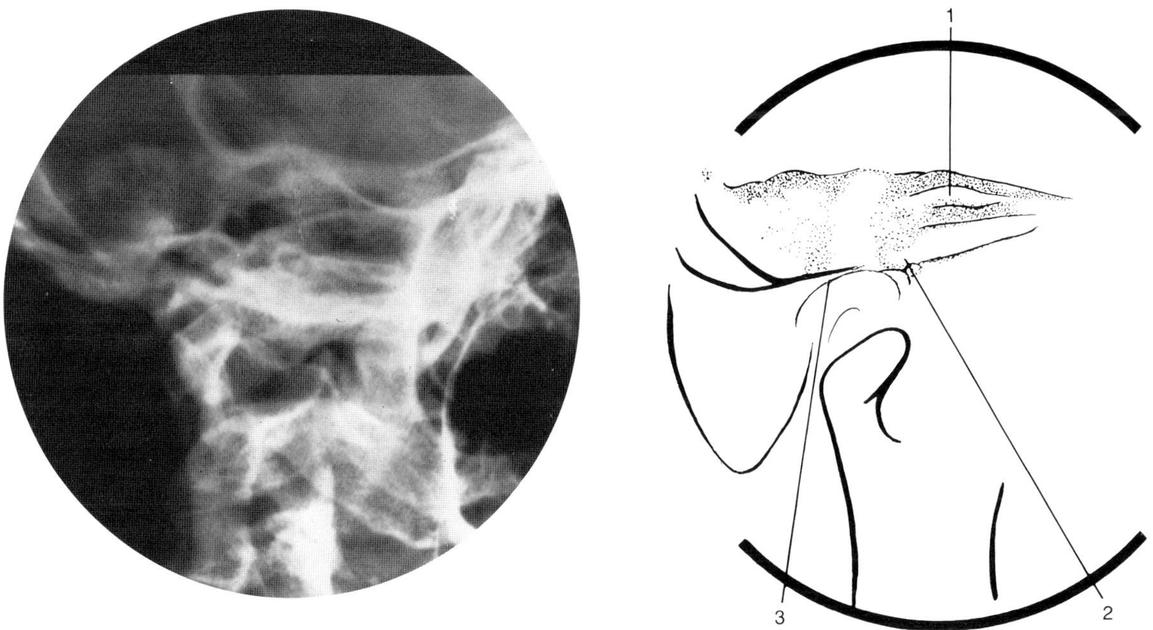

Fig. **223** **Acute total inner ear osteitis with a small antral cholesteatoma.** A radical mastoidectomy has been carried out. There is already reossification of the labyrinthine block. 1. Internal meatus, 2. Carotid canal, with complete resorption of the osteitic cochlear centers, 3. Jugular venous bulb with thrombosis. The patient died

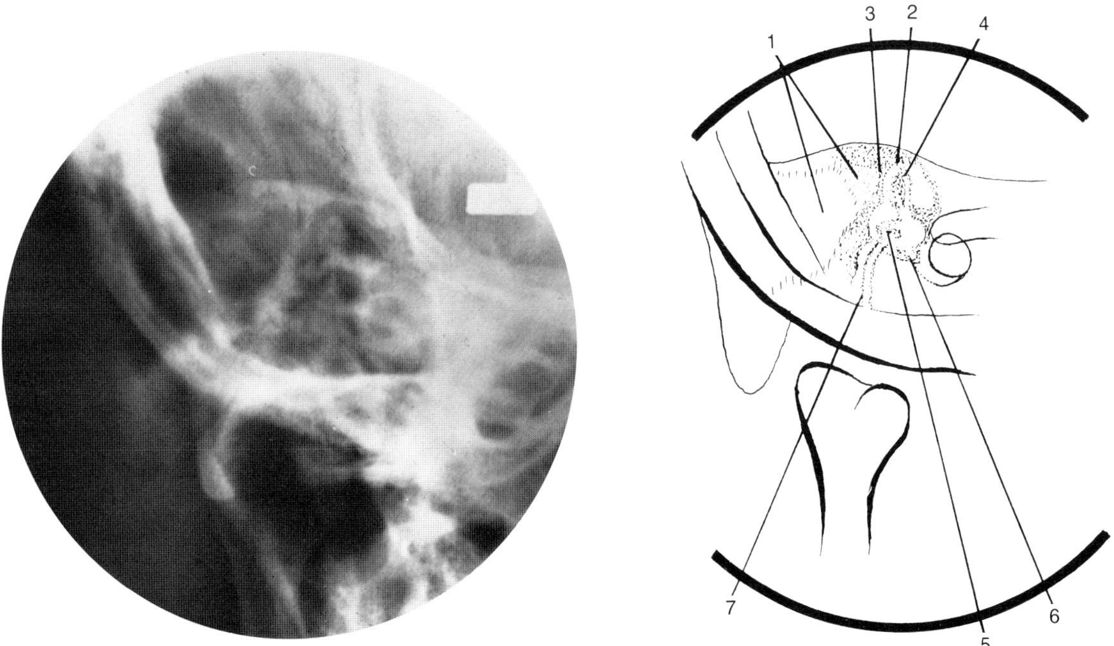

Fig. **224** **Chronic otitis media five weeks after a radical mastoidectomy with simultaneous early acute total osteitis of the inner ear.** 1. Operative cavity, 2. Early osteitis of the entire labyrinthine centers, 3. Bony partition wall between the operative cavity and the cavity of the inner ear osteitis, 4. and 5. Remnants of the anterior and lateral semicircular canals, 6. Osteitis of the basal turn, 7. Facial canal

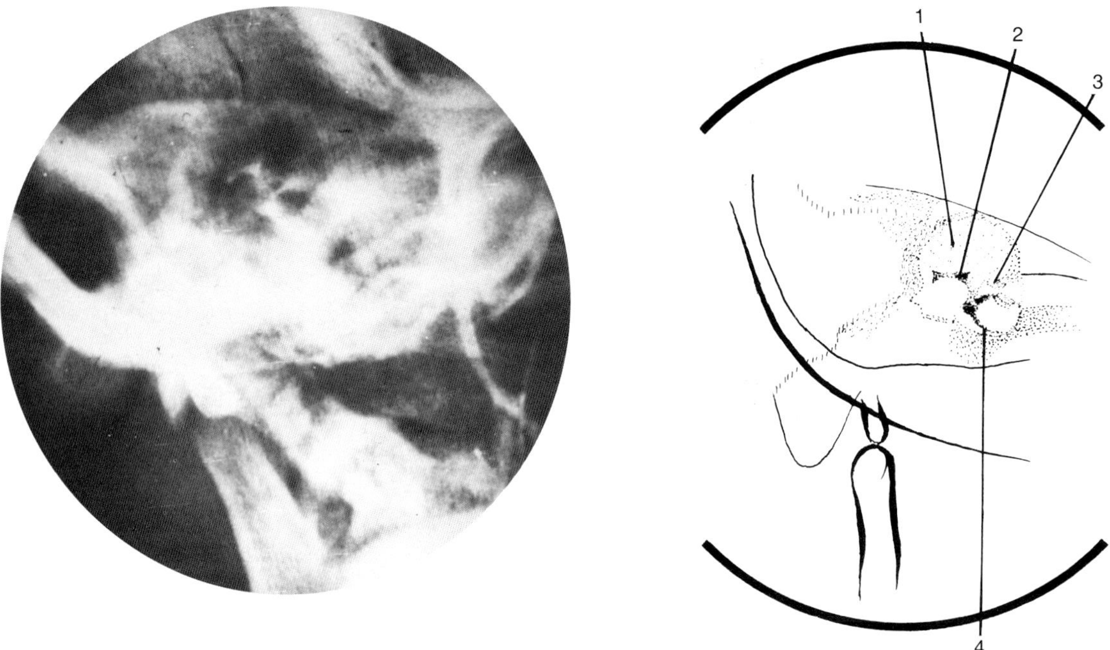

Fig. **225   Progressive acute total osteitis of the inner ear, seven weeks after Fig. 224.** 1. Positive fistula sign; destruction of the entire inner ear with the bony party wall to the radical mastoid cavity and the fundus plate of the internal meatus. 2. Osteitic remnants (not a sequestrum) of the superior, thick vestibular wall. 3. Defect of the bony fundus plate of the internal meatus. 4. Remnants of the cochlear capsule

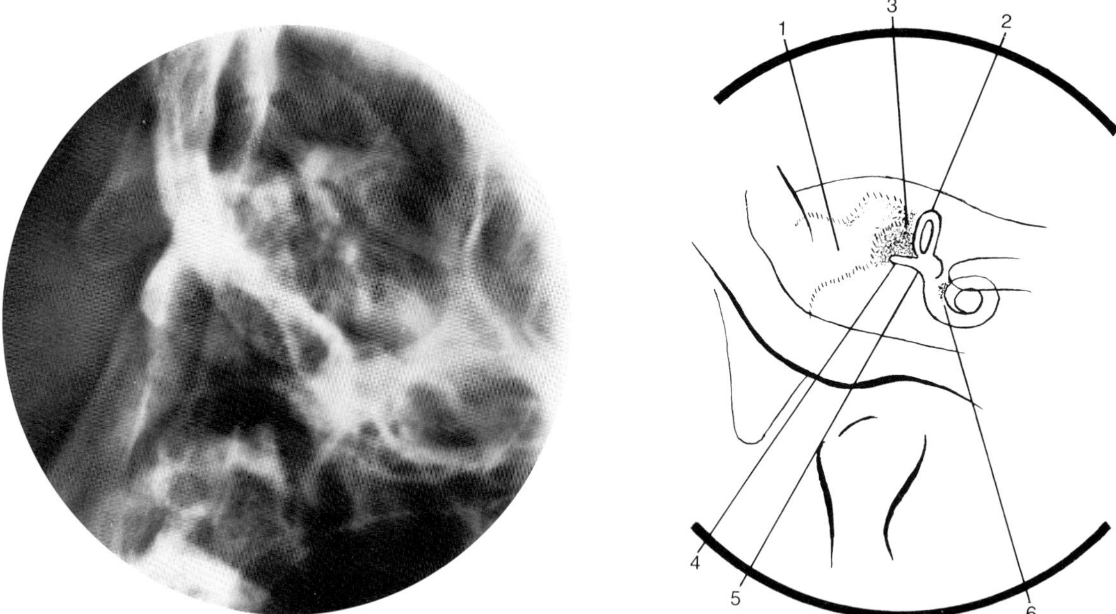

Fig. **226   Healing of acute total inner ear osteitis of the patient shown in Fig. 225, ten months after its onset.** 1. Operative cavity, 2. and 4. Anterior and lateral semicircular canals, 3. Reossification of the labyrinthine block, 5. Vestibule, 6. Cochlea with basal turn

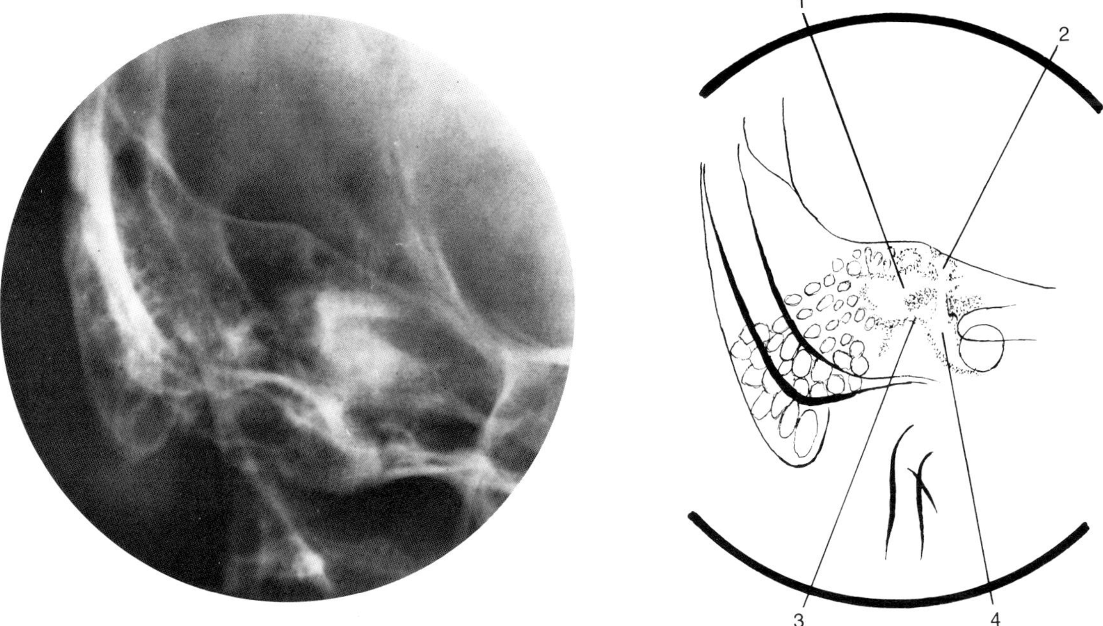

Fig. **227   Acute total osteitis of the inner ear in acute otitis media.** 1. Para-antral destruction, 2., 3. and 4. Acute osteitis of the anterior semicircular canal, of the lateral semicircular canal and of the vestibule and the basal turn

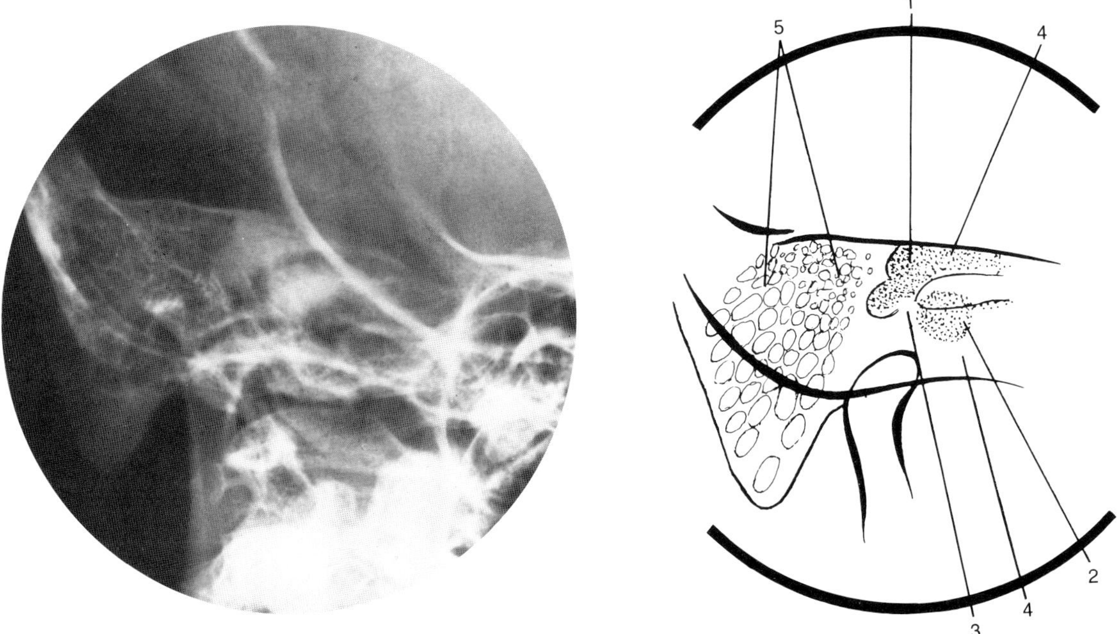

Fig. **228   Spontaneous healing after acute otitis media with osteitis of the inner ear.** 1. Bony scarring of the labyrinthine block, 2. The cochlea after acute total osteitis of the inner ear, 3. Lucency at the site of the vestibule, 4. Spongiosity of the resorbed paralabyrinthine pneumatization, 5. Completely undamaged mastoid and para-antral pneumatization

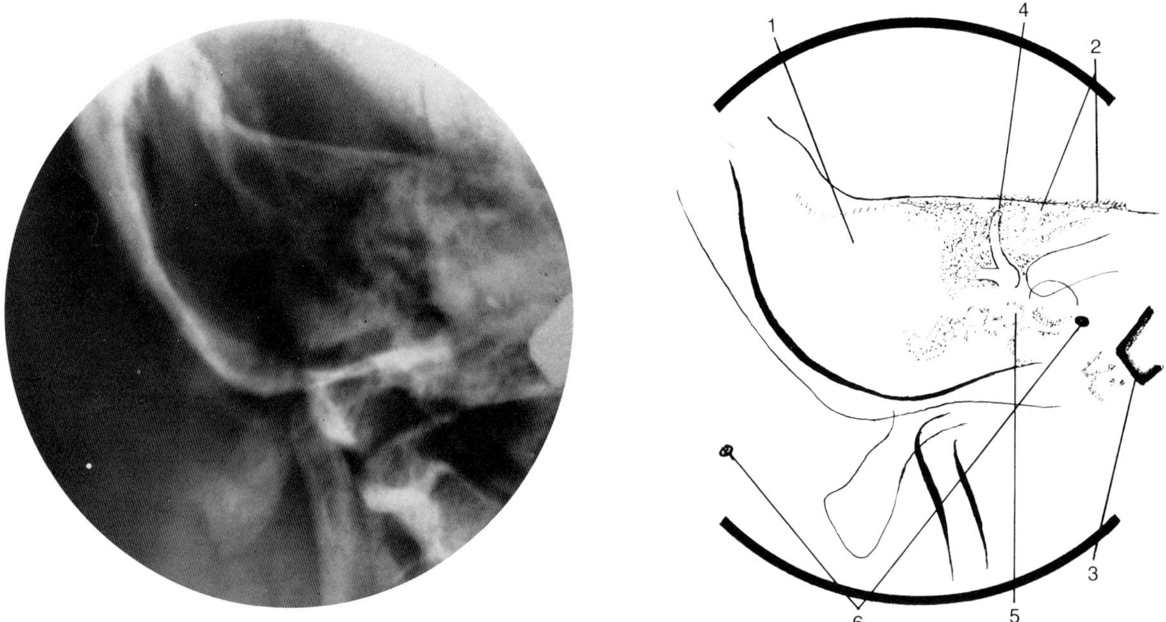

Fig. **229** **Chronic osteomyelitis of the temporal bone without osteitis of the inner ear,** extending into the petrous apex, due to damage by a grenade. 1. Operative cavity, 2. Reactive thickening of the spongiosa and the cortex of the pyramidal apex, 3. Splinters of the grenade, 4. Bony contours of the vestibule and semicircular canals well maintained, 5. Defect of the basal turn of the cochlea, 6. Metal splinter. No osteitis of the inner ear

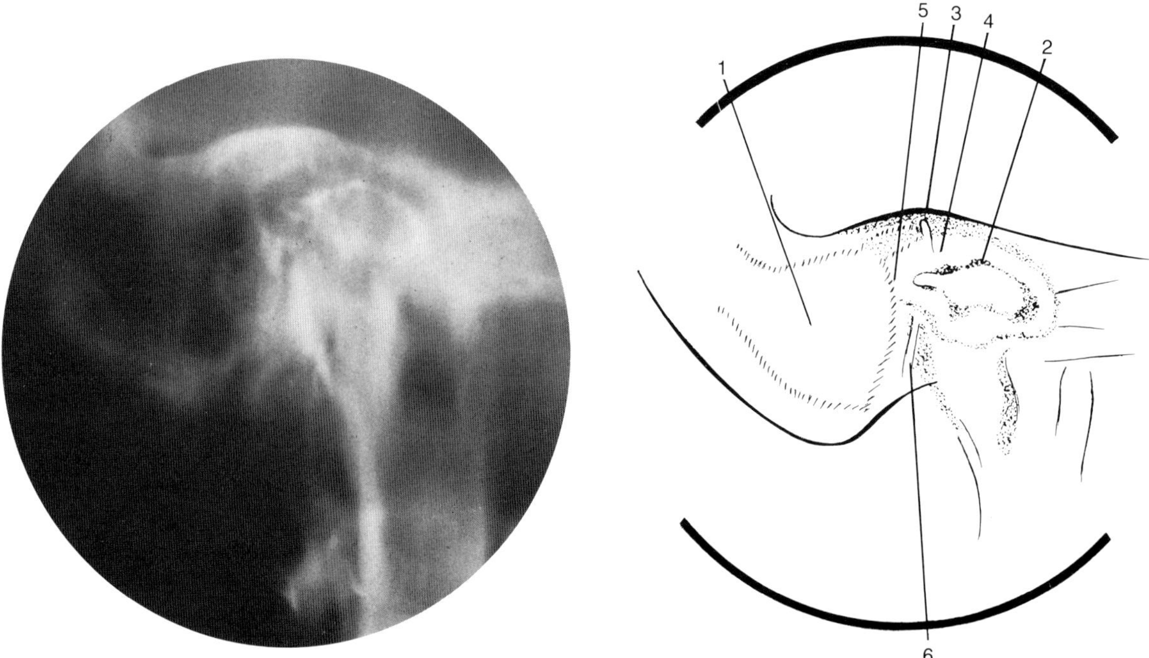

Fig. **230** **Total sequestration of the entire bony inner ear due to a small antral cholesteatoma, as shown on a tomogram.** 1. Radical mastoid cavity, 2. and 3. Sequestrum of the entire inner ear, with the exception of the dome of the semicircular canal (the arcuate eminence) extending along the subarcuate tract. 4. Broad necrotic layer, 5. Bony partition wall between the operative cavity and the necrotic layer, 6. Facial canal. Function of the nerve was unaffected

Basis of the Indications for, and Technique of, Operation for Cholesteatoma

Healing of chronic middle ear inflammation with preservation of the interdependent structures of the mesohypotympanum, epitympanum and antrum demands accurate knowledge of the type and extent of the lesion at the start of the tympanoplasty.

Three inspection openings are created at decisive points to allow a decision to be made at the start of the operation about the retention of the epitympanum:

1. At the junction of the meso- and epitympanum (*upper control window*).
2. In the aditus (the *aditus control window*).
3. In the sinus tympani between the hypotympanum and the mastoid process (*lower control window*).

Since its introduction in 1951, the diamond burr has made it easy to open the *facial-chordal* maximally for access to the sinus tympani. This creates access to the middle ear behind the lateral wall of the epitympanum and the posterior wall of the bony meatus, and behind the malleus and incus along the lateral semicircular canal as far as its ampulla. This allows:

1. the stapes crura to be broken in the presence of ankylosis without detaching the tympanic membrane in the presence of a posteriorly lying semicircular canal fenestration, with preservation of the epitympanum and the other ossicles;
2. the canal of the facial nerve to be exposed in its entire length and the sheath to be slit. (An operative film of this was demonstrated at the International E.N.T. Congress in Washington in 1957; live demonstration for K. Kettel, April 18, 1955.)

This new type of otomicrosurgical access was incorporated into tympanoplasty in 1951. Irrespective of whether a postaural or endaural skin incision has been used, access is always gained by the transmastoid transantral route, i.e., indirectly from the periphery of the pneumatic system, instead of directly at the point of origin of the disease. The great differences in the proportions of iatrogenic recurrent cholesteatomas depend on how rapidly the individual surgeon decided to adopt the open technique. The size of the cholesteatoma, its growth in depth, and extent of destruction cannot be determined from the size of the perforation and the local findings (Figs. **130–134**). The etiological, nosological and anatomical evidence described on p. 3 ff. are more important.

Small perforations of the pars flaccida with crusting constitute a definite indication for osteoplastic epitympanotomy. Clear persistent, noninflamed thickenings of Shrapnell's membrane suggest that either a circumscribed subacute seromucinous otitis media *or a primary occult cholesteatoma* is hidden in the supratubal protympanic compartment, whereas the mesohypotympanum is entirely free, and the eustachian tube is open.

Conductive deafness may not be noticed even by intelligent adults. Attention is then only drawn to an effusion in the compartments of the epitympanum by a small subsidiary event, such as persisting abnormal pressure after flying. Because every therapeutic effort is ineffective, an epitympanotomy provides the most conservative, most rapid and most reliable explanation. A concealed, noninfected white pearl about 2 mm in diameter may be found, with minimal contact with the internal surface of Shrapnell's membrane, from which it can be elevated easily and safely (Fig. **101**).

Such minimal findings are fairly common throughout life. More severe degrees determined by extent, inflammation and structural defects are clinically important. Lateral cholesteatomas are the ones which most frequently erode the lateral wall of the epitympanum, often with a still-functioning ossicular chain. Anterolateral and posterolateral cholesteatomas form the ideal group in which the matrix can be best displayed and completely removed and *in which a Type I reconstruction can be carried out.*

Operation for Inflammatory Acquired Cholesteatoma

An osteoplastic epitympanotomy for a primary cholesteatoma is governed by the processes that have determined the disease. Because the prospect of healing and of preservation of function of the middle ear is better the smaller the cholesteatoma and the less the destruction, an early operation is indicated. In almost 50% of cases, the ossicular chain can be retained. Usually a completely normal external ear and meatus are the end result of the operation.

The thickness of the squamous bone correlates very closely with the height of the epitympanum. If the squamous temporal bone lies very low because the middle cranial fossa is deep, the epitympanum is also low. The intracranial cortical bone is always hollowed out as much as possible to achieve height around the labyrinth. So long as the cholesteatoma is still small, circumscribed and not adherent, it can be elevated from the mucosa reliably under high magnification. If amputation of the head of the malleus and resection of the body of the incus are unavoidable, the surgeon is faced with the following decisions:

- Should he bridge the neck of the malleus and the crura of the stapes and reconstruct the ossicular chain as a Type II tympanoplasty in a closed epitympanum?
- Is thorough dissection of an empty tympanum with building up of the stapes to form a deep Type III more reliable and indicated on audiological grounds, in order to prevent new adhesions and ensure good aeration as far as the antrum?
- Can a paralabyrinthine residual cholesteatoma either in front of or behind the anterior semicircular canal be excluded with certainty, and is a Type III tympanoplasty with a shallow tympanic cavity therefore advisable?

The last technique permits the tympanic membrane graft to cover only the mesohypotympanum as far as the temporal part of the facial canal. Beyond that, a split skin graft covers the broad subtegmental groove along the wall of the petrous pyramid and the tympanic part of the facial canal. The postlabyrinthine rhomboid and the antilabyrinthine trigone thus remain accessible both for inspection and instrumentation, and remain clean. Any retention at this point leads to epidermal irritation, formation of granulations and stenosis at the entrance into the paralabyrinthine defect. An extending pyramidal cholesteatoma in front of or behind the labyrinth poses a problem which is very difficult to solve.

50 years ago *secondary acquired cholesteatoma* was more frequent than the primary lesion. It only later invades the epitympanum, the antrum and mastoid to produce the well-known complications arising in both cranial fossae. *However, there is little tendency to penetrate around the labyrinth.*

A dry central perforation is usually present with a concealed cholesteatoma and little suppuration. However, the mucosa is often very diseased and the cholesteatoma masses and parts of the matrix are often mixed with exuberant polypi and debris from the ossicles. An associated subclinical but active osteitis is likely to destroy the cortical bone of the middle and posterior cranial fossae.

Because of life-threatening disease of the dura and the wall of the lateral sinus in the middle and posterior cranial fossa, a radical mastoidectomy was previously unavoidable *in order to expose the perisinous and extradural foci along the sinus and the tegmen until healthy tissue was reached.* A chisel or a drill was used, and later the diamond burr. In addition to sacrificing the posterior and superior meatal wall, the *lateral wall of the mastoid process* must be completely resected as far as the middle and posterior cranial fossae. *The open tip of the mastoid process then lies deeper than the meatal floor.* As a result all external bony walls of the mastoid process are lost, and laterally it is covered only by galea. The very wide meatus remains open externally, and subject to reinfection. These patients require lifelong supervision by an otologist.

The same situation holds today if a recurrence in the epimesotympanum after a tympanoplasty with the closed technique renders removal of the wall and the posterior meatal wall necessary. Elimination of a chronic phlegmon of the galea and obliteration of an overlarge cavity are dealt with on p. 99 ff.

In the presence of a small antrum and minimal pneumatization with no extension to the two cranial fossae, the endaural exposure of the epitympanum and antrum was previously an advantageous solution. Epidermization then followed rapidly on healthy bone. Limited cavities of this type were spontaneously dry and open to inspection. This purely endaural approach to the dura and sinus is never satisfactory for eradication of complications, and is far too dangerous.

Transmastoid radical operations, and tympanoplasty with an "open" technique and the endaural approach (such as tympanoplasty with a "closed" technique) have been superseded in every case by osteoplastic epitympanotomy with retention of the meatal wall, even if widespread lateral exposure of the mastoid is necessary. The surgical solution to the problem in the epitympanum in secondary acquired cholesteatoma is similar to that for primary inflammatory cholesteatoma.

In order to operate on the primary acquired cholesteatoma so that the middle ear heals and at the same time retains its function, it is necessary to classify the cholesteatoma immediately after elevation of the bony lid, based on inspection, before any surgical procedure begins. The thin matrix is freed from the inner side of the bony lid with a straight or angled round knife whilst the lid is being elevated, without tearing the matrix. After drilling down this inner cortex with a diamond burr, the bony lid can be reinserted, provided that it is not permeated by roots of the cholesteatoma or by osteitis; in such cases it must always be discarded. A replacement can be created from plasticine mixed with bone dust from the squamous bone, pressed widely and firmly onto the edges of the temporal bone at the end of the procedure. Ossification then proceeds from the edge, although much more slowly than the fine bone layer of the epitympanic lid, which is reossified within a few weeks. The plasticine disc ultimately becomes fibrosed centrally, where it has insufficient contact with bone.

The small *anterolateral* cholesteatoma, initially lying flat between the lateral epitympanic wall and the ossicles, is only slightly inflamed. It is easily exposed and offers good prospects for closed removal. Excision of the anterior half of Shrapnell's membrane because of an epidermized perforation and later repair, if necessary, is easy. If it extends posteriorly, an anterolateral cholesteatoma displaces the air cushions between the epitympanic wall and the ossicles and fills this space compactly, on occasion together with tightly compressed, fleshy granulations if the mucosa is inflamed.

If the matrix of the anterolateral cholesteatoma has not only reached the lateral surface of the head of the malleus but also has found a way around the anterior mallear ligament and the mallear fold medially and anterosuperiorly, then the cholesteatoma is no longer completely visible after the elevation of the bony lid. The matrix adheres to the anterior wall of the protympanic recess and to the union of the petrosquamous and petrotympanic fissures (which can be recognized in a radiograph as a fine frontal arch), and to the thin tegmen of the middle cranial fossa close to the greater petrosal nerve and especially to the depression at the antelabyrinthine trigone. The spongiosa is very loose and very vascular at this point. According to Hansen (1971), the internal and external carotid arteries anastomose at this point (see anteromedial cholesteatoma on p. 108). The *anterior paralabyrinthine* cholesteatoma develops from this point.

The anterolateral cholesteatoma can develop in three directions, each of which leads to its own individual complications:

1. The matrix impinges on the *mesotympanic side of the tensor tympani fold and from there extends into the ostium of the eustachian tube.* Flakes of cholesteatoma and debris may be almost completely absent, but the matrix leads deeply into the bony eustachian tube. It must be removed completely to create a closed middle ear. Access is extended by resection of the tensor tympani muscle and its canal. Complete mucosal cover is necessary. In favorable cases, the mucoperiosteum from the antral wall of the labyrinth is available for a free graft; otherwise a free split lip graft is used.

In exceptional cases, thick-walled paratubal cells lead from the tubal ostium to the hypotympanum close to the carotid genu and can be invaded by matrix.

2. In the case of small cells, or in the very delicate spongiosa of the zygoma, matrix can create an extensive, poorly demarcated cavity and break through defects in the cortex, locally or extensively. From there, it spreads further as a shallow, very extensive cholesteatoma lying between the bony cortex of the base of the skull and the dura. The defect can extend as far as the temporomandibular joint. These en plaque cholesteatomas extending close to the foramen spinosum demand removal of matrix from the floor of the middle cranial fossa by drilling or extensive excision of the dura, and plastic repair after trephining of the temporal bone. These conditions usually require a tympanoplasty Type III (shallow).

3. The anterolateral cholesteatoma whose matrix grows round the head of the malleus reaches the dangerous antelabyrinthine trigone, which is directly related to the first genu of the facial nerve and the geniculate ganglion. The anterior paralabyrinthine cholesteatoma develops from this point.
Anteromedial cholesteatoma poses the same danger. It extends around the tendon of the tensor tympani muscle, along the anterior wall of the protympanic recess to the tegmen tympani and to the medial side of the head of the malleus.

A small, entirely localized, anteromedial cholesteatoma typically erodes the head of the malleus on its anteromedial side. This erosion can scarcely be seen in the closed technique, but may nonetheless have destroyed contact between the incus and malleus so that the lever system is disrupted. Cholesteatomas in this position are not only concealed by the incus and the malleus, but are also unreachable in operations via a postauricular approach.

Matrix either of an anterolateral or anteromedial cholesteatoma medial to the head of the malleus poses a high risk to the medial wall of the protympanic recess. For a long time, therefore, both authors resected the head of the malleus to achieve the necessary view and to prevent residual cholesteatoma. Initially, Type I tympanoplasty was not used, although it appeared to be a very favorable method of reconstruction. Often, inspection after destruction of the ossicular chain showed that this step had been unnecessary. A further advance was achieved when it proved possible and safe *to remove the anterior face of the head of the malleus in the presence of a completely mobile ossicular chain as far as the prolongation of the contour of the neck of the malleus, (occasionally, its superior curvature also) and yet to retain full contact with the incus.* Dissection was easily carried out in a longitudinal direction on the anterior wall of the head of the malleus with a new, very sharp diamond burr at a high rate of revolutions (about 80,000). The head of the malleus does not appear to move at relatively high magnifications (16×). Transmission of mechanical or acoustic trauma is not to be feared, since bone conduction loss does not occur, or else recovers rapidly.

The medial malleoincudal fold between the ossicles and the labyrinthine wall forms a natural posterior limit of *anteromedial cholesteatoma.* Even if the cholesteatoma extends along this anatomical structure to the incus, the fold can still often be recognized in histological sections (Fig. **194**).

Posterior cholesteatomas (both lateral and medial) are usually due to retraction and thus demonstrate a shallow matrix. Small cholesteatomas with only slight epidermal irritation behind the epitympanic wall are often solely to be recognized with an angled endoscope. This is also true of anterior cholesteatoma: eradication in the early stages is a relatively minor procedure which prevents interruption of sound conduction, slow extension of the cholesteatoma into the aditus, antrum and mastoid, and the formation of a fistula. The surgeon who wants to be sure about the pathological findings in order to prevent a later iatrogenic cholesteatoma due to retraction, will only drill down the bony wall of the epitympanum unwillingly. For preference, he will carry out an osteoplastic epitympanotomy, which requires only slightly greater effort.

A defect of the long process of the incus is common. The lever system is then reconstructed by a Type II tympanoplasty by drilling suitable receptor surfaces on an allogenic handle of the malleus or incudal process with the diamond burr to form a strut between the stump of the incus and the stapes, which is glued on both sides and covered with fine fascia (p. 94).

Osteoplastic epitympanotomy has created conditions which facilitate a timely operation on a pathological basis, particularly for concealed epitympanic cholesteatoma. These lesions include the nowadays quite common *primary inflammatory acquired but occult cholesteatoma with no sign of a perforation, as well as deep invaginations which are scarcely suspected of being cholesteatoma, even with the angled endoscope.*

Tailored Operation for Cholesteatoma

If all cholesteatomas are picked up and operated on prophylactically in a manner determined by their point of origin, about half of all primary acquired cholesteatomas of the epitympanum do not extend beyond the aditus and the entrance to the oval window niche.

To ensure safe dissection, the epitympanic bony lid should be extended beyond the antrum for *all cholesteatomas*, and should then pass upward again beyond the lowest point of the tegmen lying over the aditus, to the level of the sinodural angle. The posterior point of danger for the petrous pyramid lies at that point, i.e., the spongiosa or pneumatization of small cells of the postlabyrinthine rhomboid between the cortex of the middle and posterior cranial fossae and the two posterior crura of the anterior and posterior semicircular canals before their confluence.

Osteoplastic epitympanotomy for posterior cholesteatoma is intended not only to deal with the cholesteatoma and its matrix reliably, but also to free the entire network of folds from progressive scar formation. Blockage of the system of folds by tympanosclerosis, and fixation by osteophytes in the small compartments in the continuation of Prussak's space, which serve as a vibration damper between the lateral epitympanic wall and the ossicular chain, must also be corrected. A careful search and probing is necessary when the bony lid is being freed from the incus because of occasional bony fixation. In this manner an uninterrupted ossicular chain regains its complete vibrational capacity.

The reconstruction of a wide tympanic cavity consisting of three levels (hypo-, meso- and epitympanum), with carefully directed postoperative aeration, offers the best conditions for healing with delicate mucosa in order to prevent further recurrence by renewed contraction. An important prerequisite is the maintainence of the air stream through the hypotympanum into the sinus tympani and the aditus. A blast of air due to activity of the eustachian tube ought not to explode into the mastoid through a large defect in the posterior meatal wall. *This is one of the decisive reasons why the bony posterior meatal wall should not be removed in either the external meatus (canal wall down) or in the posterior tympanotomy approach.*

A high jugular bulb compromising aeration of the hypomesotympanum, leading to recurrence of atelectasis and retraction and, therefore, to retraction cholesteatoma, is discussed on pp. 42 and 144. Lateral extension of the hypotympanum by displacing the tympanic membrane graft in a groove in the meatal floor are also discussed at that point. There is a theoretical possibility of achieving sonoinversion of the windows by surgery. Whether the hearing results for healed cholesteatoma are any better than those for an in-the-ear hearing aid remains doubtful.

Cholesteatoma in the Mesohypotympanum

Epitympanotomy permits an assessment of the extent of the matrix of every primary acquired cholesteatoma from the epitympanum in the *three possible directions* (mesohypotympanic, mastoid and pyramidal) so that the operation need not be more extensive than dictated by the extent of the disease. The nondiseased part of the middle ear system need not be exposed further than the mucosal inflammation demands. The operation for cholesteatoma is thus tailored to the individual pathological findings. The three directions of extension named above should be assessed, beginning with spread in a *mesohypotympanic direction*. If the disease is a pure mucosal inflammation arising from the ostium of the eustachian tube and the tensor folds, and passing through the inferior aeration pathway to the hypotympanum and the sinus tympani, it should be treated as such.

If a very thin epidermal matrix extends over the promontory and through the lower aeration pathway as well as over the *inner surface of the pars tensa*, then the pars tensa must be freed from the tympanic stria out of the annulus fibrosus, in order to inspect it. It may be that the matrix can be freed by meticulous dissection from the collagenous fibrous layer so that the pars tensa is maintained; this is very often unsuccessful. It must then be sacrificed and a large, possibly total, graft must then be inserted to replace it. The same also applies to total epidermization of the medial wall of the middle ear by the completely atrophic pars tensa.

Removal of the thin matrix from the medial wall of the middle ear, from the promontory and from the hypotympanic aeration pathway is tedious. Bony edges are drilled down with a diamond burr, but the endosteal layer on the promontory and in the entrance to the oval niche is preserved if possible, because epithelium then grows in more rapidly. An unimpeded view into the depth of the sinus tympani and the facial recess is essential. If no local tissue is available for the epithelium, satisfactory conditions for the lining of the air-containing space and a very wide middle ear are created by a suitable im-

plant of split-thickness lip or amnion. The bony lid is reintroduced to create as much space as possible, even if the epitympanum is empty. Favorable conditions are then available for the creation of a new sound conduction system at a second operation, after epithelialization is complete. The stapes, the stapedial stumps and the oval niche covered with a fine matrix are the major problem, and a very rare indication for a two-stage operation (p. 176).

Matrix which has extended deeply into the round window niche seldom lies on the membrane. Between the two lies a small cyst with relatively healthy mucosa, as over a smooth footplate of the stapes. The wall of the round window niche must be levelled off by approaching from the promontory, to allow the matrix to be elevated so that the remaining narrow niche is not blocked by connective tissue. Mucoperiosteum from the semicircular canal or other tissue is laid on the round window membrane to encourage epithelialization. If possible, a fringe of the subiculum remains standing at the edge of the sinus tympani so that it leads the air streaming through the hypotympanum to the round window membrane in a physiological manner.

A deep funnel almost always runs along the hypotympanum parallel to the inferior edge of the promontory from the hiatus of the round window niche. If the matrix grows into this funnel, or if it is filled with granulations, it should be opened sufficiently by smoothing, using an approach from the promontory and hiatus.

A high jugular bulb often rises at this point up to the entrance to the niche. Its bony covering is very delicate. It cannot be displaced, and the hypotympanum can only be extended in a lateral direction. A high genu of the internal carotid artery can project into the hypotympanum; in this case, the bony wall of the canal is replaced by a fibrous, nonpulsating plate. Thick-walled, deep bony niches can be present over the carotid genu under the ostium of the eustachian tube, representing the rudimentary attachment of the anteroinferior cell tract. Care must be exercized with the drill or curette at this point.

Cholesteatoma in the Mastoid

Often posteromedial epitympanic cholesteatoma extend through the aditus into the mastoid process without involving the hypotympanum. *They can be exposed by a tailored approach along the tegmen of the aditus and the antrum.* Most patients with prolonged suppuration only present when a complication arises. The proportion with an extensive cholesteatoma is therefore large. On the other hand, if patients in the higher social classes present to the otologist because of minimal symptoms, the great majority have limited disease and little destruction. They can be dealt with by an operation which preserves function. However, even large, relatively uninfected mastoid cholesteatomas can exist for many years without being noticed.

Antral and mastoid cholesteatomas are mainly the result of *posteromedial cholesteatomas* beginning with deep invaginations at the handle of the malleus around the processes of the incus, extending upward along the facial canal medial to the ossicles where they turn backwards posterior to the medial malleoincudal fold. If they encounter a *Körner's septum*, their extension in this direction is blocked and they turn into the facial recess and the tympanic sinus. Because these cholesteatomas not only surround the ossicles very quickly but also erode them, there is little prospect of retaining the incus or the head of the malleus. The *epitympanum* is then empty. It is urgently necessary to free the anterior segment of the middle ear of all matrix; for example, by drilling the pyramidal process and by extending the entrance into the tympanic sinus along the descending course of the facial nerve.

Cholesteatoma matrix which lies on the cortical bone of one of the cranial fossae can be removed reliably, rapidly and easily by polishing with the diamond burr. The same principle applies as before; namely, that the operation proceeds from the aditus and the antrum and is tailored to the needs of the individual patient. Air spaces with healthy epithelium are conserved, and ventilation is achieved through the aditus as in classical antrotomy or mastoidectomy. If there is reason to clear the mastoid process, all cell groups are dissected out. There are two possibilities:

1. to allow natural aeration and ingrowth of epithelium into the wide mastoid process;
2. to obliterate the mastoid, including the wide antrum, with a firmly compressed plasticine plug to prevent adhesions and retention.

The sheath of an exposed facial nerve can be freed of matrix by careful strokes with the diamond burr in the long axis of the nerve.

Cholesteatoma Matrix on the Sinus and Dura Mater

Removal of matrix which adheres to the wall of the sinus or dura formerly caused no problem because the cavity remained open into the meatus after a radical procedure and after using an open technique. Nowadays, the matrix is eradicated to avoid a very wide cavity and to retain a posterior meatal wall. If the matrix is thick, papillomatous and inflamed, it can often be easily peeled off. A thinner, flatter, less infiltrating matrix is removed reliably with the largest diamond burr at a slow rate of rotation.

If there is any doubt, the suspicious area should be excised and closed, using a robust autogenic material and human biological glue; it might need to be secured with plasticine. The technique is as follows: *Firstly*, the field is extensively exposed until healthy tissue is reached on all sides, and the sinus wall or dura are freed from the inner layer of cortical bone. *Secondly*, a robust graft (for example, of periosteum) and glue are prepared. *Thirdly*, the healthy sinus wall is closed securely superiorly and anteriorly by packing with compressed cotton wool between the cortical bone and the wall of the sinus. As a result of its moisture content, the compressed cotton wool swells markedly and compresses the sinus. The sinus should not be transfixed, because: 1. the surrounding tissue is inflamed; 2. the patency of the contralateral sinus has not been tested; and 3. a perisinus abscess is not present, so that the sinus is not obstructed by a mural thrombus and should remain patent after the temporary tamponade. The wall is excised to the limit of the matrix. A periosteal graft is introduced subcortically into the deep defect after which the cotton wool is removed carefully beginning at the superior end, taking care to avoid air embolus. The defect is glued immediately. Further periosteal grafts with adhesive externally extending widely over the surrounding bone are fixed to the healthy surrounding sinus wall with a few 4/0 sutures. Because the remaining mastoid walls have previously been cleaned carefully of matrix remnants with the diamond burr, it is now possible to press the plasticine plug firmly against the bone in the tip of the mastoid process.

The procedure for matrix adherent to the dura in Trautmann's triangle or to the tegmen tympani and antri is similar. As much CSF as possible is drained through a fine incision, and a plasticine plate is then introduced under the cortical bone to prevent a prolapse, and is covered on its tympanic surface with fascia.

Rapid, Progressive and Recurrent Cholesteatoma in Childhood

The cholesteatoma cavity in all young patients is only slightly infected, and usually limited by the bony structures, so that the operation can be carried out following the same rules as for tympanoplasty in older patients.

In the early years of life the immunological resistance is still incompletely developed, and the mastoid process is still in the phase of growth and shaping of its spongiosa. The polypoid mucosa, the proliferative inflammation, and the marked irritation of the germinative cell layers of the matrix cause a cholesteatoma of the antrum to penetrate in an uncontrolled manner into the still very loose spongiosa of the mastoid. Remnants of this granulation tissue are the cause of recurrence. The best protection is wide exposure of the mastoid via a lateral approach. The necessary clearance of the spongiosa to the extreme anatomical limits of the cortical bone can be easily carried out, irrespective of whether the structure is suspected of being cholesteatoma or not. Very little mucosa is preserved. The plasticine permits reduction in size of the very wide, infected mastoid cavity up to the level of the facial spine. A large antrum should remain open for functional reasons.

Labyrinthine Fistula (Figs. 231–232)

Erosion of the lateral semicircular canal without cholesteatoma arises exactly at the point where one of its sources of arterial blood supply from the stylomastoid artery reaches the inner ear capsule and ends in the enchondral capsule. The matrix and perimatrix destroy the isolated labyrinthine dome without osteitis, or affect the inner ear, the perilymph membrane or the endolymphatic sac. Elevation of the matrix is the last procedure and is carried out without trauma. Cover with healthy fascia is adequate, especially if the epitympanum and the ossicular chain are retained, because in this case the fistula cannot be damaged by manipulations in the absence of a radical mastoid cavity. Furthermore, we know from many fenestration procedures for otosclerosis that although gentle manipulation can cause dizziness, it does not cause permanent damage.

A *mass of cholesteatoma* granulations springing from a bony edge affected by osteitis may penetrate the lumen of the labyrinth. It must then be drilled out toward both sides as well as in the long axis from the ampulla, using a diamond burr. A generous fenestration is created until the lumen is almost completely exposed by springing its edges (for example, with a suitable excavator as used in fenestration surgery). Even then the function of the inner ear is not necessarily lost. In order to close off the interior securely in the presence of a circumscribed endolabyrinthine cholesteatoma, without it

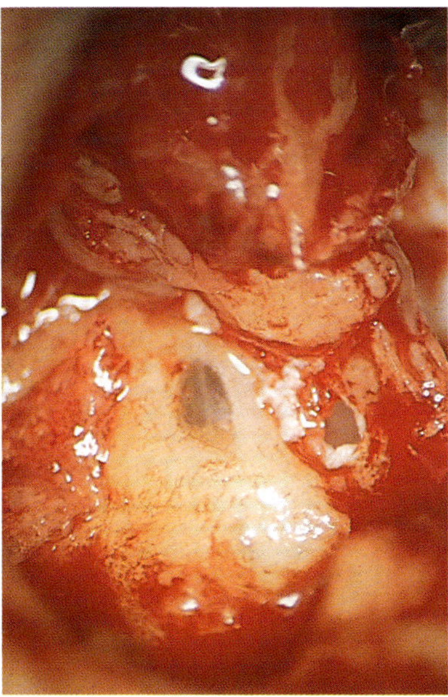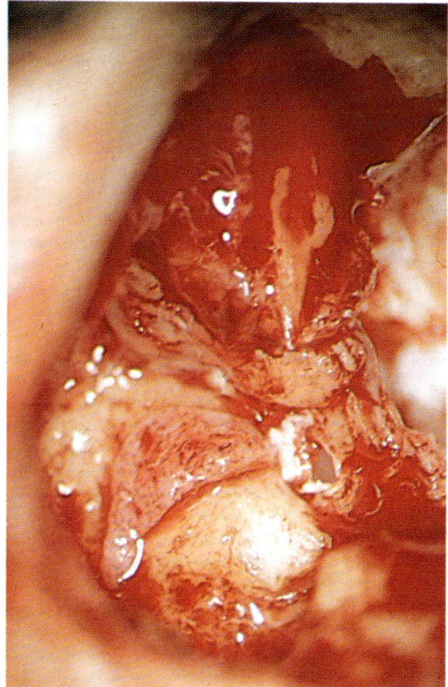

Figs. **231** and **232** **Chronic middle ear inflammation with a large secondary cholesteatoma and erosion of the lateral epitympanic wall.** Osteoplastic exposure of all middle ear spaces. After careful elevation of the cholesteatoma matrix over the lateral semicircular canal, a large fistula close to the ampulla came into view, which had been suspected from the endoscopic view before this operation (see Fig. **144**). The fistula was covered with fascia, which was sealed laterally to the bone with fibrin glue

being eroded by connective tissue externally, a small curved bone or plasticine plate covered with fascia is laid over the lumen.

This typically longstanding stationary fistula due to the resorption of the lateral semicircular canal does not constitute one of the progressive forms of paralabyrinthine osteitis.

Operations for Para- and Retro-labyrinthine Cholesteatomas of the Middle ear

Because middle ear cholesteatomas penetrate the paralabyrinthine constriction only anterior and posterior to the arcuate eminence, it is important to ascertain their position and extent before the operation begins, particularly of occult primary inflammatory acquired cholesteatomas. Only their narrow, circumscribed entrance can be recognized during epitympanotomy. Preoperative radiographs including plain films in Wullstein's, Chaussée III or Schueller's view satisfy the diagnostic requirements. The most satisfactory CT scan is the axial view, but it does not demonstrate the paralabyrinthine involvement. Therefore an additional coronal view is necessary to distinguish clearly between delicate spongiosa and bone defect.

Space for the lateral extension of paralabyrinthine cholesteatoma is not available. The neighboring cortical bone of the surface of the petrous pyramid is often eroded earlier than the labyrinthine canals. Only after it has transgressed the paralabyrinthine constriction can the cholesteatoma extend in a retrolabyrinthine direction between the inner ear, the internal meatus and the carotid canal toward the petrous apex. In extreme cases (Fig. **222**), the middle ear cholesteatoma reaches such a size that the entire apex is destroyed, and only a few structures of the bony internal ear remain. Even then two functions of the inner ear and that of the facial nerve can be relatively well preserved. The cortical bone of the two surfaces of the petrous pyramid is, to a large part, resorbed. The dura and the carotid artery lie free, covered by matrix.

It is impossible in the long run to maintain small cavities of paralabyrinthine cholesteatoma free of scales, keratin, and other debris from the epitympanum, using suction from the meatus through a funnel drilled in the antelabyrinthine trigone or the postlabyrinthine rhomboid. The matrix does not remain uninfected, but continues to develop. Furthermore, lesions of the surface due to manipulations and granulations lead to scar tissue stenosis. Any cavity which cannot be inspected is the site of origin

of recurrence. Exposure and clearance must be achieved surgically by a simultaneous approach from *lateral and above*. A preliminary osteoplastic epitympanotomy decisively shortens and extends access to the inner ear by removal of the lateral epitympanic wall and the squamous bone as far as its inner cortical layer. The lever action of the ossicles is scarcely ever to be retained, although it can be during decompression of the facial nerve because of entrapment by a fracture inside its labyrinthine segment.

The supra-auricular incision should be extended superiorly, followed by division of the squamous bone on all sides by osteoplastic trephine using the cutting and diamond burrs. This is carried as far as the dura, initially that of the tegmen tympani and antri along the labyrinthine block and beyond that, over the temporal squama, so that the temporal squama can be lifted off after freeing on both sides of the arch in the lateral as well as the basal plane. In this manner, the cholesteatoma is exposed in continuity in the paralabyrinthine constriction.

Drainage of suppuration of the petrous pyramid in impending meningitis was attempted for a long time using the endocranial extradural route. Holmgren proposed this route in 1917 for fenestration of the anterior semicircular canal in the arcuate eminence. H. L. Wullstein carried out this endocranial extradural fenestration for stapes fixation in chronic middle ear suppuration in 1951, i.e., before tympanoplasty, and thus demonstrated sonoinversion of both inner ear windows. This access, now called "middle fossa approach", has become more usual for surgery of the internal auditory meatus.

The facial nerve lying anterior to the arcuate eminence serves as a landmark for opening of the paralabyrinthine constriction from the cortex. Behind it lies the attachment of the superior petrosal sinus, which must be released to expose the cortex of the posterior surface if a posterior paralabyrinthine cholesteatoma is present. As much CSF as possible is drained by a small stab incision in the dura over the temporal lobe in order to provide space. This point is closed by adhesive or fine sutures at the end of the operation.

The matrix is stripped off the easily visible walls of the cavity and also from the exposed dura using a polishing or a diamond burr. If the matrix cannot be freed from the dura, the latter must be excised and repaired. Periosteum is pushed into the cranial fossa to close the defect, adhesive is applied to it and a second layer of periosteum is glued from outside. If the neighboring bone can be freed of matrix reliably using the diamond burr, the paralabyrinthine defect is filled with plasticine. A CSF fistula must not be present. Commonly, either the anterior or the posterior crus of the semicircular canal is eroded widely with sharp edges (osteitic granulations are absent and, therefore, membranous labyrinthitis also). Then it is drilled down right at the beginning in an attempt to maintain the function of the inner ear, i.e., using a technique without bone dust and irrigation/aspiration. After the arcuate eminence has been demonstrated, a very sharp flat chisel is used to cut through the anterior crus, preferably with one stroke, followed by the posterior crus with a further cut. Fascia is immediately glued over it for closure. If the cholesteatoma has opened the cochlea medial to the facial nerve, it is impossible to be sure that it is free of cholesteatoma, even using the angled endoscope. Despite the loss of hearing, exenteration of the labyrinth can scarcely be avoided.

Immediate trephining of the middle cranial fossa in a lateral and basal direction carries the risk that the intracranial pressure forces the bony lid into the middle ear after suture of the galea over the temporal bone. To prevent this, a plasticine plate is laid on the floor of the middle cranial fossa and fixed anteriorly and posteriorly to the temporal bone.

The *posterior paralabyrinthine cholesteatoma* borders on both cranial fossae from the arcuate eminence to the medial edge of the endolymphatic sac and as far as the internal acoustic porus. If it is allowed to extend over a long period, it becomes a deep basal pyramidal cholesteatoma and threatens to break through into the semicircular canals and into the vestibule from a superomedial direction.

The situation of the *anterior paralabyrinthine cholesteatoma* is complicated by the course of the facial nerve and the proximity of the internal carotid artery. Indeed, the labyrinthine part of the nerve serves as an anatomical landmark for opening the cortex of the petrous pyramid as far as the dura of the middle cranial fossa and the carotid artery with a diamond burr, and of reaching the pyramidal apex, bypassing the ampulla of the anterior semicircular canal lying over the cochlea and in front of the fundus of the internal auditory meatus. The bony surfaces can be freed of matrix with the diamond burr. The facial nerve and the carotid artery must also be cleared of matrix, in order to be able to close the cholesteatoma cavity with plasticine. The dura of the middle and posterior cranial fossae is thus securely closed against a CSF leak. Freeing and transposition of the facial nerve provides no advantage. An inflammed papillary and very thickened matrix which can be peeled off the ganglion and the labyrinthine course of the facial nerve is the exception. It can be removed with great security and care

using the polishing burr, initially using the larger diamond burrs on the broad surface, and thereafter with the small burrs along both sides where the matrix extends onto neighboring bone. The results are checked with the angled endoscope. A mild paralysis of the nerve recovers in a few weeks.

The same procedure can also be applied to the internal carotid artery. The bony canal is drilled down beyond the limit of the cholesteatoma. The healthy wall of the internal carotid artery is thin within the bony eustachian tube and surrounded by a venous plexus, which picks up the pulsation. The venous plexus becomes thrombosed, due to the prolonged pathological effect of the cholesteatoma, and the arterial wall becomes very thickened. Pulsation is scarcely visible, and it is therefore possible to eradicate a delicate matrix from this wall easily, using the diamond burr. On the other side of the paralabyrinthine constriction, the retrolabyrinthine cholesteatoma is divided from the artery as far as the foramen lacerum by the internal auditory meatus and the gasserian ganglion. There the dura can be incised and repaired as far as the foramen spinosum, followed by filling with very soft plasticine, so that no circumscribed pressure is exercised on the nerve.

The same procedure can be extended to cholesteatoma of the petrous apex. The eroded bony wall of the internal meatus can be removed as far as the neighboring facial nerve and the superior vestibular nerve. The angled endoscope again is useful in orientation. Pyramidal cholesteatomas extending further have probably eroded into the inner ear; they must be resected and the facial nerve transposed. More extensive procedures such as subtotal petrosectomy (Fisch 1985) have no place in a monograph on tympanoplasty devoted to healing of the petrous pyramid and maintainance and improvement of hearing.

Finally, the osteoplastic lid is re-inserted and screwed into place with miniplates, and protected from the middle ear by fascia. This is followed by reconstruction of the epitympanum, using a Type III tympanoplasty with a deep tympanic cavity and a high columella.

Once healing is complete, radiological views, including CT scans, are necessary for monitoring the course of the disease over many years.

Congenital parasellar epidermoids (cholesteatoma), especially those in the cerebellopontine angle invading the petrous apex, are discussed on p. 164 ff.

Conclusions: Complications of cholesteatoma due to spread by the mastoid route are very much more common than those due to spread by the petrous pyramid. Mastoid complications can almost always be controlled by surgery and antibiotics. All paralabyrinthine cholesteatomas, even those in the early stage and those which are symptomless and appear to be free of infection, demand radical eradication. Function of the inner ear is always at risk, either due to an unexpected injury or due to unavoidable partial resection of the inner ear capsule. For this reason, an epitympanic cholesteatoma whose matrix reaches the medial wall is always to be regarded as an initial stage of a paralabyrinthine cholesteatoma. The longer the treatment is delayed, the more difficult it becomes.

Conductive Deafness of Inflammatory Origin

The pathology of four diseases and their functional effects on the fine structure of the middle ear have not yet been dealt with. These are:
- subacute otitis media and middle ear fibrosis;
- ossicular fixation and tympanosclerosis;
- otitis media with effusion, and cholesterol granuloma;
- tympanic membrane atrophy, retraction atelectasis and adhesive processes.

Subacute Granulating Otitis in the Epitympanum (Figs. 233–234)

The treatment of acute otitis media by antibiotics avoids the suppurative stage, but the disease may persist in a subacute form, affecting the mucosa and its folds. The resulting scar tissue compromises the lever system. In addition to mild swelling of the pars flaccida, there is a slight conductive deafness so long as the edema of the folds is very lax and the obstruction of the ossicles is slight. These changes arise at the places where the function of the pneumatic system is most complex, i.e., tympanic diaphragm and the compartments of the epitympanum. As the inflammation is only suppressed, but not eradicated, a mass of inflammatory infiltration remains. The folds are adherent, and the epitympanic cushions are unrecognizable. The epitympanum can no longer be aerated, even with excess pressure (see Fig. **251**). The epithelium is lost, due to compression lasting for many weeks. Adherence of the granulation tissue to the surface, and connective tissue metaplasia of the stroma are the early phases of adhesion and retraction. Occasionally, a slight secretion into the mesohypotympanum drains spontaneously with restitution of the function of the tube. So long as the stroma of the folds is lax and edematous and the tubal function has returned to normal, the deafness is not serious and indeed, the hearing may appear normal for a long time. However, the conductive deafness may be very pronounced from the inception of the disease, especially if marked mucosal swelling or secretion obstruct one or both windows. The disease progresses to a very severe form when scar tissue sets in, possibly with alarming, even if insignificant, serous labyrinthitis. Patients often complain of a marked feeling of fullness in the ear, but scarcely ever of pain.

Before the era of antibiotics, an entirely different form of subacute otitis media, usually without perforation and secretion but with severe deafness, was feared: after a clinically silent phase lasting several weeks, severe life-threatening complications affecting one or both cranial fossae could present with no prodroma. The organism was usually a pneumococcus, and the illness sometimes referred to as a pneumococcal mastoiditis. Radiography of the usually well-pneumatized bone showed increasing destruction of the mastoid process and the petrous apex. A full mastoidectomy was necessary. The *posterosuperior* cell tract in the postlabyrinthine rhomboid was easy to open, whereas the *posteroinferior* cell tract was difficult to find. Pachymeningitis followed penetration medial to the sigmoid sinus below the ampulla of the posterior semicircular canal, superior to the jugular bulb and limited anteriorly by the facial nerve.

In mucosal otitis the three levels of the middle ear, although closed to sound pressure transformation, can be left unopened, provided that there is no acute danger of osteitis of the inner ear and the petrous apex arising from the antelabyrinthine trigone and spreading via the *anterosuperior* cell tract, or from the hypotympanum via the *anteroinferior* cell tract along the internal carotid artery. (The latter can be drained along the artery by Ramadier's operation). In the latter event, all middle ear structures must be removed in the early stage. Because marked proliferation of granulations, rather than suppuration, was the characteristic of this form of otitis media, subsequent adhesive processes around the ossicles could not be prevented effectively by antrotomy.

The chronic forms of severe, protracted inflammation of the folds block the epitympanum anterior to the aditus. The cause of *aditus block* (Richardson 1963) or of *occlusion aditus* (Bollobas

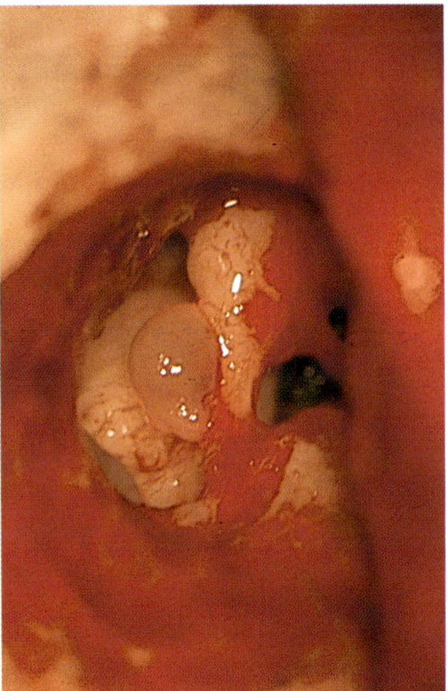

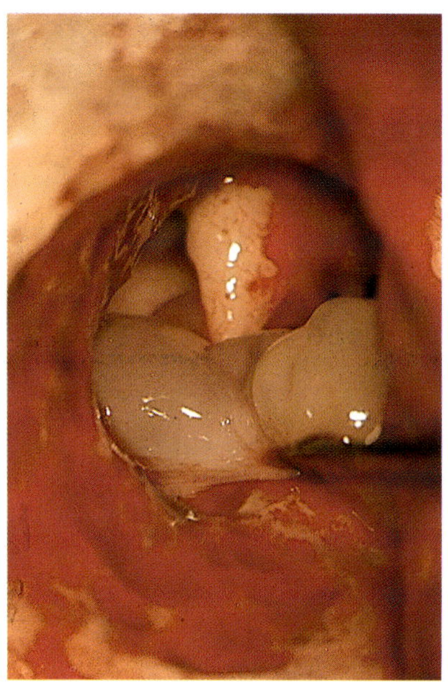

Fig. **233**   **Adhesive otitis media.** Osteoplastic epitympanotomy. The aeration and drainage of the posterior segment has been interrupted by a mucosal polyp which developed in the incudal fossa medial to the body of the incus. The polyp hinders the movement of the ossicular system and is the cause of recurrent effusions. A further mucosal polyp can be seen in the depth of the antrum

Fig. **234**   **Adhesive otitis media.** Osteoplastic epitympanotomy. The large mucosal polyp has been pulled out of the depths of the antrum with the double forceps, and divided at its pedicle in the incudal fossa

1971), i.e., the interruption of the ventilation of the retrotympanic spaces, is not to be sought in the aditus but rather in the *tympanic diaphragm* and the lateral epitympanic cushions.

Papillary retraction and invagination cholesteatomas can arise as a result of prolonged inflammation. Operative findings at osteoplastic epitympanotomy for severe mucosal and mucoperiosteal infiltration show that the aeration and drainage disorder of the middle ear at this stage usually no longer lies in the eustachian tube, which is usually found to be patent.

In the end stage of this subacute form of otitis media, even intensive antibiotic treatment does not succeed in aerating the almost sterile adhesions in the epitympanic compartments. The posterior middle ear segment thus remains excluded from ventilation and drainage. Ventilation tubes in the mesohypotympanum have no effect on this posterior obstruction. The continuing absence of reaeration is characterized by increasing opacity in Schueller's view (compared with the well-developed pneumatization of the opposite side) as well as by the absence of further cell formation according to the developmental phases during pneumatization.

Every epitympanum would heal with restoration of the air-containing compartments if the air penetrated into the clefts, either spontaneously or by active insufflation. Instead of this, the classical histological picture of contraction of the massive interossicular adhesions and irregular hollow spaces follows over many years. The only method of preventing this development is timely treatment, including division of the adhesions and the removal of granulations, preserving the mucosa along the natural aeration pathways of the middle ear.

The pathology of nonspecific granulating inflammation of the folds is the same in infants as in adults. As the operative findings in the epitympanum have shown, the head of the malleus and incus are indeed undamaged, but lie embedded in granulation tissue, with no remaining air spaces. Both the tympanic cavity and the antrum appear to be almost free of disease. Osteoplastic epitympanotomy can be carried out reliably and successfully even in a three- or four-year-old child.

Middle Ear Fibrosis

The cause of this unusual reaction of the middle ear mucosa has not yet been explained. Histology shows a tissue rich in connective tissue and occasional sclerosis, but free of inflammation, with few glands and atrophic epithelium. The history reveals a feeling of fullness in the ear and deafness increasing over many years. Otalgia is unusual, and occasionally of gradual onset. The position and color of the tympanic membrane are almost normal, although the membrane may sometimes be slightly thickened with fine scar tissue but no perforation. For a long time it was believed that middle ear fibrosis mainly affects the mesohypotympanum and the epitympanum less so. Because an ossicular defect is virtually never present, surgery was restricted to the mesohypotympanum and antral inspection. Elevation of the tympanic membrane showed that the middle ear no longer had a lumen but was filled with lax or thick, fibrous connective tissue strands (Fig. **235**).

This condition causes a marked conductive deafness and possibly an apparent sensorineural deafness due to obstruction of the two inner ear windows, causing disorders of impedance, with or without an abnormal stapedial reflex. Forced inflation of the tube produces only a slight, slow bulging of the tympanic membrane as an indirect response to the increased pressure in the tympanic ostium of the tube.

Osteoplastic epitympanotomy has shown that the same adhesions and membranes in which the ossicles are embedded fill all clefts of the epitympanum; the ossicles almost never show a defect. Middle ear fibrosis is therefore an absolute indication for osteoplastic epitympanotomy. An attempt at blind release of sclerosing noninflammatory masses behind the closed lateral epitympanic wall via an antrotomy carries the risk of severe trauma of the inner ear. The contours of the ossicles are initially indistinct, even with a complete view of the entire epitympanum. The fibrotic fibers and masses retract if they are dissected apart. It may be advisable to interrupt the ossicles temporarily at the incudostapedial joint before dissection, to protect the inner ear.

If no mucosa is available in the epitympanum and on the ossicles for regeneration, the question arises as to whether the head of the malleus and the body of the incus should be amputated because the ossicular chain is no longer capable of vibration, and the tendency to new adhesions is so marked that the prognosis for hearing is very unfavorable.

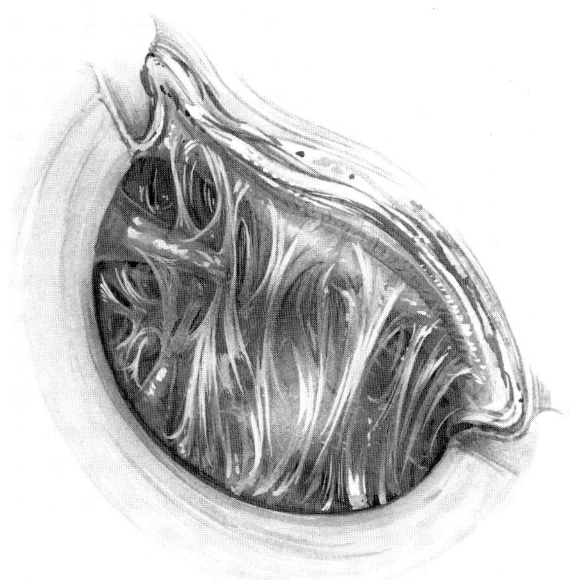

Fig. **235** **The mesotympanum as shown after elevation of the tympanic membrane**, filled with grey, thick inflammatory tissue forming cords and membranes. The mucosa is completely absent (H. L. Wullstein 1968)

The denuded epitympanum is covered with a mucosal substitute to create a Type III tympanoplasty with a deep, capacious tympanic cavity connected to the antrum after stapedial build-up. This demands lateralization of the bony lid. The prospects for orderly aeration of a classical Type III tympanoplasty with a shallow tympanic cavity are unfavorable. The tympanic ostium of the bony eustachian tube can be enclosed in the middle ear fibrosis.

The hearing result for middle ear fibrosis depends on careful and long-term aftercare. Initially, tubal inflation by the endoscopic endonasal route should be carried out daily, beginning two to three days after the operation. It may be advisable to introduce postaural drainage from the antrum externally, in order to allow repeated inflation under pressure. Repeated instillation of electrolyte solutions containing cortisone for about two weeks may also be advisable.

Ossicular Fixation (Figs. 236–243)

Osteophytic fixations are almost exclusively the local result of superficial mucoperiostitis and osteitis at neighboring points; for example, between the tegmen and the anterior surface of the protympanic recess, between the stapes and the wall of the niche and between the incus and the medial epitympanic wall. They cause extensive interference with the vibration of the ossicular chain. The mucosal disease has often healed a long time earlier. Almost without exception, they can only be found with the help of osteoplastic epitympanotomy, which enables the function of the freed ossicular chain to be reconstituted. The osteophytes are completely removed with a suitable diamond burr to prevent recurrence. If the site of fixation lies on the medial surface of the ossicle, partial removal or even temporary resection and reimplantation of the incus may be necessary.

Postinflammatory calcification or even *ossification* of the tendon of the stapedius and tensor tympani muscles may occur simultaneously or independently. Adhesions regrow after simple division. The pyramidal eminence or cochleariform process should be removed because the muscle function is lost, due to disease.

Massive, longstanding adhesions, extensive fibrosis and calcification surrounding the ossicles can form a single mass which fills the epitympanum but which can be removed with a drill or diamond burr. The sound transmission system then is of no further use. Modeling follows in such a way that the air flow is conducted via the two aeration pathways to the windows and then via the aditus into the antrum after the epitympanic bony lid has been replaced. A deep tympanic cavity with a high columella is the goal of this reconstruction.

These massive adhesions can also be divided successfully from the wall and the ossicles to restore satisfactory vibration and free air-containing clefts under exceptionally favorable circumstances. In other cases it is advisable to remove the head of the malleus and the body of the incus, to create a Type III tympanoplasty with a high columella and a retained epitympanic air space.

Tympanosclerosis was termed "middle ear sclerosis" from the time of von Tröltsch (1881) to Zöllner (1963). Since the time of Politzer (1983), it has been distinguished histologically from otosclerosis. It was included by Lempert (1945) as clinical otosclerosis in the indications for labyrinthine fenestration. Only exceptionally was the operation indicated for stapedial fixation. H. L. Wullstein (1952) included it logically in the indications for

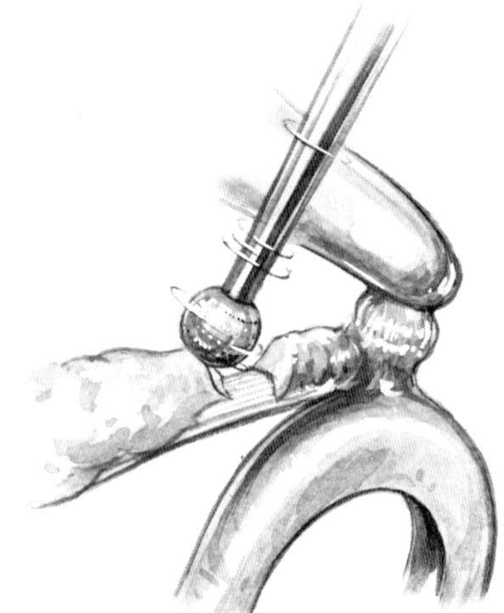

Fig. **236 Removal of osteoid from the stapedial tendon.** The bony deposits surrounding the tendon are removed down to the tendon with a fine diamond burr, and the tendon is divided if necessary with a sickle knife (H. L. Wullstein 1968)

tympanoplasty under the term "tympanosclerosis." Tympanosclerosis, confined to the tympanic cavity, had been known for a long time. Osteoplastic epitympanotomy has clearly shown that its site of predilection and extent correspond to the folds (Fig. **239**). The extremely sensitive stroma within the folds reacts in the form of abnormal connective tissue metabolism; this has been the subject of many morphological studies. The plaques form during episodes of localized inflammation or during recurrent inflammation surrounding the ossicles; often they demonstrate layers. Fixation of the ossicle may be slight and circumscribed and yet lead to complete immobility of the ossicular chain. This type of concealed focus is only found during the operation. It lies particularly between the head of the malleus and the anterior wall of the epitympanum or the tegmen tympani.

An operation without osteoplastic epitympanotomy, designed to improve hearing, is doomed to failure in the presence of massive scarring of the epitympanum. A shallow tympanoplasty with a stapes columella does not achieve satisfactory hearing results in the presence of the poor mucosa and aeration. The same principles as in otosclerosis also apply to scar tissue fixation of the stapes in the oval window niche (see below).

Eradication is difficult in the presence of complete involvement of one or both ossicles in the epitympanum. All the layers of a tympanosclerotic plaque can occasionally be removed entirely, leaving

Fig. **237 Osteoplastic epitym-panotomy.** The arrow shows fixation of the head of the malleus to the tegmen tympani and the anterior epitympanic wall by osteitis

Fig. **238 Osteoplastic epitym-panotomy, showing the same patient as in Fig. 237.** After complete removal of the mass of osteitis, the wound surface on the ossicles is covered with a mucosal graft taken from the aditus ad antrum, to prevent renewed fixation

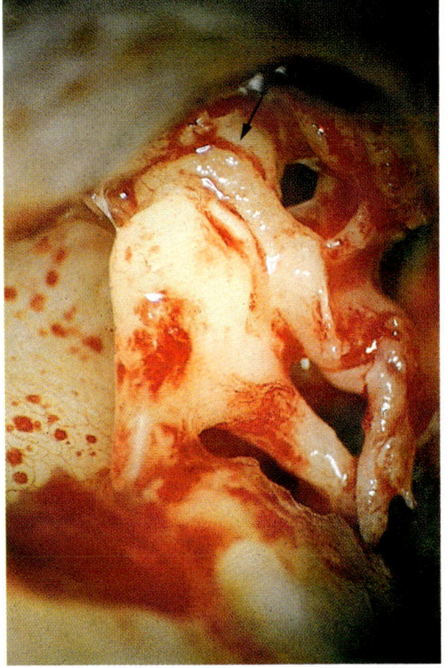

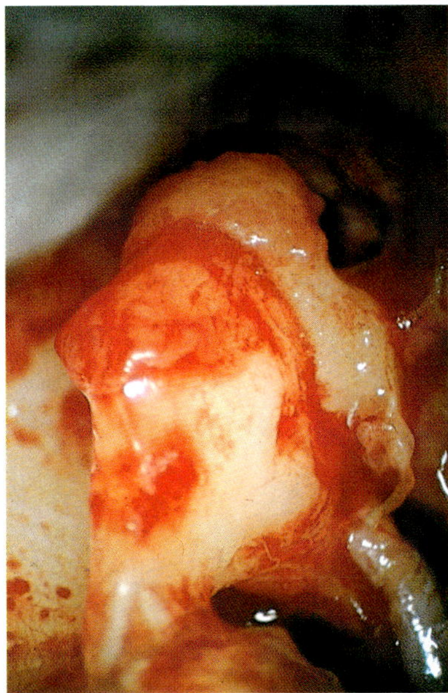

237   238

the bone exposed. Sufficient healthy mucosa to allow rapid regrowth from surrounding tissue is only available in small defects. In other cases mucosal grafts from the tegmen tympani or the labyrinthine wall of the antrum should be considered. If the result even then is unsatisfactory, a Type III tympanoplasty with a high columella, a deep tympanic cavity and an empty epitympanum is recommended for improvement of aeration and sound pressure transformation.

Temporary division of the incudostapedial joint is also advisable in a Type I procedure because the ossicular chain is manipulated during separation of the tympanosclerotic plaques. The lentiform process springs laterally and must be refixed to the head of the stapes. A small plaque around the stapes can be easily removed to restore function to the stapes. If the stapes is walled in and the niche filled up, removal of the stapes is to be preferred. It may be reduced in size with the diamond burr and then reimplanted. Care must also be taken that the walls of the niche re-epithelialize, irrespective of which stapedial replacement is used.

In contrast to otosclerosis, the function of the incus in tympanosclerosis can be defective, either due to difficulty in restoration of the vibratory ability of the ossicular chain or to a defect in the chain. It is then impossible to suspend the replacement stapes; furthermore, a reliable surface for placement of a high columella in the oval window is not available.

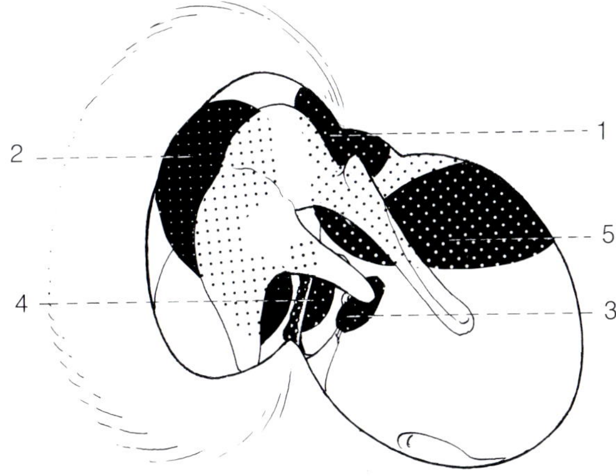

Fig. **239 Sites of predilection of tympanosclerosis:** 1. Between the head of the malleus and the facial wall of the protympanic recess; 2. between the malleus, incus and tegmen tympani; 3. oval window niche; 4. occasionally, at completely isolated small sites, for example, in the interossicular folds close to the oval window niche and the stapes; 5. recessus supratubalis and orifice of the Eustachian tube. (H. L. Wullstein 1968)

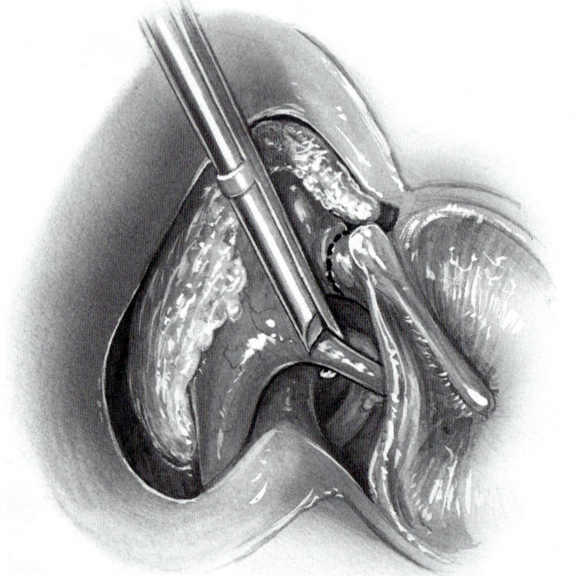

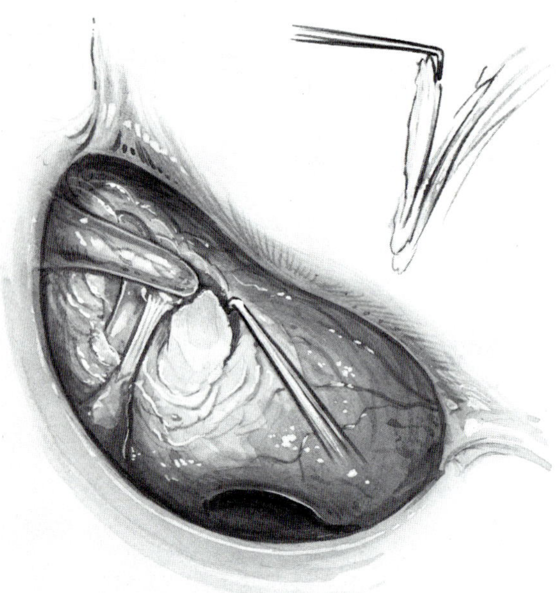

Fig. 240 Tympanoplasty for tympanosclerosis in the epitympanum. There is broad fixation of the malleus or incus or of both. The neck of the malleus and the long process of the incus are divided in preference to dissection and mobilization of the chain, which has uncertain results. No attempt is made to create a Type I or Type II tympanoplasty with preservation of the lever action in the epitympanum, and sound conduction is created using a Type III (deep) tympanoplasty with build-up of the stapes (H. L. Wullstein 1968)

Fig. 241 Removal of a tympanosclerotic mass from the oval window niche. The mass of tympanosclerosis is loosened layer by layer with a sickle knife or a small hook, and removed (H. L. Wullstein 1968)

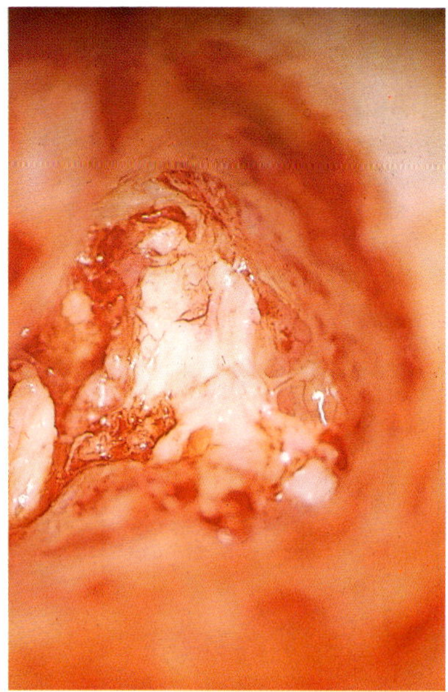

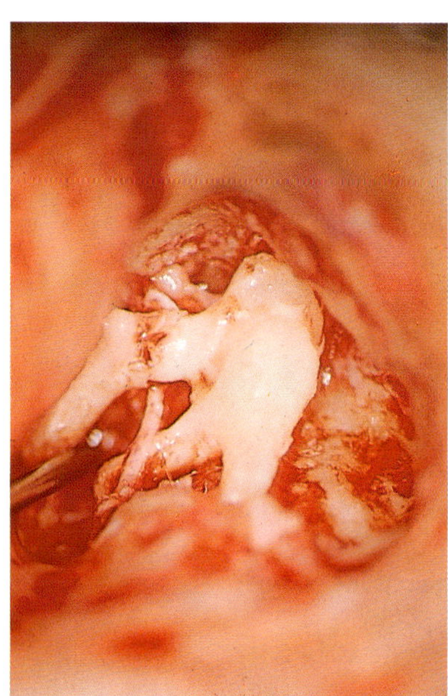

Fig. 242 Severe tympanosclerosis in the epitympanum with an embedded ossicular chain

Fig. 243 The same patient as in Fig. 242 showing the situation after very cautious removal of the tympanosclerotic mass in layers from the surface of the ossicle. At a second stage, after healing of the repair of the tympanic membrane, the sclerotic fixation of the annular ligament is dealt with by a stapedectomy

242

243

There is also a danger that the high columella forces the membrane closing the window into the vestibule, even so far as to contact the utricle. This can happen immediately or later, due to increasing scar tissue contraction of the tympanic membrane graft. This event severely impairs cochlear function and induces severe tinnitus. Healing and improvement of hearing are then best achieved by a two-stage operation, and by a three-stage procedure in the presence of chronic middle ear inflammation with a perforation of the tympanic membrane (p. 176).

However, a one-stage stapedectomy is permissible if the middle ear is free of inflammation and the tympanic membrane is intact; for example, in isolated tympanosclerosis of the stapes. If the incus is absent and a Type III tympanoplasty with high columella is inevitable, the columella can be prevented from sinking into the vestibule as follows: the denuded wall of the niche is covered with a robust membrane; for example, doubled, compressed temporalis fascia vaulting over the wall of the niche beyond the facial canal and the wall of the promontory so that it adheres to them firmly. It is glued to the walls carefully with fibrin adhesive. The graft is firmly fixed so that it can tolerate a columella after interposition of a small slice of periosteum the same size as the stapes footplate.

Otitis Media with Effusion: Cholesterol Granuloma

The extent and sequelae of recurrent otitis media with effusion can only be understood if both the eustachian tube and the system of epitympanic folds are taken into account in the clinical picture. This book is not the place to consider the pathomorphology of otitis media with effusion in any depth. It is much more important to discuss the principles which contribute to an understanding of the excessive and recurring reaction of the middle ear. Furthermore, the operative procedures which are advisable to prevent the late sequelae of progressive and severe middle ear or inner ear deafness due to immobilization of the ossicles by fibrous and sclerotic scar tissue must be discussed. The worse the regenerative capacity of the mucosa, the more difficult it is to eliminate these sequelae by surgery.

The initially very mild inflammation of the eustachian tube and tympanic cavity spreads from the tympanic ostium rapidly and easily to the neighboring folds. They react more vigorously than the tissue of the rigid periosteum of the walls of the middle ear, with serous infiltration of the delicate stroma and permeability of the thin epithelial layers, producing a profuse serous transudate or exudate into the lumen of the tympanic cavity. The secretion arising from these extensive mucosal surfaces, particularly from the folds in the narrow epitympanum, flows into the hypotympanum. If clearance is unsatisfactory due to the small number of ciliated cells and inhibition of their activity, the increased activity of the goblet cells and the newly formed glands in the still partially opened eustachian tube stimulates the secretory cells to produce copious amounts of nonpurulent mucus. Furthermore, if drainage through the tube is obstructed, the mucus becomes more and more thickened to form a clear but very tenacious viscous plug, which is sucked into the wide ostium of the tube by the swallowing act, but is not carried away.

The exposure of the child to attacks of airborn infection happens at a time when transmitted maternal immunity has expired but the child's own immune resistance is only slowly developing. Between the ages of two and eight, the lymphatic immune system undergoes exuberant development compared with other organs which are developing more slowly (Fig. 6). This discrepancy between the biokinetic growth processes and the onset of maturity causes the serious immunological response of the infant, which must be treated with extreme care and understanding.

Apart from the very mild bacterial infections, other immunological reactions, biochemical stimuli to bacterial breakdown products, and autonomic regulation mechanisms (for example, on the mucosa of the eustachian tube and middle ear) need to be considered in the genesis of protractive or recurrent hyperergic epitympanitis (Kumazawa 1975, Wullstein 1985).

A temporary abnormality of air pressure, due to incomplete and intermittent mechanical obstruction to rapid refilling of air at the tubal torus, is a clear noninfective cause for sudden effusions. Severe but brief reduction of pressure (for example, in landing in an aircraft), often produces a brisk mucosal transudate, particularly from the mucosal folds, within minutes, but it is not recurrent or persistent. Its resolution is determined by how quickly the effusion can empty from the compartments.

If the folds are well formed, almost no effusion develops because of the free air exchange between the middle ear and the antrum. But if they are thickened due to catarrh, or are adherent, then the variations in air pressure are often very slowly compensated for (Figs. 55, 56). A single clinical observation over many decades can contribute more to the understanding of this feature than many measurements on patients.

During childhood the senior author suffered numerous attacks of severe purulent acute otitis media in one ear only. It underwent repeated spontaneous perforation or required repeated paracentesis, and on one occasion almost required mastoidectomy. He suffered repeated tubal middle ear catarrh in the other ear, with deafness but without perforation. The pneumatization was very extensive on both sides and the cells delicately developed. The tympanic membrane had few residual scars. In later life, during every landing in an aircraft, a copious *middle ear effusion in the less diseased ear* developed within a few minutes during the last 300–500 meters of the descent. It caused symptoms on swallowing for the next four or five days as a result of cicatricial folds impeding the equalization of air pressure. The ear with profuse suppuration in the mastoid process never showed the slightest effusion because the pus draining from the antrum had destroyed the air pockets, and the air pressure was transmitted directly to the antrum.

The sequel of repeated effusions of this type is fibrosis, initially slight but later marked, in the stroma of the folds. The folds become thickened, and more and more adherent, stiffened and scarred. They lose their delicate function in sound appreciation. For example, transients are no longer heard, due to lack of damping of vibrations and rapid decay of the after-vibrations. The isthmus of the compartments is closed, localized retention cysts and papillae from the basal cell layers develop profusely. Serious persisting disturbances of function are initiated, including tympanosclerosis and even cholesteatoma.

Osteoplastic epitympanotomy is indispensible for *cholesterol granulomas* with retention cysts, newly formed lymph follicles and signs of early tympanosclerosis. It is particularly indicated for *chronic hemorrhagic seromucinous middle ear inflammation (idiopathic hemotympanum or blue drum)*.

Ultimate healing is to be expected *if the secretions can drain continuously from all clefts of the epitympanum, and the ossicles are thoroughly aerated.*

Atrophy of the Tympanic Membrane, Retractions, Atelectasis and Adhesive Processes

The site and nature of disturbance of aeration between the eustachian tube and the aditus should be determined as far as possible from the appearances of the tympanic membrane before and during inflation and deflation. Fibrotic scars and atrophy in the pars tensa associated with hyalin and calcified deposits are the sequelae of previous myringitis. If they do not interfere with function, they do not require surgical correction. However, they require supervision to monitor the progress of the conductive deafness.

Retractions, Atelectases and Adhesive Processes as a Result of Seromucinous Middle Ear Otitis Media with Effusions
(Figs. **244–254**)

The most circumscribed form of visible atelectasis is that of Prussak's space, an indication of adhesions, on occasion, of all the small compartments between the lateral bony wall and the ossicles. They are mainly aerated from the posterior isthmus; their re-aeration is difficult. A slight, direct irritation of the tensor fold can also induce isolated adhesions at this point.

Retractions caused by inflammation of the tensor and mallear folds which advance slowly but progressively may be limited to the space *anterior to the neck of the malleus* and lead to massive scarring with indrawing extending as far as the superior folds running from the head of the malleus and the incus to the tegmen tympani. There is a risk of fixation of the malleus to the tegmen by osteitis (Fig. **237**) or the development of an anterolateral and more particularly, of an anteromedial retraction cholesteatoma.

Retraction *behind the neck of the malleus and lateral to the incus* is induced by the marked cicatricial effect of the folds which form the lateral epitympanic air cushions at that point. The final result is a posterolateral retraction cholesteatoma lying between the inner side of the lateral epitympanic wall and lateral to the body of the incus.

Retraction pockets *between the neck of the malleus and the tympanic segment of the facial nerve*, i.e., medial to the incus in the fossa incudis, are determined by scar tissue stenosis of the medial folds lying at that point in the epitympanum, and the persisting low pressure in the antrum. They cause the most frequent form of posteromedial retraction cholesteatoma.

Further local action is exerted on the posterosuperior quadrant of the pars tensa in the presence of well-developed folds in the facial recess running to the posterior segment of the oval niche and to the stapes. The result is the *typical, sharply demarcated atrophy of this quadrant* with the most severe degrees of retraction and adhesion. It advances medial to the incus along the lateral semicircular canal and

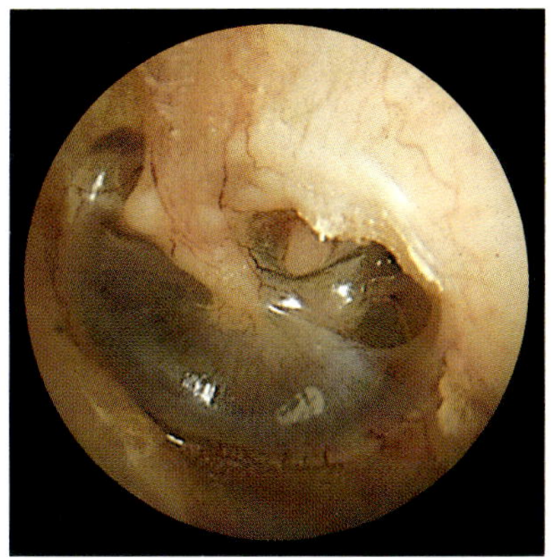

Fig. 244   Otitis media with effusion and retraction of the atrophic tympanic membrane: 1. pars flaccida in the anterior segment and 2. the pars tensa in the posterosuperior quadrant. Spontaneous Type III tympanoplasty. View with a straight 4-mm, 0° endoscope

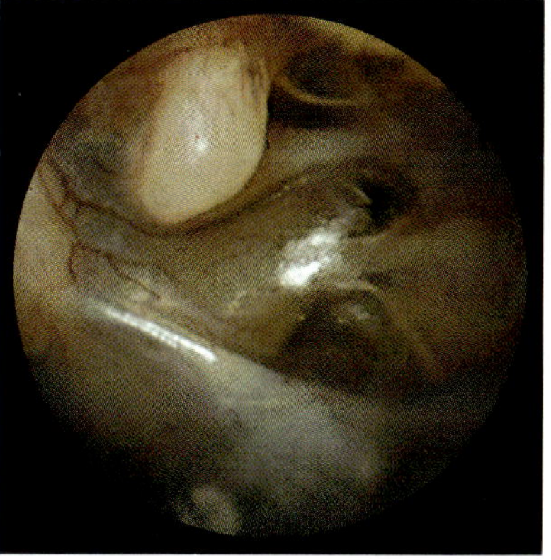

Fig. 245   Otitis media with effusion and retractions of the atrophic tympanic membrane. View into the depth of the posterosuperior quadrant of the pars tensa. The sinus tympani and the round window niche, the intact incus, the stapedial joint, the stapedial tendon and the pyramidal process are clearly visible. Several secretory vesicles are to be seen above them and in the recesses of the sinus tympani and the round window niche. 4-mm, 30° angled endoscope

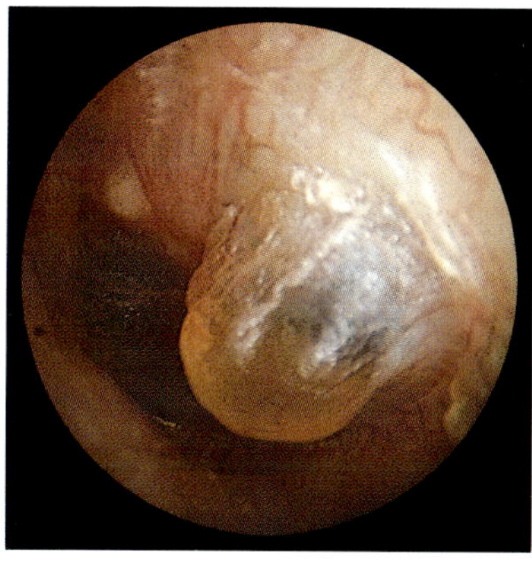

Fig. 246   Otitis media, with effusion and retraction of the atrophic tympanic membrane. The retraction of the posterosuperior quadrant is prolapsed by active, titrated insufflation via a tubal catheter. It is filled with serous secretion. The retraction has simultaneously stretched the pars flaccida, and the lateral epitympanic air cushions are filled with air. This is evidence that the posterior tympanic isthmus is open

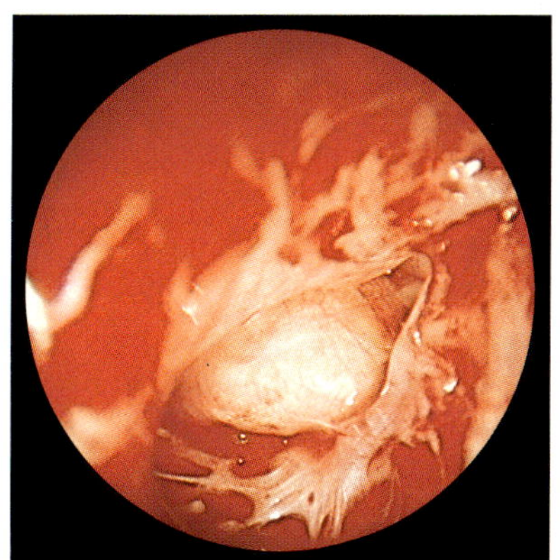

Fig. 247   Otitis media with effusion and retraction of the atrophic tympanic membrane. Operative endoscopy. The closed meatal skin tube is released together with the retraction of the pars tensa. Superior inspection with the straight 4-mm, 0° telescope. Numerous fine adhesive bands run obliquely over the entrance to the round window niche and to the subiculum. There are adhesions to the chorda tympani, the stapes, the stapedial tendon and the facial canal

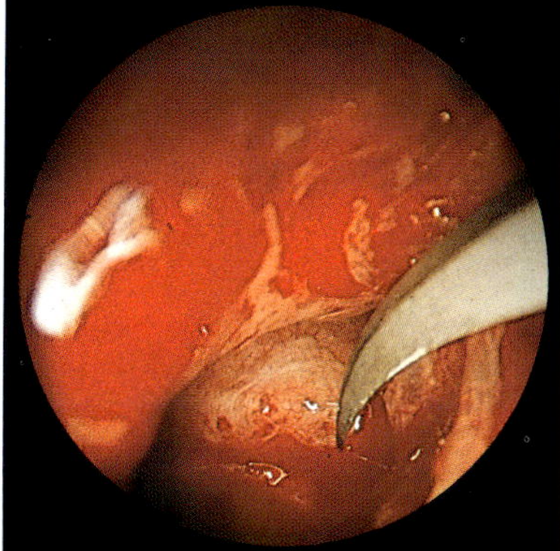

Fig. 248   Otitis media with effusion and retraction of the tympanic membrane. Operative endoscopy. The adhesions are released and the granulations are removed, the aeration and drainage pathways dissected with great care from the remaining middle ear mucosa and the intact fully mobile ossicular chain, using a straight 4-mm, 0° telescope and a fine sickle knife, and later, a fine double-cupped forceps

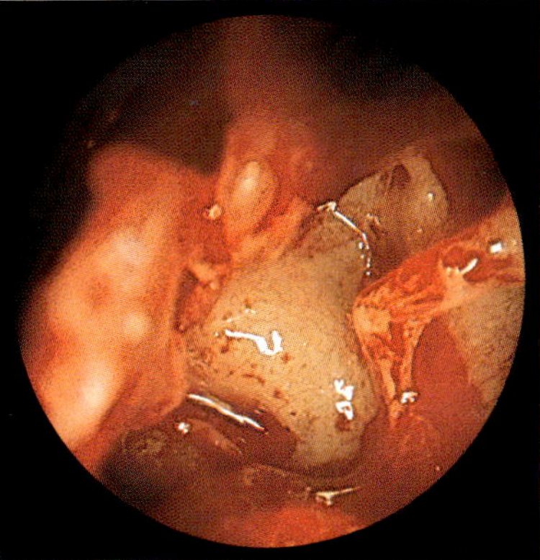

Fig. 249   Otitis media with effusion and retraction of the tympanic membrane. Operative endoscopy. The site after dissection and before reinforcement of the tympanic membrane with fascia and return of the closed meatal skin tube. Meatal packing and atraumatic step-wise closure of the supra-auricular skin incision follow

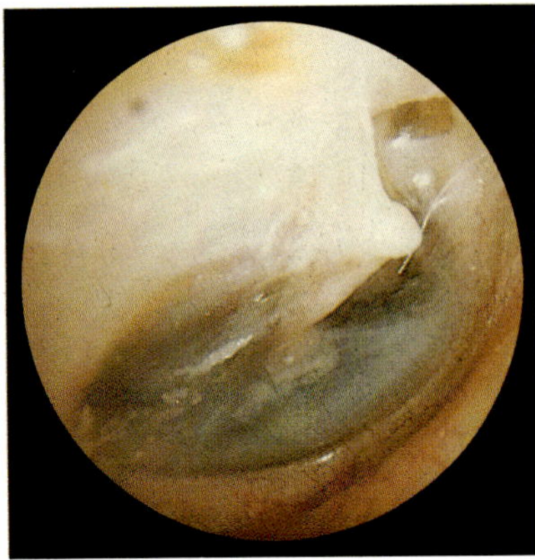

Fig. **250** **Adhesive otitis media.** Middle ear filled with yellowish-brown fluid. Retraction of the pars flaccida adherent to the neck of the malleus. Early atrophy of the collagen fiber layer can be recognized in the pars tensa

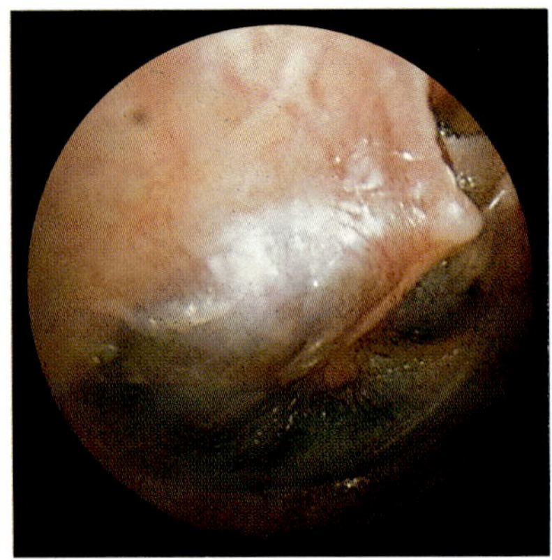

Fig. **251** **Adhesive otitis media, showing the same ear as in Fig. 250 after active and titrated insufflation with a tubal catheter.** The retraction of the pars flaccida remains adherent, a sign that the lateral air cushion does not contain air, and that the mucosal folds at the site are inflamed and adherent. There is a risk of development of an epitympanic retraction cholesteatoma. The posterosuperior quadrant of the pars tensa has protruded markedly after filling with air. A fluid level can now be clearly recognized in the mesohypotympanum on each side of the umbo

leads to the development of an antral cholesteatoma.

The tympanic diaphragm may undergo scar tissue retraction in its entire length. Superficial retraction of the two superior quadrants of the pars tensa as far as the facial canal is possibly accompanied by degeneration of the collagen fibers in this segment and adhesion of the atrophic Shrapnell's membrane, causing an increasing postinflammatory and atelectatic disorder of *all aeration pathways*. The pars tensa achieves contact with the promontory and the supratubal recess, the retraction pocket then extends into the sinus tympani and the hypotympanum. Finally, only the thin free epidermis of an atrophic adherent tympanic membrane remains over the tympanic ostium of the tube. The rest is adherent to the promontory and the upper and inferior aeration pathways. This remnant moves on the slightest increase of pressure by the Valsalva maneuvre, evidence that the entire eustachian tube is normal and that it opens into the tympanic cavity. If such a development is anticipated, it should be prevented by osteoplastic epitympanostomy.

The adhesion must be sought and released at its previously diagnosed point of origin. As in chronic seromucinous effusions and tympanosclerosis, it is critically important *to eliminate the disorder of aeration at its point of origin* before it causes progressive adhesions and mucosal atrophy.

Closure of the eustachian tube itself leads to deep retraction and complete adhesion of the atrophic pars tensa over the entire mesohypotympanum, extending as far as the ostium of the eustachian tube. The end of the indrawn sac cannot be seen, even with a 30° endoscope, because the air becomes completely absorbed so that the atrophic membrane extends deeply along the walls of the ostium.

The reciprocity due to opening and closing on swallowing, both whilst awake and asleep, with the intervening resorption phases, is the basic prerequisite for the coordinated action of the eustachian tube and the middle ear. Every therapeutic procedure must therefore be so designed that the function of this regulatory mechanism is maintained.

There are two anatomical reasons for the blockage of a ventilative air flow. One lies in the eustachian tube; the other, in the tympanic diaphragm. This theoretical background forms the basis for therapy. Successful treatment of otitis media with recurrent effusion, at any age, requires treatment of concomitant rhinitis and sinusitis, which in young children is no less important than adenoidectomy under endoscopic control. Exceptionally, large, deep-lying tonsils narrow the nasopharynx and the opening to the tube on swallowing. The motility of the tubal torus should be tested carefully in conjunction with that of the soft palate, looking for an occult cleft. Antiallergic treatment should be considered.

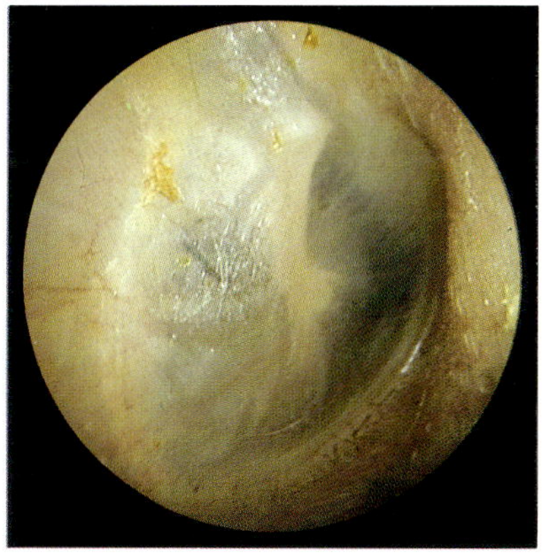

252

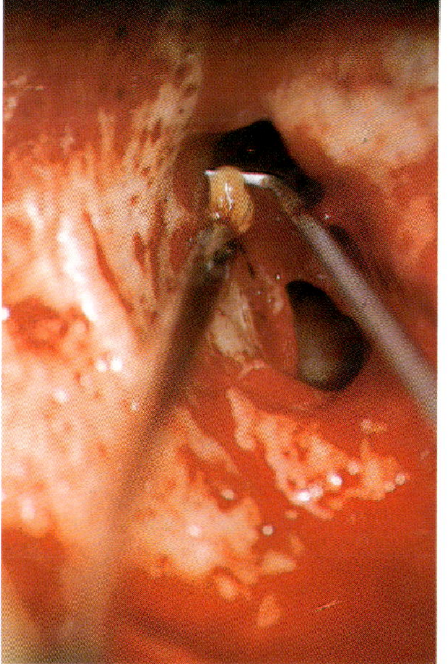

253

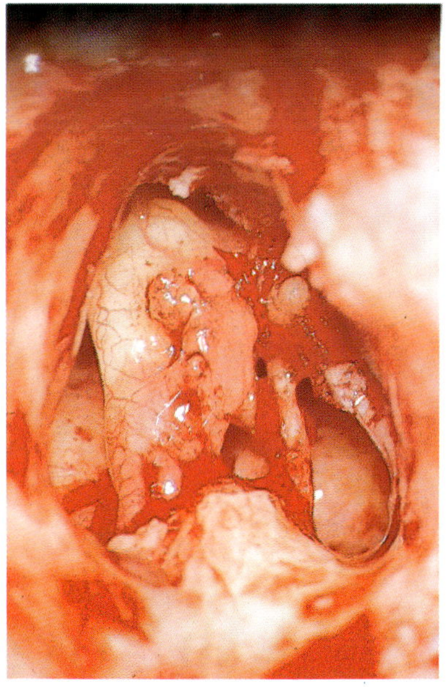

254

Fig. 252 The same ear as in Figs. 250–253, three months after operation. The tympanic membrane is in a normal position, Prussak's space contains air, and the pars flaccida and pars tensa are healthy

Fig. 253 Osteoplastic epitympanotomy of the same ear as in Figs. 250 and 251. The closed meatal skin tube and the tympanic membrane, together with the retraction of the pars flaccida, are freed, elevated and pressed onto the anterior meatal wall. A superior middle ear inspection has been carried out. The small choles-

terin cysts are removed from Prussak's space with a sucker and a 90° needle. The chorda tympani is also freed from adhesions and granulations

Fig. 254 Osteoplastic epitympanotomy of the same ear as shown in Figs. 250–252. After removal of the bony lid, the fibrous granulation tissue is removed. The inflamed folds of the lateral epitympanic air cushions are spread apart, with preservation of the neighboring mucosa. Dissection of the region of the tympanic diaphragm and exposure of the entire aeration and drainage pathways follows

Local treatment is limited initially to daily endoscopical toilet of the nose and the nasal passages, followed by inhalations (aerosol with vibration, pressure blast) and to paracentesis to allow aeration after aspiration of the effusion. The latter is almost always successful in children but, in adults and in some adolescents, catheterization of the eustachian tube with active insufflation is the therapy of choice.

The most successful and noninvasive treatment of children is a month's holiday in the high mountains. The most preferable areas are those with a dry climate at a height of 3,500–4,500 ft. in full sun, protected from the wind. In the morning the child should go up in a lift to about 7,500 ft., inducing a rapid change of pressure. The child should remain at this height for several hours, still protected from the wind, but in the sun. Soon after midday the child walks downhill again, thus undergoing gradual reverse action on the aerodynamic system.

Large towns with an unfavorable climate need a childrens' home with these characteristics during the months when winter sports are not possible.

Extensive surgical procedures are only to be considered for repeated brief recurrences. The introduction of ventilation tubes is easy and very popular, but the following three points should be remembered:

1. *This form of treatment does not treat the underlying disease.* Serous and mucous secretion cannot drain through the middle ear ventilation tubes. Exchange of air through the tubes leads only to equalization of pressure in the mesohypotympanum and the meatus and in no way affects the interaction between pressure in the anterior and posterior middle ear sectors. The meatal air differs from that previously processed by the nasal turbinate and the mucosa of the eustachian tube. In addition, the changing internal pressure due to tubal activity is absent. Most important of all, the ventilation lies in

the first narrowing of the middle ear system, but anterior to the second constriction. The drainage of secretion from this point is possibly facilitated if the secretion is not so viscous and is less copious. However, the epitympanic compartments are not aerated. The seromucinous effusion and the inflammatory degeneration of the walls endangers the mechanics of the most delicate part of the middle ear system for the later years of life. Furthermore, damage to the cochlea is a possibility, recognizable in its mildest form by an early loss at the higher frequencies between 10,000 Hz and 20,000 Hz, which cannot be diagnosed with current conventional audiometers (Wullstein and Wullstein, Schlitt, 1985).

2. *Iatrogenic sequelae can occur.* The frequent clinical sequelae of middle ear ventilation include purulent otitis media, atrophy and perforation of the tympanic membrane, scars and iatrogenic cholesteatoma of the pars tensa. So long as the physiological equalization of internal pressure has not been restored, there is no guarantee that the function of both sectors of the middle ear has returned to normal.

3. *The final results on the pathology and function of the middle ear of the abnormal and interrupted development are not fully known for several years.* The immediate improvement of hearing is good because the temporary obstruction to sound conduction is relieved. The results several months or years later are usually no better than those without the use of ventilation tubes. There is concern about the ultimate outcome many years later because of the danger of scar tissue and sclerotic lesions of the folds. If the result after the first introduction of the middle ear ventilation tube is good and remains so, then it may be suspected that it was used too soon and unnecessarily. If the ventilation tube must be introduced a second or further time, then the doubts for the maintainance of a good effect in the distant future are even greater. Procedures directed at the cause might be more suitable and less troublesome than the introduction of ventilation tubes together with prophylactic use of antibiotics in high doses, which are regarded in many centers as necessary, but which also lead to resistance.

Our body is so created as to heal wounds and to release living forces which contribute to recovery. This also applies to the operative trauma of an adequate size, but not to paracentesis because the damage is too minimal. In this case, the site is the epitympanum. Mastoidectomy is not the right procedure, either on local or pathological grounds.

A more minor operation which can be considered is *irrigation of the epitympanum* to allow aspiration of the mesotympanum. It is carried out from the opened antrum (antrotomy) after release of Shrapnell's membrane (upper cavity opening) through the same supraauricular incision. The folds, which are also thickened and adherent, are parted, and the interossicular clefts cleared (operative endoscopy is illustrated in Figs. **247–249**). Whether the necessary aeration of the epitympanic compartments has been achieved satisfactorily cannot be assessed immediately with certainty. If necessary, this operation can be extended as an epitympanotomy.

A more logical surgical method is a planned osteoplastic epitympanotomy, which makes antrotomy unnecessary. In the hands of an experienced surgeon, it is scarcely more invasive than the procedure named above. It permits precise assessment of the character of the disease of the folds, breakdown of the individual adhesions, clearance of early granulations, mucopolypoidal reactions, and secures air exchange as far as the antrum (Figs. **252–253**). *The planning of the operative procedure* is determined by the following criteria:

- What were the otoscopic and endoscopic findings of the tympanic membrane immediately before the operation?
- Does the pars tensa *together with* the pars flaccida move sufficiently with a simple Valsalva maneuver, or only after active tubal inflation with the catheter? (This demonstrates how far and in what manner the epitympanic compartments are refilled with air via the tympanic isthmi.)
- Does the pars tensa move, whilst the pars flaccida remains indrawn, showing that the epitympanic compartments are blocked and not actively refilled with air?
- Does the atrophic indrawn part of the pars tensor remain adherent or does it bulge out, with or without a content of secretion?
- Has the effusion dispersed into the middle ear space or partially emptied into the eustachian tube, or has it been sucked back into the epitympanic spaces because of its viscous-elastic properties?
- Does the Toynbee maneuver cause immediate indrawing of the atrophic atelectatic tympanic membrane, accompanied by simultaneous subjective worsening of hearing?
- Does emptying of the middle ear proceed as rapidly as refilling with air?
- What is the hearing threshold, between 8 and 10 kHz, and between 18 and 20 kHz?
- What is the shape of the impedance curve?
- What was the appearance on Schueller's view and axial views of the skull of the paranasal sinuses especially the ethmoid sinuses?

The Operation (Figs. 255–264)

After access has been obtained as always along the temporal squama and with release of the Shrapnell's membrane, the antrum is opened through the retromeatal cribriform zone, and access is extended with the diamond burr as far as the short process of the incus. If endoscopy from this point as well as via the anterior inspection opening shows that the compartments are only loosely obstructed, vigorous suction is applied on both sides, followed by inflation and further suction. This is followed by irrigation with Ringer's solution or a suitable disinfectant. If tubal inflation before the operation was difficult, which is unusual, a tube is placed in the antrum for a short period of postoperative local treatment with Ringer's solution. Shrapnell's membrane must be carefully replaced. The effect of the meatal packing does not extend beyond 48–72 hours. Beyond this time the air content must be checked by inflation of the eustachian tube and the removal of the tube from the antrum (see Figs. 255–260).

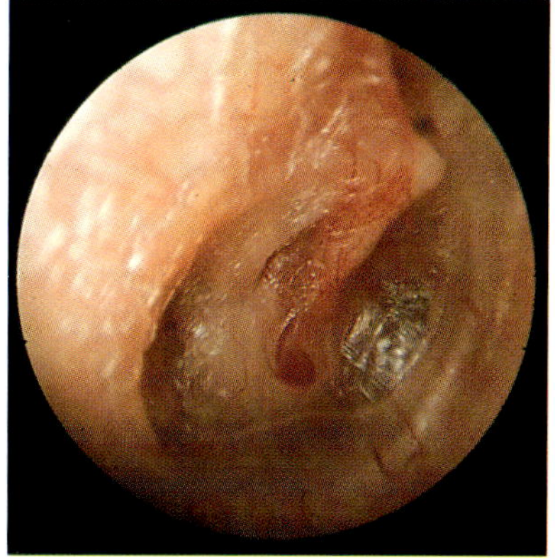

Fig. 255 Otitis media with effusion and atelectasis. The tympanic membrane moves with the Politzer maneuver, and the secretion collects in the hypotympanum. The middle ear cavity is pumped empty with the next swallowing act. The atrophic tympanic membrane collapses progressively in the absence of reserve air in the posterior segment of the middle ear, and an adhesive process begins to develop

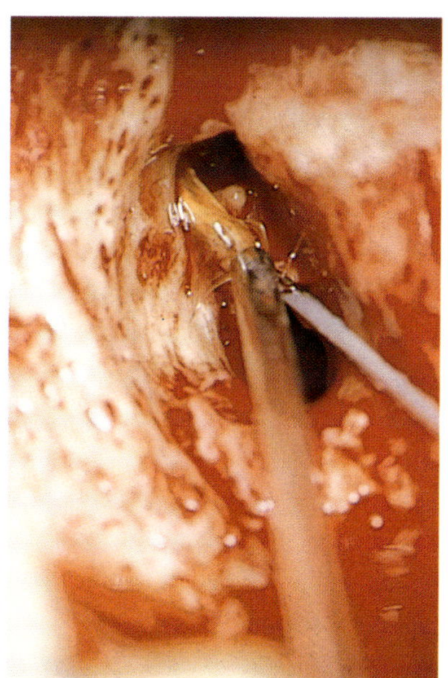

Fig. 256 Otitis media with effusion and atelectasis, showing the same ear as in Fig. 255. A superior middle ear inspection at the beginning of an epitympano-antromastoidectomy. Thickened, yellow, and very viscous secretion is being sucked out of Prussak's space

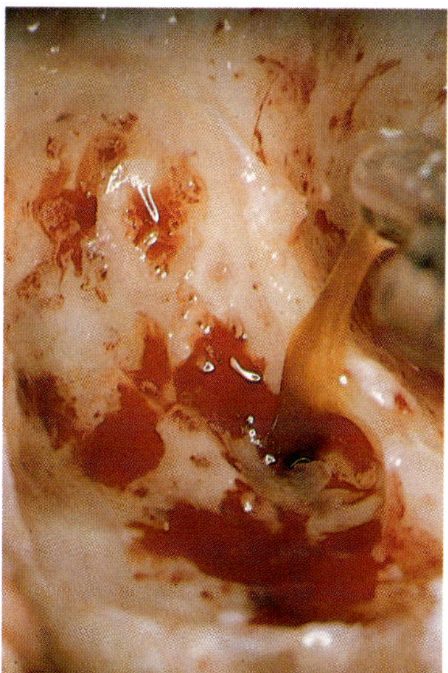

Fig. 257 Otitis media with effusion and atelectasis, showing the same ear as in Figs. 255–256 undergoing epitympano-antromastoidectomy. Eradication of the diseased mastoid cells begins in the retromeatal cribriform zone and posterior to the suprameatal spine. The thickened mucosal secretion is sucked out after opening the first cells

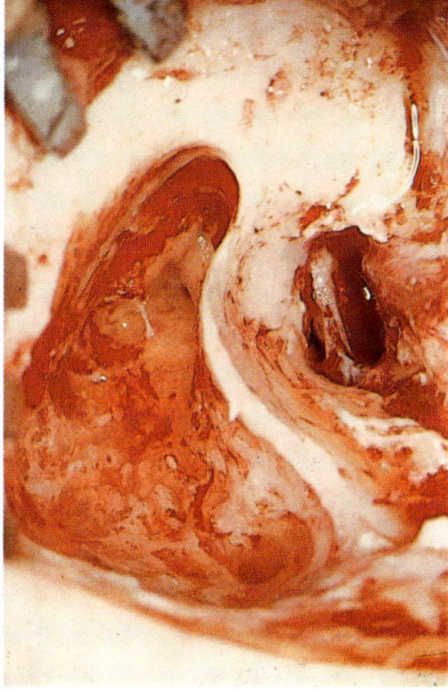

Fig. 258 Otitis media with effusion and atelectasis, showing the same ear as in Figs. 255–257, undergoing epitympano-antromastoidectomy. The cell system of the posterior sector is almost completely cleared. Endoscopic inspection of the second constriction via the tympanic and epitympanic routes follows (Figs. 259, 260)

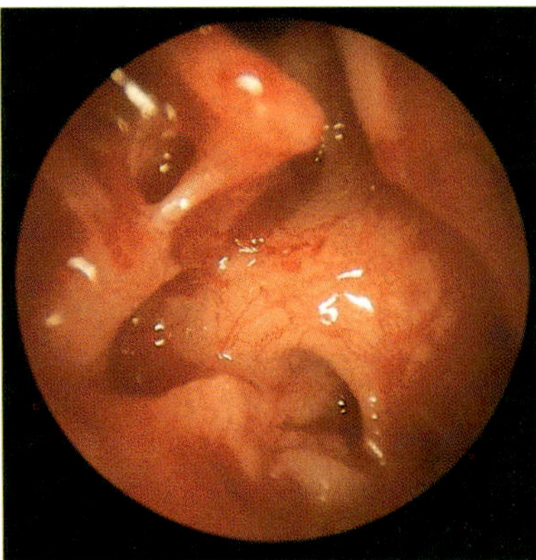 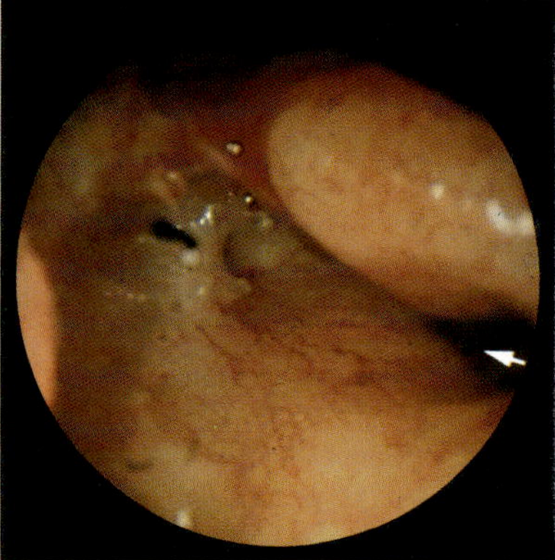

Fig. **259   Otitis media with effusion and atelectasis. Operative
endoscopy** of the same ear as
shown in Figs. **255–258** undergoing epitympano-antromastoidectomy. An anterior view through a
straight 0°, 4-mm endoscope. Evaluation of the second constriction
on the tympanic side around the
long process of the incus, the
stapes with its tendon shows swollen folds and adhesions. The entire
region of the diaphragm is obstructed, but the round window niche is free. The mucosa in the mesohypotympanum is swollen but
well vascularized and with no polypoid swelling on the surface. The
sinus tympani is divided by the styloid prominence and the chorda
tympani into a posterior and a
lateral sinus

Fig. **260   Otitis media with effusion and atelectasis. Operative
endoscopy.** Retrotympanic inspection of the second constriction with
a 4-mm, lateral 30° endoscope, introduced into the epitympanum and
giving a view of the free aeration
and drainage pathways between
the ossicles and the lateral semicircular canal and the facial canal, as
far as the stapes, which is marked
with an arrow

If the ossicles are embedded in granulations in the epitympanum, the operation should be continued as an osteoplastic epitympanotomy. If the radiographs show that the region around the aditus and the antrum is denser than the opacity of the mastoid, the surgeon will usually elect to carry out an epitympanotomy immediately. The entire tegmen and the ossicular area are freed of granulations, using the sickle knife, the curved or the angled needle and fine suction tubes. The greatest care is exercized to retain any surviving mucosa to assist in healing. The middle ear spaces are filled with gelatin sponge (pledgets of gelfoam impregnated with Ringer's solution, an antibiotic and possibly cortisone). Inflation also begins in these cases two to three days later. This procedure is only slightly more difficult, but is more reliable with respect to long-term functional results and prevents any iatrogenic lesions (Figs. **252–253**).

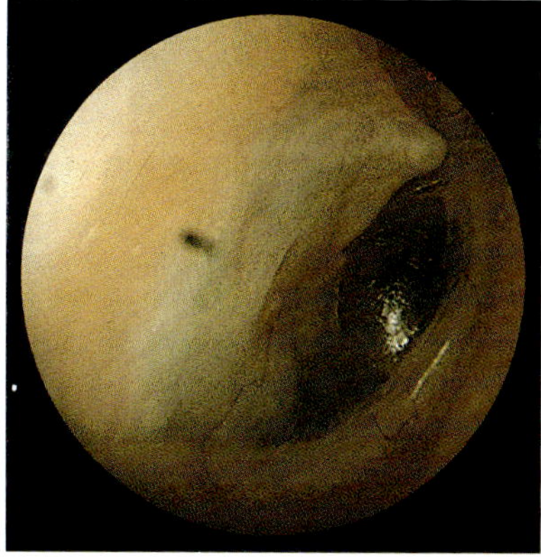

Fig. **261 Condition twelve months after operation.** The reinforcement due to interposition of the fascial graft in the posterior pars tensa can be clearly recognized. The middle ear is well aerated, and the eustachian tube functions normally

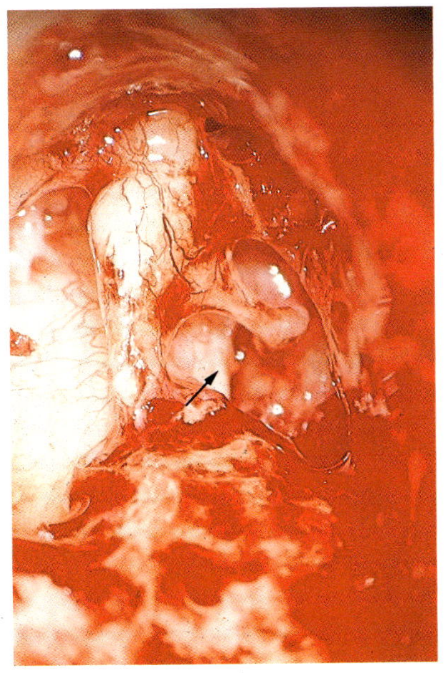

Fig. **262 Osteoplastic epitympanotomy and stapedectomy for clinical otosclerosis** with a prolapsed facial nerve in its horizontal course (marked by an arrow) widely exposed over the oval niche and the stapes. View after division of the incudostapedial joint and removal of the stapedial crura

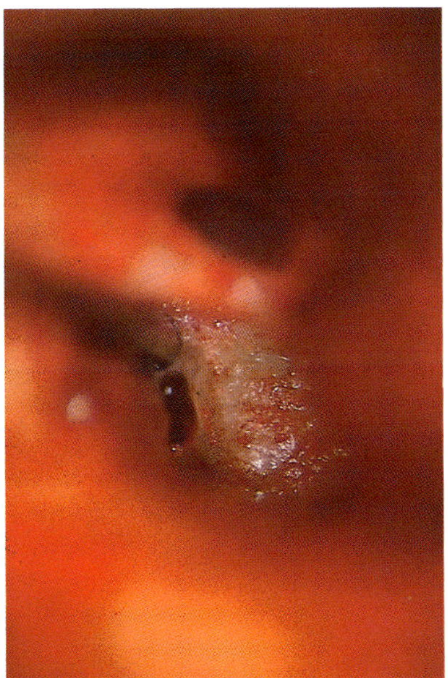

Fig. **263 Osteoplastic epitympanotomy and stapedectomy.** A newly created window (with a fluid level) on the promontorial wall of the niche. Medial to this lies the exposed facial nerve

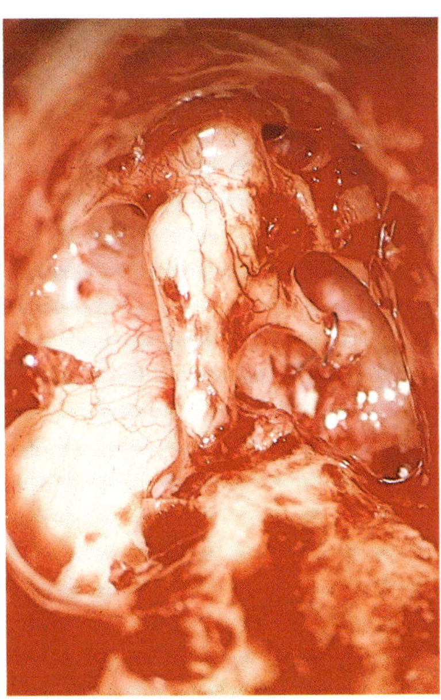

Fig. **264 Osteoplastic epitympanotomy.** After covering of the window, the steel wire prosthesis is inserted and its loop fastened to the long process of the incus above the lentiform process

The Eustachian Tube

The course of the eustachian tube running below and within the base of the skull becomes increasingly complicated in animals higher up the phylogenetic scale. The relation of the length of the sphenoid to the basisphenoid with the basiclinoid affects the angulation of the sphenoid and the relationships of the middle to the posterior cranial fossa, thus also affecting the eustachian tube. The bony eustachian tube develops from a series of centers inferior to the middle cranial fossa. The bony eustachian tube plus a part of the tympanic plate joins the cartilaginous plate in the sulcus of the pharyngotympanic tube on the inferior surface of the base of the sphenoid, the transitional zone between the stiff part of the tube and the expansible part. This area can be well demonstrated by inflation of the cartilaginous part on a computer tomogram; for example, in a search for tubal polyps in the part of its course lined by glandular mucosa.

The superior wall of the bony eustachian tube with the canal of the tensor tympani muscle is separated by a thin bony wall from the middle cranial fossa close to the inferior wall of the sulcus for the greater petrosal nerve. Its inner wall forms the carotid canal. This is the region of close contact of the squamous bone and the tympanic plate of the temporal bone with the sphenoidal spine, the petrous crest, the petrosquamous and petrotympanic fissures, as well as the soft tissues of the infratemporal fossa. Pneumatization along the bony tube is found in mammals; it is most developed in the human.

The cartilaginous part of the eustachian tube has an extensive, rich lining of ciliary and goblet cells and is surrounded by mucous glands and lymphoid follicles. The concentration of goblet cells and ciliary cells decreases from the nasal cavity to the middle ear. It is particularly at risk from chronic inflammation of the neighboring ethmoidal cells: secretions flow from this sinus over the inferior turbinate to the ostium of the tube. Therefore, every treatment-planning of tympanoplasty begins with thorough assessment of the ducts of the sinuses, the pharyngeal ostium of the tube and Rosenmueller's fossa during opening and closing, using rigid endoscopes of various angles. The flexible endoscope provides a view in depth of a large part of the course of the cartilaginous tube with the help of inflation.

When the eustachian tube opens momentarily to allow refilling under normal physiological conditions, only a small quantity of air, which is processed by the mucous cells of the hypotympanum, is required for the mesohypotympanum. The air of the anterior segment slowly restores the reservoir in the posterior segment. Little further mucosal activity is necessary posterior to the tympanic diaphragm; thus, the mucosa is extraordinarily poor in accessory structures at that point, and no debris is produced.

Disorders of Tubal Function
(Figs. 265–267)

The tympanogram provides little information about the pathology of the *epitympanum* during assessment for tympanoplasty because of the close collaboration between the eustachian tube and the anterior and posterior segments of the middle ear.

The tympanogram curves measuring a system's impedance show the sum of various values of middle ear pressure change and sound wave resistance: The series of factors involved apparently relate more to those closer to the tympanic membrane than to those distant from it.

Kumazawa et al. (1974) have confirmed that the peaks differ between successive measurements, first passing from high pressure to low pressure (the "forward" measurement, as usual) and then from low pressure to high pressure (the "backward" measurement); in his view, the average value is to be regarded as definitive.

The tympanic membrane moves very sluggishly in an external direction in the presence of a thick, *mucus effusion* of the *anterior segment*. If the anterior sector is healthy, but the posterior segment is completely filled, the pars tensa moves normally, but Shrapnell's membrane follows with a very slug-

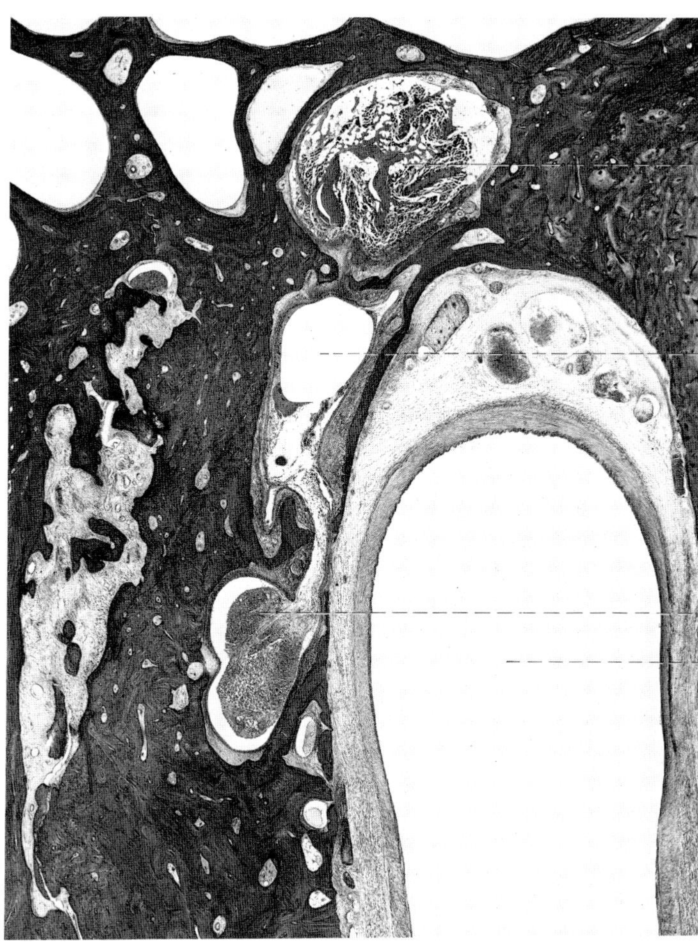

Fig. **265** **Relation of the eustachian tube and the paratubal cells to the carotid canal in the temporal bone** (H. L. Wullstein 1968)

gish external movement. The sudden air stream then strikes the tympanic membrane in the anterior segment. The tympanic membrane can only bulge very slowly because the middle ear is filled with viscid secretions, since air or watery secretions which can readily escape into the antrum are not retained in the epitympanum.

Kumazawa et al. (1974) have differentiated impedance measurements by their tubo-tympano-aerodynamogram, which records the after-vibrations of the tympanic membrane. These are very informative about the two middle ear segment. In this test, the air, which can be measured by deviation of the tympanic membrane, penetrates to the window niches of the *anterior* segment. This air builds up in front of the diaphragm because the isthmus is not equally patent for rising and falling pressure. According to Kumazawa, the steep rise a−b in the curve (Fig. **267**) is the time of ingress of air, and lasts about 0.5 sec. After the tube closes, the increased air pressure due to the Valsalva manoeuver falls from b−c, but not to the initial atmospheric pressure. A slightly increased level (c−d) remains

until the next swallow (d−e). It appears that the modest persistent increased pressure is too weak to hold the cartilaginous tube open until equalization is completely achieved.

The following hypothesis can be put forward: if the patient does not swallow, the fall of pressure from c to e proceeds slowly. The quantity of air necessary for refilling flows gradually into the *posterior* middle ear segment through the tympanic diaphragm, and the necessary congested pressure is equalized via the spaces of the entire mastoid process. This gradual refilling in the posterior segment affects the pockets of the folds, particularly the small ones between the head of the malleus and the lateral bony wall, including the visible Prussak's space.

Six disorders of tubal function can be defined, 4 intrinsic and 2 extrinsic.

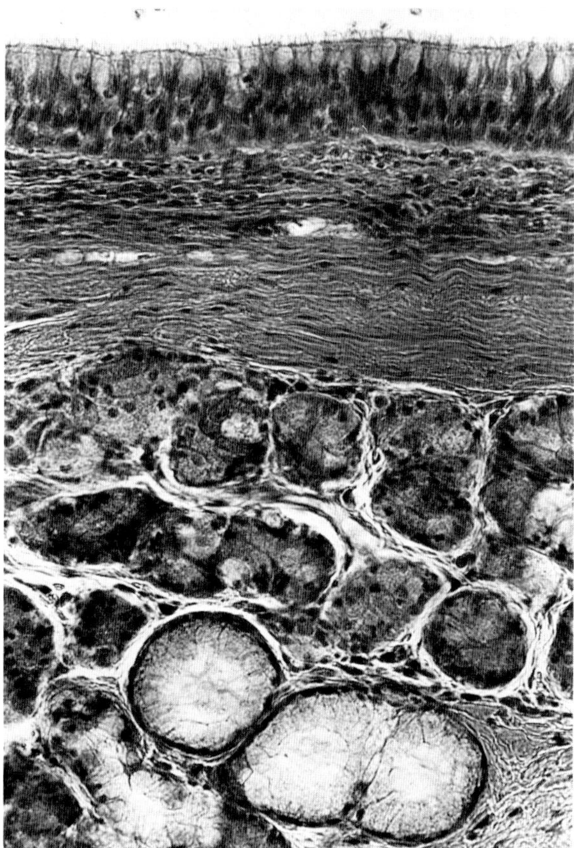

Fig. **266   Mucosa of the cartilaginous tube** (370 × magnification). Multilayered ciliated epithelium with goblet cells and rich acinous glands (H. L. Wullstein 1968)

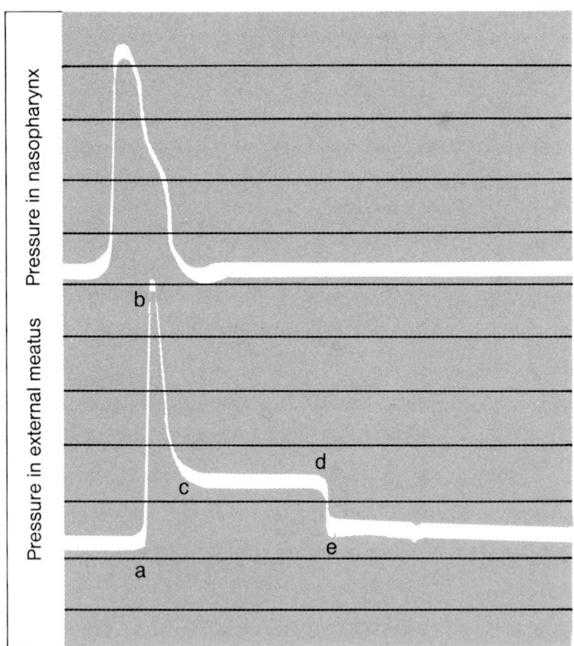

Fig. **267** Upper: **Pressure in the nasopharynx.** Lower: **Pressure in the meatus** (Kumazawa 1974)

Intrinsic Obstructions

1. Partial or total blockage of the *tympanic ostium.* Massive chronic mucosal inflammation extends from the supratubal recess and the start of the hypotympanum (i.e., the sacculus of the promontory, the bony recess in the inferior mesohypotympanic aeration pathway at the level where the carotid canal lies close to the inferior edge of the promontory) into the ostium of the tube. It can be reduced easily by pricking and sucking on compressed cotton wool. Polyps should be removed. Small or medium-sized polyps lying medial to the ossicles may remain hidden from view in the closed technique. This is also true of polyps on a pedicle in the protympanic recess and may also apply to unusually large polyps which function as valves at the opening of the eustachian tube and may even be sucked inside it.

The *tympanic ostium* is seldom completely obstructed due to *ossification* and *formation of osteophytes.* Provided that disease is confined to the distal end, the bony segment can be reopened successfully using the diamond burr. It is helpful to look for the canal of the tensor tympani muscle and to resect the muscle in its entire length, which is indicated in any case because of the chronic myositis. The open lumen of the bony eustachian tube is reached in short stenoses (care is needed for the internal carotid artery). The absent mucosa must be replaced as after clearance of the bony ostium of cholesteatoma matrix. Healthy mucoperiosteum from the labyrinthine wall may be used if it is present, or a nonkeratinising split mucosal graft from the lip applied to any available original tissue from the tubotympanic mucosa. Amnion may be used for small defects.

2. Atresia of the bony and cartilaginous segment of the tube.
Atresia of the *entire bony tube* and *connective tissue atresia of the cartilaginous tube* are difficult to correct. Attempts to bypass the atresia by exposing the bony tube through the middle cranial fossa or by diverting the air through the accessory nasal sinuses have been unsuccessful. Reconstruction is possible using an osteoplastic epitympanotomy with cover by an arch of plasticine glued with mucosal substitute to achieve early aeration as far as the antrum.

3. Inflammation and constriction of the bony and cartilaginous segments; the patulous tube due to mucosal atrophy.
Chronic mucosal inflammation of various grades of severity within the bony eustachian tube almost always heals, even very edematous swellings with a

tendency to form polyps, mucosa with deep inflammatory infiltration, and mucoperiostitis with chronic disease of the peritubal cells in the bony tube. The greatest diameter of these peritubal cells can exceed that of the lumen of the tube.

Inflammation in the *cartilaginous* tube affects not only the epithelial layer, producing increased goblet cels, but also the mucosal glands of the submucosal layer and especially the peritubal lymphoid follicles. It is therefore resistant to treatment. The extent of the ossification of the lumen of the bony tube can possibly be demonstrated by axial CT scans, but that of the cartilaginous tube can only be demonstrated with simultaneous inflation of the tube by Valsalva's maneuver.

Reliable evaluation of the inflammatory swelling can be achieved during the operation, if necessary, by gentle catheterization of the tube. The resistance serves as an index of the intensity and length of the inflammatory swelling. At the juction of the bony and cartilaginous tubes there is a danger, in marked stenosis, that the semirigid probe can penetrate the subcranial vascular sheath along the internal carotid artery and pass into the soft tissues of the neck.

4. Functional disorders and blockage of the tubal torus, and adhesions of the nasopharyngeal ostium; the patulous tube due to congenital anomalies.

Transnasal endoscopy with rigid or flexible systems is indispensible for assessment of the tubal torus and the surrounding nasopharynx, beginning with a search for remnants of the adenoid in Rosenmueller's fossa and for cicatricial stenosis of the cartilaginous eustachian tube. The latter is usually due to an excessive adenoidectomy. Previously it was often due to syphilis, and nowadays is frequently caused by tuberculosis of the nasopharyngeal mucosa. Tuberculosis heals with chemotherapy, but does require prolonged follow-up because of the persistent marked tendency to form further cicatritial stenosis, which renders a reconstructive procedure on the tubal torus not only difficult but also of very doubtful value. Exceptionally, a viral papillomatosis can extend from the nasopharynx to the middle ear via the eustachian tube.

Inspection with the endoscope has improved the early diagnosis of carcinoma deep in the tubal torus. It can only be distinguished from tuberculosis by biopsy.

Treatment of Chronic Salpingitis in Chronic Middle Ear Inflammation

Occasionally, however, rarely, this disease can heal spontaneously without treatment in the course of years. Local outpatient treatment may achieve temporary success, but whether this is long maintained is very uncertain. Permanent healing is achieved by tympanoplasty because the natural aeration of the closed aerodynamic system is restored. *For this reason, H. L. Wullstein (1952) has insisted on a one-stage operation for chronic middle ear inflammation since the introduction of tympanoplasty.*

Treatment of chronic tubal inflammation requires endoscopic assessment of the ostia of the nasal sinuses, particularly the anterior and posterior ethmoid sinuses, and elimination of chronic rhinosinusitis.

Postoperative treatment of the eustachian tube, like that of the middle ear, should be restricted to a few days. This is particularly true of local antibiotic treatment. The agent should be determined by culture and sensitivity tests, and should be administered from the middle ear and from the eustachian tube using catheterization with active insufflation. Prolonged preoperative treatment is unsuccessful and causes increased sensitization of the mucosa and reduction of the powers of resistance of the tissue.

Drainage of secretion from the tubal torus can often be observed with the endoscope after treatment of the middle meatus of the nose. If a chronic ethmoid inflammation does not heal rapidly with local conservative treatment, an ethmoidectomy is indicated. Measurement of the tubal resistance (first described by Zoellner in 1942) using the impedance meter is very useful for demonstrating restored tubal function, but inflation is difficult. The prerequisite for this is a well-executed tympanoplasty.

The recognition and treatment of chronic salpingitis using the special flexible nasopharyngeal endoscope, with inflation of the cartilaginous eustachian tube, facilitates local diagnosis and treatment. Preoperative endoscopy should be carried out for every profuse secretory mucopolypoid otitis media because mucopolypoid inflammation can extend along the entire length of the eustachian tube. The deep effect of the infection is limited to the spaces with bony walls, so long as periostitis and osteitis have not developed. In contrast, in the cartilaginous eustachian tube, there is a phlegmonus inflammation due to chronic inflammation of the gland acini, the peritubal soft tissues and the lymph follicles. The endoscopic view shows not only the severe chronic infiltrating swelling and suppuration of the mucosa, which may at some points be polypoidal, but also plaque-like swelling of the severely infected lymphoid follicles. A single careful diagnostic probing of the eustachian tube during the operation serves to squeeze the secretions from the mucosa, and even tear off a polyp, but an impression of the intratubal conditions is not obtained.

After careful opening of the mucosal swelling, pricking and sucking of the edema through a compressed surgical cotton wool plug and removal of polypoid mucosa from all segments of the middle ear, a plastic catheter is introduced into the tympanic tubal ostium, and the area is thoroughly irrigated with disinfectant.

This is followed by the introduction of a broad-spectrum antibiotic effective against pyocyaneus, proteus and coli, as well as an electrolyte solution to fill the middle ear cavity. At the end of the operation, the eustachian tube is irrigated energetically several times, firstly using disinfectant, followed by a saline solution and then filled in its entire course with an antibiotic-electrolyte solution. Finally, the middle ear spaces are filled with gelatin sponge. As demonstrated above, the marked local effect is lost within two to three days.

Excessive deflation is the result of lowered tubal resistance or of a temporary or longstanding open tube. In many people this happens occasionally under certain circumstances. The cartilaginous tube may have been too lax since youth, due to an unsatisfactory return to the closed position. On the other hand, it may be the result of marked atrophy of the mucosa and its accessory structures, and inadequate formation of mucus in later life. The film of mucosal secretion consists of a gel layer, an interpolated surfactant and a sol layer. If the walls of the lumen are expanded, the film is no longer sufficient for the walls to adhere in the resting position during increased breathing and especially during speech, causing autophony. Phases of inadequate production of secretions and deficient closure are common after resolution of a nasopharyngeal catarrh and are signs of an early mucosal atrophy. It may be that autonomic influences play a role. Such an atrophy arises on one side only, if the tubal or middle ear catarrh was usually unilateral in earlier years. Kumazawa (1985) has shown that obstruction is caused by sympathicomimetic action and reduced by parasympathicomimetic effects.

The symptoms of longstanding autophony may be reduced by submucous injection of paraffin into the entrance to the tubal torus, but this has now been abandoned because the dose is too difficult to calculate and the material is not tolerated. If too much is injected, the resistance to inflation becomes too great and its sequelae then replace the auto-

phony and continuous deflation. If the risk of infection of the middle ear due to the temporarily patent tube can be demonstrated to be very great, especially in children, a natural form of treatment is a holiday at the seaside, with saline and iodine breezes. Exhausting sunbathing in hot, airless conditions is injurious.

Extrinsic Obstructions

5. Extratubal compression arising in the middle cranial fossa.
Intracranial extratubal obstruction can be caused by neoplasms in the greater wing of the sphenoid because the bony eustachian tube lies immediately under its floor. The most frequent lesions are meningiomas (which are to be regarded pathologically as fibroblast hamartomas of the dura), benign and malignant tumors of various types, and osteodystrophy.

6. Compression arising in the infratemporal, pterygopalatine and retromaxillary fossae.
Obstruction of the cartilaginous tube *from the inferior side* is caused by benign and malignant tumors in the infratemporal, retromaxillary or pterygopalatine fossae. Apart from the conductive deafness, the clinical picture is dominated by pain in the second or third divisions of the fifth cranial nerve, particularly if the tumor is malignant. The pain is localized to the middle cranial fossa, the parietal region, or the teeth; unfortunately, the toothache is misdiagnosed for a long time by neurologists or dentists.

A CT scan of the base of the skull is urgently indicated for every early disorder of aeration of the middle ear with a suspicion of an extrinsic obstruction and especially in the presence of persisting pain or trismus.

A long-term perforation in the anteroinferior quadrant is indicated for permanent obstruction of the middle ear due to extrinsic blockage, especially if it is due to a malignant tumor.

Tympanoplasty in Trauma of the Temporal Bone

Trauma to the temporal bone, ranging from circumscribed and concealed lesions to serious open compound fractures, is primarily a surgical problem. This chapter describes the use of tympanoplasty to restore the function of the middle ear. Procedures for reconstruction of the facial nerve do not fall within the limit of this monograph. Plasticine, consisting of a mixture of pentacalcium hydroxide triphosphate and biological tissue glue, constitutes a major advance, sealing the fracture site and, in so doing, promoting healing.

Isolated Fresh Injuries of the Tympanic Membrane

(Fig. **268**)

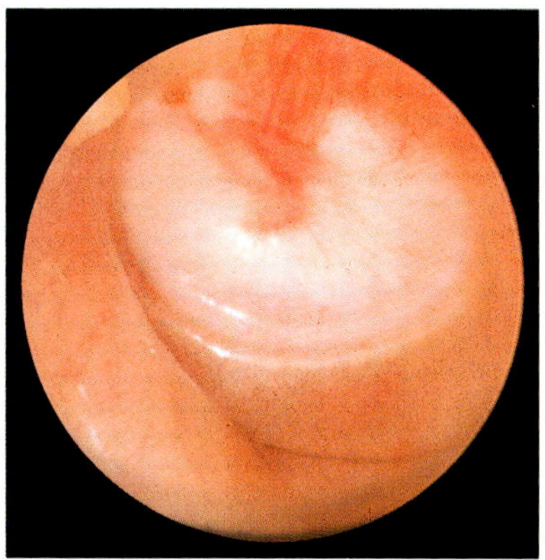

Fig. **268**   **Posttraumatic cholesteatoma**

Even large noninfected tears heal spontaneously. If the edges of the cutis have become rolled inward, they must be rolled out again and maintained in this position by the introduction of a gelatin sponge. Tears which do not heal spontaneously develop eventually into a round perforation; they must be closed by tympanoplasty. However, small perforations with healthy collagenous fiber framework extending to the edges of the perforation can be induced to heal spontaneously by mild stimulation (with 5% or 10% silver nitrate, for example). All traumatic perforations are closed, observing the rules already laid down for inflammatory lesions.

The problem is rendered more complex if the acoustic trauma causes subluxation of the ossicular chain: occasionally an incudostapedial dislocation is visible through the perforation. In this case the hearing does not improve when a patch is laid over the perforation, and the ossicular chain must be reconstituted surgically by osteoplastic epitympanotomy, either at the same time as the perforation is closed or after spontaneous healing.

Delay is advisable if the injury is associated with acoustic trauma of the cochlea, to allow the inner ear to recover before it is exposed to further trauma (the noise of the drill, for example).

Simultaneous acoustic damage to the middle and inner ear can be very serious. The sequelae include severe sensorineural deafness or complete deafness on both sides, and bilateral tears of the tympanic membrane, possibly complicated by middle ear infection. A tympanoplasty is urgently indicated; it will also make the wearing of a permanent hearing aid possible. Such trauma is typical of mine and grenade explosions, in which bilateral blindness often occurs because the injured person was hit while bent forward, walking, in search of explosive material. The only communication with the outside world for such a patient is then through a remnant of hearing in one ear, with complete deafness of the other ear.

Shattering of the Mastoid Process and the Squamous Temporal Bone; Temporal Bone Injury due to Foreign Bodies (Shot) (Figs. 269–271)

Shattering of the mastoid process due to local trauma requires wide exposure by a retrosuprauricular exposure and debridement of the mastoid process, preferably extending to the two cranial fossae. Dural injuries and CSF fistulae are nowadays localized most reliably using the microscope. Careful irrigation and suction, and filling with gelatin sponge are necessary. If the fracture extends into the posterior meatal wall, a simple solution is the replacement and reconstruction of the bony meatal wall, using the shattered fragments embedded in a plasticine disc with careful wide contact to the bone and cover with fascia (Fig. **91**). If too little mucosa remains, the inferior part of the mastoid cavity can be completely filled with plasticine and closed off from the remaining antral cavity by fascia. If the medial wall and the apex of the mastoid process are also fractured and no longer provide an attachment for the sternocleidomastoid muscle, they should be removed.

Fracture lines of the temporal bone, particularly in children, have the remarkable property of expanding if the dura protrudes through them and pulsates. The immediate surgical goal must be the stimulation of ossification. Plasticine can also be used for this purpose; it is pressed onto the cortical bone to bridge the defect and produce abundant ossification of its edges.

Closure of a dural tear and a CSF fistula in the tegmen tympani with maintainance of the ossicular system is achieved by an osteoplastic epitympanotomy, which provides a view of the traumatized region and all the ossicles. This procedure shortens and widens access to the floor of the middle cranial fossa as far as the arcuate eminence. A bone strip is drilled out of the temporal squama, superior to the tegmen tympani. It should be wide enough and long enough to allow the dura to be elevated from the floor of the middle cranial fossa beyond the arcuate eminence. A stab incision is now made to release the CSF. Prolapsed brain should be replaced carefully and held in place by a solid allogenic or xenogenic membrane; for example, lyophilized dura or "Neotymp", glued over the defect. If a wide bone defect is present, it is filled with plasticine. The epitympanic wall is then replaced and the external auditory meatus reconstituted.

This otosurgical procedure, carried out immediately after shock has been controlled, is much less invasive than neurosurgical procedures in which the temporal lobe is elevated. A premature intracranial procedure in this type of fracture can lead to a fatal relapse into shock.

Dural tears of the posterior cranial fossa are rarer. If they lie medial to the sinus in Trautmann's triangle, they should be closed by a plasticine plate with fascia glued over it. Dural tears lateral to the sinus should be sutured and glued; they can be covered by the postauricular galea. More extensive lesions should be treated by a procedure similar to that for the middle cranial fossa.

Small injuries to the sinus which can be controlled by packing within the mastoid process, or those which only ooze, are closed by suture of the walls, leaving the sinus patent. This is most simply achieved with suture and adhesive, using double layers of fascia or periosteum and massive plugging of the mastoid cavity with plasticine under pressure. Severe bleeding from the sinus must always be closed if there is an opportunity to do so; first, anterior to the jugular bulb (taking care to prevent air embolus) and then superior to the sinus.

The most thorough treatment is to inspect *fresh deep fractures, fracture lines and defects of the posterior meatal wall* from the mastoid, and to fill out the contour of the meatus as appropriate with plasticine. A skin defect in the meatus is then closed with fascia or full-thickness skin glued into place.

A *fresh open fracture line* carries the danger of infection. After elevating the skin-periosteal sleeve via a postauricular incision, the projecting edges are smoothed with a diamond burr. The cell system is opened wide enough to permit evaluation of the extent of the fracture line, bleeding and infection. The cortical bone is closed as described above.

Old fracture lines in the posterior meatal wall may be closed, or communicate with the pneumatic system; they carry the danger of an atypical traumatic cholesteatoma due to ingrowth of skin. They can be eradicated with ease from the mastoid process.

Fractures of the petrous pyramid due to external violence, especially shot and grenades, are common in wartime. They penetrate the cochlea and remain hidden in the petrous pyramid close to the internal carotid artery if they do not splinter the sphenoid bone, reach the center of the base of the skull and cause death.

In a healthy middle ear these injuries are initially sterile. In the early stages it is permissible to cover the depth of the bony canal with plasticine, containing an antibiotic depot, after debridement of the wound. It cannot become infected as cover with soft tissue can. Because the factors causing osteitic para-

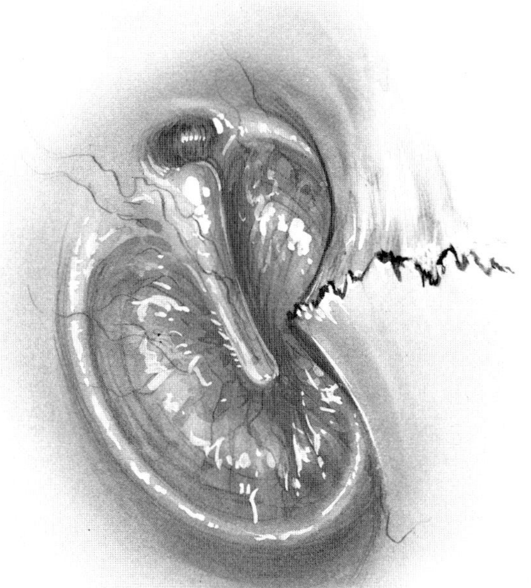

269

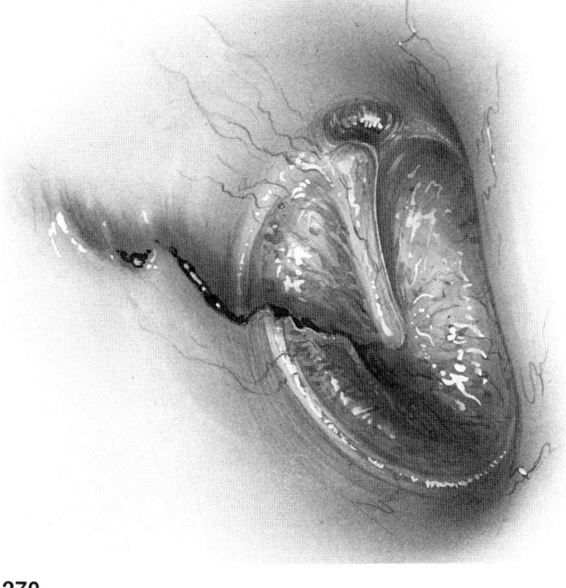

270

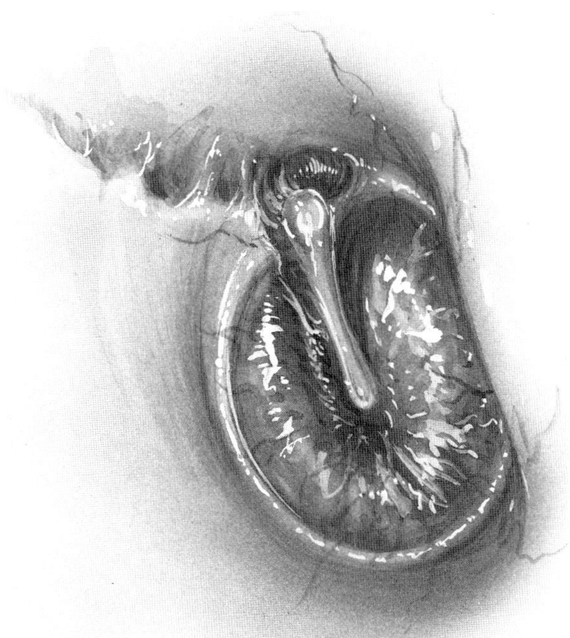

271

Fig. **269** **Fracture of the anterior meatal wall.** The bony fragments narrow the meatus from in front. The meatal skin over the fracture line has been torn, but the tympanic membrane is undamaged (H. L. Wullstein 1968)

Fig. **270** **Fresh fracture of the temporal bone.** The fracture line runs through the posterosuperior meatal wall. The meatal skin, the fibrous annulus and the tympanic membrane are torn (H. L. Wullstein 1968)

Fig. **271** **A longstanding fracture of the temporal bone** opening from above into the lateral epitympanic space and reaching the pars flaccida of the tympanic membrane (H. L. Wullstein 1968)

labyrinthitis are absent in such cases, subsequent *total inner ear osteitis does not occur*, but widening of a semicircular canal alone, due to *chronic endostial osteitis; prolonged osteomyelitis of the temporal bone may occur if the middle ear does not heal immediately*. Closed fractures of the petrous pyramid with loss of the inner ear function are not an indication for operation.

Fracture lines in the *anterior meatal wall*, usually with marked posterior dislocation, must be smoothed with the diamond burr after elevation of the periosteal sleeve so that the entire tympanic annulus is visible in the tympanomeatal angle. A cleft-like defect of the wall is unimportant; it is also filled with plasticine. The often associated fracture of the mandible inferior to the condyle must also be exposed and treated.

Linear Fractures

The classical subdivison into longitudinal and transverse fractures is clinically justified because the first usually damages the middle ear and mastoid, whereas the latter do not. However, they ought not to be regarded either causally or pathologically in such a contrasting manner. Computed tomography has shown that fractures of the petrous pyramid extend from the petrous bone to the temporal squama and vice versa. This happens in indirect fractures due to the mechanical stress on the temporal bone and its complicated strut system based on the principle of lightweight construction. It is known from the anatomy of the temporal bone where the weak points of this lightweight construction lie.

Longitudinal fractures in the bony wall of the middle ear require reconstruction of the spaces, and of continuity of the sound conduction apparatus after rupture, dislocation or fracture of the parts of the ossicular chain. If possible, a Type II tympanoplasty should be done and, if not, a Type III procedure. The typical fracture lines lie in the posterior and superior walls:

- purely posteriorly, on occasion through the canal of the facial nerve; or
- running obliquely posterosuperiorly into the periantral spaces; or
- superiorly through the wall of the epitympanum into the temporal bone.

Removal of splinters in the first type is followed by drilling along the course of the fracture line, with decompression of the facial nerve and the chorda tympani and filling of the large defect with a plasticine plug. A similar procedure is carried out for the second type of fracture.

In the third type, infracture of the lateral wall of the epitympanum with damage to the ossicular chain must be expected, requiring cover at that point. The bony epitympanic wall is cut as usual and then removed in two pieces. The fragments are embedded in a plasticine plate so as to ensure contact with bone at two points at least upon replacement subsequent to the completion of all necessary manipulations in the epitympanum.

Damage to the ossicular chain, including fracture of the long process of the incus due to infracture of the epitympanic wall, is treated initially by an attempt to splint the crus by glueing on a fine strip of autologous bone material. If this does not succeed, a Type III tympanoplasty with a deep tympanic cavity is carried out after resection of the incus and the head of the malleus, and filling of the empty protympanic recess with plasticine to guarantee a non-turbulent airstream to the aditus. The stapes is built up, if possible, to contact the neck of the malleus.

The lenticular process can be torn from the head of the stapes by a downward blow on the incus. Repositioning is then necessary, with bridging of the resulting fine gap, because the released long process of the incus is distorted laterally. A suitable small piece of cartilage from the tragus, or more simply plasticine, is introduced and fixed by glueing a very small piece of fascia over it.

If the blow was more robust, both stapedial crura may be snapped off on the wall of the promontory. The most reliable results are achieved by a replacement of the stapes and the insertion of a small piece of connective tissue which has been previously placed on the footplate to ensure against perforation and to achieve a solid tissue union. Any type of alloplastic replacement material or an allogenic stapes of suitable size relative to the footplate may be used. It is fastened to the lenticular process in the manner described above.

The malleus and incus can be displaced inferiorly into the mesohypotympanum and may even be catapulted into the external meatus. An epitympanotomy is then necessary to allow placing of one or both ossicles in the correct anatomical position. Bridging and fixation at the contact points then follow, using delicate glued strips of fascia. Because the mucosa is healthy and delicate, there is little risk of extensive adhesions which could impede sound transmission.

Trauma with or without a fracture line in the temporal squama can cause a marked springing of the roof of the middle ear, leading to dislocation of the malleus or incuse or of the long process of the incus from the head of the stapes (Figs. **273–274**). Suitable access for repositioning can only be achieved by osteoplastic epitympanotomy.

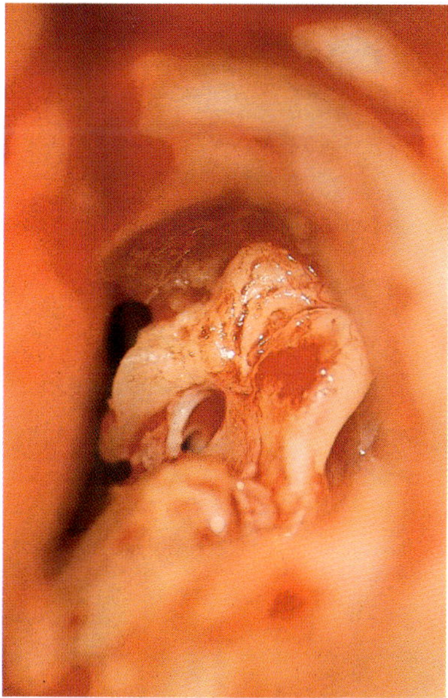

Fig. **272   Acoustic trauma with tearing of the tympanic membrane and dislocation of the ossicles at the malleoincudal joint**

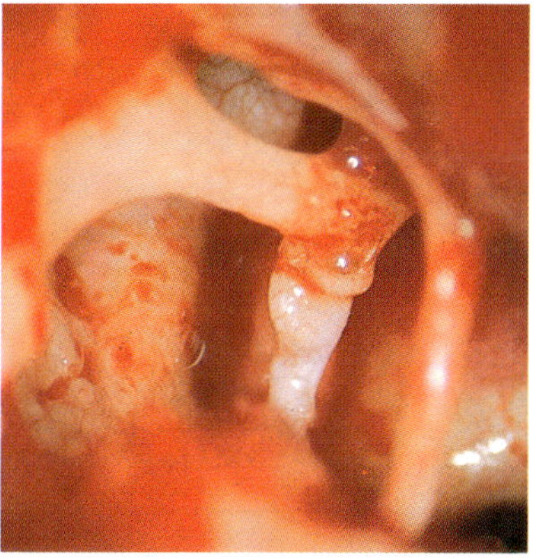

273

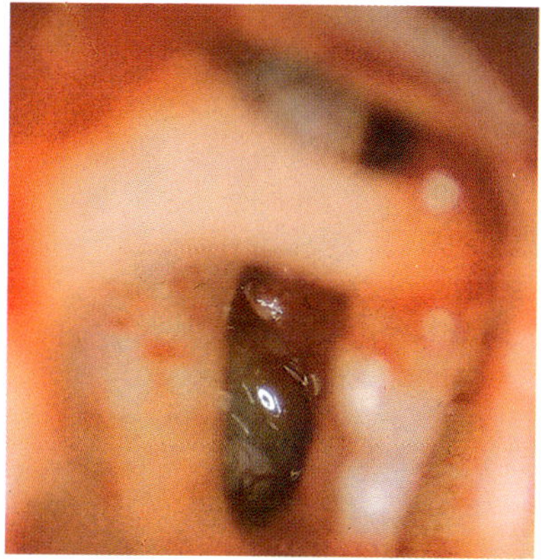

274

Figs. **273–274   Transverse temporal bone fracture.** Osteoplastic epitympanotomy, subluxation of the incudostapedial joint and fracture of the footplate

Fractures and the Facial Nerve
(Figs. **275–277**)

Bleeding into the nerve sheath, bruising and tears can result from fractures in the temporal bone. These traumatic lesions require immediate surgical correction. They can be subdivided into the following anatomical types (Bebear 1984):
1. in the region of the ganglion (35%);
2. superior to the origin of the chorda tympani (40%);
3. inferior to this point (25%).

Lesions in the region of the ganglion. Evidence of a fracture in the labyrinthine course of the nerve is only an accidental finding on plain films, but it is certain to be found on CT scans. The fracture line lies partly in the thin floor of the middle cranial fossa and causes a contusion in the region of the ganglion or in the margin of the foramen of the facial nerve in the fundus plate of the internal auditory meatus. This leads to entrapment of the nerve. This lesion of the nerve may be combined with an epitympanic dislocation of the ossicles, requiring exposure of the entire course of the nerve. The operation therefore begins with an osteoplastic epitympanotomy. Simultaneous exposure of the superior surface of the petrous pyramid was discussed under the procedure for an anterior paralabyrinthine cholesteatoma. Temporary opening of the epitympanum renders operative access at this point much wider and shorter than before. An extensive osteoplastic resection of the temporal squama, as for an operation on the internal auditory meatus, is not necessary. An osteoplastic extension of the opening to the middle cranial fossa superior to the ossicles gives sufficient space to allow the nerve to be followed as far as its exit from the internal meatus, using fine diamond burrs, straight and angled picks, and round or sickle knives. This opening is subsequently closed with plasticine. A tear of the nerve requiring repair is not to be expected at this point without fracture with loss of function of the inner ear. If the inner ear is indeed dead, a much wider surgical field, extending into the mastoid process, is created by resecting the inner ear and sacrificing the middle ear spaces.

Lesions superior to the origin of the chorda tympani. Serious damage may occur in the tympanic and mastoid course of the facial nerve above the origin of the chorda tympani, mainly in wide fractures close to the posterior tympanic spine, possibly extending into the inner ear. A limited procedure (see above) is only permissible if the surgeon is certain of the pathological findings.

Lesions inferior to the origin of the chorda tympani. Facial nerve lesions of this type are usually very severe and the nerve may even be torn due to splintering and bruising. Extensive exposure extending into the soft tissues of the neck and the insertion of a nerve graft may be needed.

If a traumatized middle or inner ear becomes infected, or if the middle ear was already chronically infected, a *chronic* temporal bone osteomyelitis or circumscribed *endosteal* osteitis of the inner ear may develop. An acute total osteitis of the labyrinth (i.e., para- and endolabyrinthine) does not develop, however, because the necessary *paralabyrinthine factors are wanting* (see p. 134). The duration of this osteitis and osteomyelitis cannot be predicted. The osteomyelitis and the chronic osteitis of the inner ear persist for months of years, so that a series of successive radiographs and, possibly, surgery are therefore advisable.

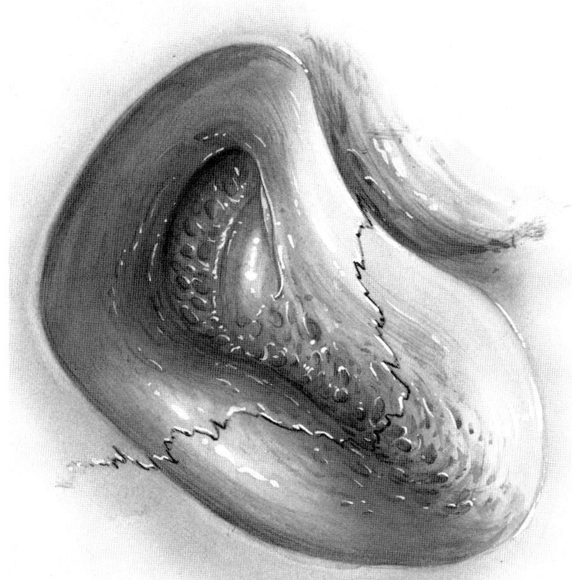

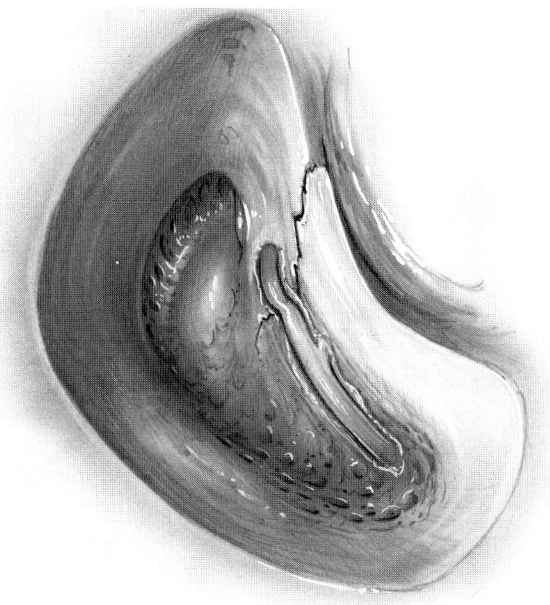

Fig. **275 Temporal bone fracture.** Transcortical opening of the mastoid process and clearance of the cell system. The fracture line runs through the anterior wall of the sigmoid sinus and opens into the posterior meatal wall (H. L. Wullstein 1968)

Fig. **276 Exposure of the facial nerve in a fracture of the temporal bone.** After a transcortical mastoidectomy and exposure of the facial nerve, the contusion of the nerve above the origin of the chorda tympani due to dislocation of the distal fragment can be seen (H. L. Wullstein 1968)

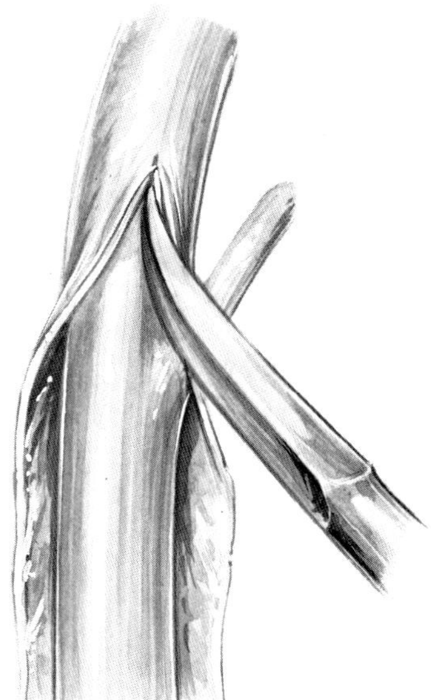

Fig. **277 Decompression of the facial nerve, showing slitting of the nerve sheath.** The connective tissue sheath of the nerve is slit with the point of the sickle knife outward from within, preserving the nerve fibers (H. L. Wullstein 1968)

Congenital Cholesteatoma, Aneurysms of the Internal Carotid Artery, Congenital Anomalies, Facial Nerve, Dysplasias

Occult Congenital Cholesteatoma of the Middle Ear versus Occult Primary Acquired Inflammatory Cholesteatoma

Congenital cholesteatoma was initially a purely clinical term for occult cholesteatomas which were visible behind the tympanic membrane (House 1953, Cawthorne 1963, Derlacki et al. 1973, 1985). A congenital origin from ectodermal embryonic remnants was also proposed by Aimi (1983). At the beginning of its development, the tympanic ring is responsible for limiting the penetration of meatal ectoderm, before Shrapnell's membrane and Rivini's notch develop.

Aimi postulated that papillary ectodermal tissue penetrates the mesenchyme of the tympanic isthmus above the level of the tympanic membrane in the fifteenth to the twentieth weeks, and is then nipped off from the developing tympanic membrane. In contrast, Mündnich (1939) concluded that the true cholesteatoma is a hamartoma of the middle ear cavity arising during the brief period of contact of the epithelium of the first branchial cleft with the tubotympanic pouch in the fourth and fifth embryonic weeks. It is thus an embryonic anomaly arising long before the formation of the external auditory meatus. This process is impossible in the pars flaccida, whose anlage appears in the fifth fetal month. Thus, congenital epidermoids are those lying behind the tympanic membrane which can be recognized in the early stage by otoscopy (McDonald et al. 1984).

In our view occult epitympanic cholesteatomas are acquired primary lesions which have not yet led to a small perforation with crusting in the Shrapnell's membrane, as explained on page 106 ff. Thus, both types of occult cholesteatoma exist. *The frequency of occult papillary epitympanic and occult congenital cholesteatoma is so far unknown.*

In order to distinguish occult *congenital* cholesteatomas in the mesotympanum from occult *papillary primary inflammatory acquired cholesteatomas* in the epitympanum, it is necessary to operate on both in the same manner, to allow analysis of the disease in its undisturbed state. This can only be achieved with osteoplastic epitympanotomy. Reliable data about the occult congenital cholesteatomas have not been reported in large numbers, and it is impossible therefore to give a firm opinion about their frequency.

Wang et al. (1974) described bilateral mesotympanic cholesteatomas in a four-month-old child. They regarded the lesion as being congenital, but only found loose debris lying behind the tympanic membrane, with no evidence of a capsule. The child had had a difficult forceps delivery and probably suffered a bilateral injury to the tympanic membranes, which had healed spontaneously and rapidly.

Congenital Intracranial Intradural Epidermoids

Epidermoids may be regarded as hamartomas of the neural tube (Bostroem 1897, Nager 1982); they are formed of a very thin, flat nonpapillary epidermis. Like middle ear cholesteatoma, they extend intradurally rather than extradurally over the surface of the brain stem and the cranial nerves and even along the base of the skull to the opposite side. For this reason a neurosurgeon may have to abandon an attempt at complete removal, and an operation for recurrence may be necessary many years later.

Like the middle ear cholesteatoma, an epidermoid of either cranial fossa forces its way into all grooves, clefts and fissures, and its clinical picture thus varies. It extends from the middle cranial fossa into the pyramidal apex between the basisphenoid, the basiclinoid and the petrous part of the temporal bone. The pathway lies between the superior sphenopetrosal ligament (which runs from the postero-inferior clinoid process to the superior petrous apex) and the inferior sphenopetrosal ligament above the fibrocartilage of the foramen lacerum close to the sphenoidal lingula.

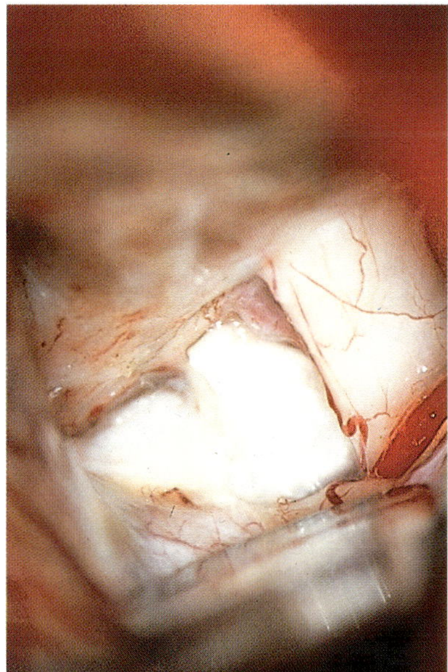
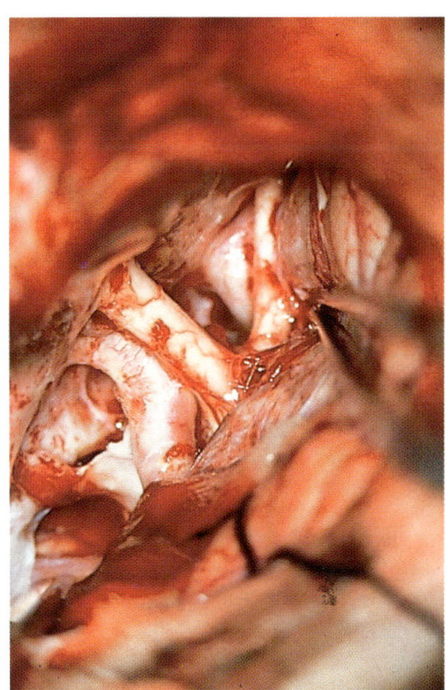

Fig. **278a   Middle cranial fossa.** Parasellar cholesteatoma, the left optic nerve and the short segment of the opthalmic artery are exposed, but the internal carotid artery is still covered (Koos et al. 1985)

Fig. **278b   View after removal of the cholesteatoma,** exposing the following: the ipsilateral and contralateral carotid artery, the optic nerve with the chiasma, the right middle cranial fossa with the third cranial nerve and, inferiorly, the superior cellebellar artery (Koos et al. 1985)

As a result, over a period of many years, gross destruction of the petrous pyramid develops, extending close to the inner ear, so that ultimately there is doubt about its genesis. As in epitympanic cholesteatomas, both inner ear functions may be long preserved in intracranial epidermoids, and they are only very slowly and imperceptibly damaged. The function of the facial nerve also remains unaffected. The demonstration of a cholesteatoma in the middle ear cavity eliminates any doubt as to its otogenic origin. This situation falls primarily in the remit of the neurosurgeon. In the extreme case a large cholesteatoma amputates the entire pyramidal apex and its cortical bone as far as the labyrinthine block; the only question arising on a CT scan or MRI is whether the lesion represents the deep extension of an epitympanic cholesteatoma. In this case the otologist should be called in for an immediate procedure or a second-stage operation (Fig. **278a, b**).

The congenital epidermoid of the posterior cranial fossa constitutes one of the space-occupying processes of the cerebellopontine angle (Fig. **279**). It can penetrate through the petro-occipital fissure into the tympanic plate.

Inspection of the pyramidal wall of the middle ear via an osteoplastic epitympanotomy is necessary (p. 134 ff.), because even detailed radiological investigations may not demonstrate the origin of an acquired (possibly occult) cholesteatoma from the

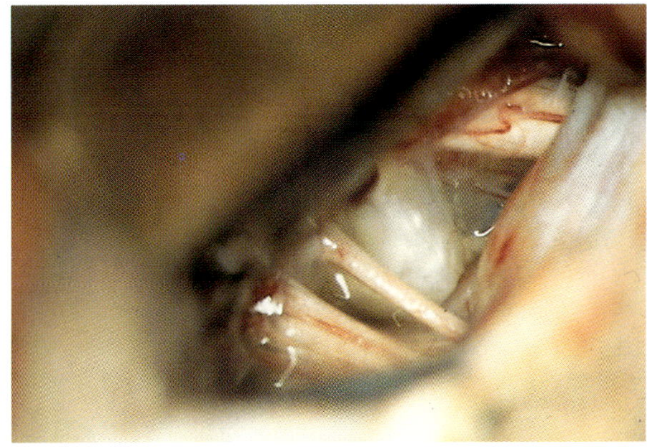

Fig. **279   Posterior cranial fossa.** Cholesteatoma in the lower part of the cerebellopontine angle. From above, downward, the posterior inferior cerebellar artery, the VII and VIII cranial nerves, the cholesteatoma, and the IX and X cranial nerves can be seen (Koos et al. 1985)

anterior or posterior points of danger on the paralabyrinthine pathway to the pyramidal apex.

When dealing with an intradural epidermoid the neurosurgeon always has precedence. He can demonstrate the site of growth and extent of destruction into the petrous pyramid. The functions of hearing, balance, taste, and facial movement need not have been compromized for long. The loss of middle ear function caused by access to the infratemporal fossa (Fisch 1985) is a severe sacrifice, particularly as the external auditory meatus is also lost, and the sensorineural deafness cannot be treated by a hearing aid, although the inner ear is still capable of function. The neurosurgeon and the otologist should consult jointly during the surgery to decide how far the neurosurgeon may go in the petrous pyramid to achieve decompression, so that the otologist may carry the operation within the temporal bone to its conclusion, sparing the still-functioning middle or internal ear. The otologist should take into account the fact that the neurosurgeon may well be considering carrying out a later, second procedure. The function of the cochlea is valueless after the infratemporal procedure because the eustachian tube must be sacrificed, the middle ear spaces are obliterated and the external meatus closed off.

The method of filling the defect in the petrous pyramid with fat, muscle, or plasticine to hold it open to allow later inspection can, on occasion, be decided after careful evaluation with the angled endoscope passed along the internal carotid artery into the foramen lacerum.

Pure cysts of the base of the skull, extending from the sphenoid into the apex of the petrous bone, may have originated from the endodermal lining of the future sphenoid sinus, which is only separated from the cyst by a thin layer of bone. In contrast to an epidermoid, total removal of the wall of the cyst is unnecessary. Long-term drainage can be provided by an ipsilateral or contralateral ethmoidectomy through the posterior wall of the sphenoid (Montgomery 1979, Schuknecht and Gao 1983).

Aneurysm of the Internal Carotid Artery

The genu of the internal carotid artery can project in a very deceptive manner into the anterior hypotympanum, where it is covered only by a very thin layer of bone. Operations have led to frightful mistakes, whether due to a far anterior jugular bulb or a chemodectoma arising from the tympanic canaliculus.

The internal carotid artery can exceptionally give rise to a spontaneous intrapyramidal aneurysm which grows extensively over many years. It is fundamentally different from the numerous, usually small, intracranial dissecting aneurysms arising at one of the numerous branching points. The latter are absent from the internal carotid artery before it leaves the foramen lacerum. On the other hand, the elastica surrounded by a venous plexus within the bony canal is relatively weak. If this weak wall extends beyond the foramen lacerum, a true aneurysm can arise, leading to widespread erosion of the petrous pyramid and even cranial nerve paralyses and exophthalmos (Figs. **280–281**). Recently, this danger has been produced by surgical exposure.

Deficient elastica *just anterior to the entrance into the bony canal* is probably the cause of *aneurysmal distention into the anterior hypotympanum* (see above).

An epidermal or intracranial cholesteatoma of the petrous apex might have exposed the internal carotid artery over a varying length along its bony canal. The matrix adheres to its wall. In congenital epidermoids it can be exposed from within the temporal bone synchronous with intracranial extradural access through the surface of the middle cranial fossa working toward the foramen lacerum, where the otological and neurosurgical procedures meet.

Eradication of the matrix by the otosurgical method, accomplished by inspection through the angled endoscope, is more effective than a neurosurgical procedure in preventing a local recurrence of the epidermoid. Obliteration of the bony defect reliably prevents an aneurysm and is more certain than obliteration with soft tissue such as muscle or fat, which undergoes scar tissue retraction and pulls away from the walls. Very exceptionally, an intradural epidermoid penetrates from the posterior cranial fossa (see above) into the pars tympanica as far as the internal carotid artery (Zehm). It remains within the basal mastoid part of the temporal bone, and affects neither the antrum nor the hearing. It is therefore removed by resection of the mastoid process and the tympanic plate, with sacrifice of the sigmoid sinus and the jugular bulb.

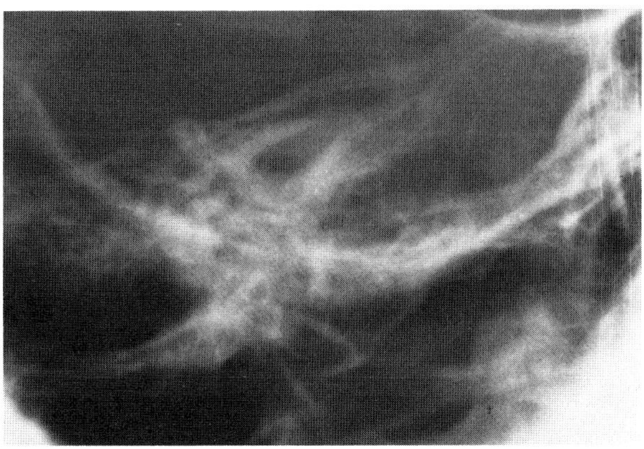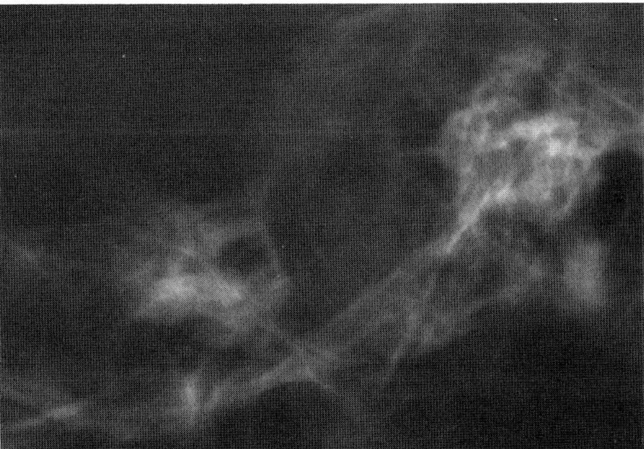

Figs. **280–281 True aneurysm of the internal carotid artery in its entire intrapyramidal course after a twelve-year observation period.** Calcification in the arterial wall (above and below). Intermittent exophthalmos, with involvement of the second to the sixth cranial nerves, regressing over several years to a slight exophthalmos

Congenital Anomalies

The development of surgical methods for treating meatal atresia and middle ear congenital anomalies was made possible by the introduction into ear surgery of not only the microscope, drill and diamond burr, but also by the advent of healing of free-standing membranes. The CT scan provides information about the configuration of any anomaly of the walls, the ossicles and the extent of the air space. Doubt may remain about the course of the facial nerve and its branches within the middle ear.

The purpose of an operation for meatal atresia and middle ear anomalies is the construction of a meatus and sound conduction using tympanoplasty Types I to V, if necessary, with the help of a fenestration.

The method used for the middle ear defect must be very adaptable. Because the operative procedures which may be considered have been extensively described in preceeding chapters, only a short explanation of the procedures for the slightest and most severe grades will be given here.

A partial but bony pars tensa, partially malformed ossicles (the most frequent form of deafness in mongolism), and concealed fixation of the stapes footplate, due to inadequate development of the annular ligament, cause unremarkable local findings. In the first case, a myringoplasty is necessary; in the second, reconstruction of the ossicular chain, and in the third, building up of the stapes or stapedectomy.

In extreme cases of atresia and middle ear anomalies, the external ear, the auricle and the cartilaginous meatus are absent. The two superior eminences are present but are almost free of cartilage; the two lower ones are similar. The temporal bone presents a uniform lateral bony surface with no indication where the meatus can be sought. The creation of the bony meatus might be thought to lead immediately to the middle ear and not first of all into the mastoid. A curved skin incision is therefore used, as for a wide epitympanotomy, with its anterior segment prolonged to the point where the site of insertion of the superior otobasion of the auricle might be throught to be on the temporal bone, anterior and superior to the temperomandibular joint. The incision is continued posteriorly in a wide arc down to the bone and prolonged further between the superior and inferior appendages to *provide a robust, far-reaching and wide cover for the anterior contour of the meatal entrance.* The incision runs inferior to the inferior appendages. A suitably large flap is thus created, which can be rotated from *below* into the meatal entrance. Care must be exercized to create a wide external meatus which has no tendency to stenose. A bony plane without anatomical landmarks is exposed.

Coronal and axial computer tomography provide information about the accompanying facial scoliosis and hemiatrophy of the mandible, the middle cranial fossa and its position, the air spaces of the temporal bone, the pneumatization of the mastoid process, and, especially, the size and depth of the tympanic cavity.

The facial nerve is the structure at greatest risk, and it is therefore looked for first. It points the way into the epitympanum. The trunk of the nerve is always undivided as it leaves the geniculate ganglion; it may therefore most reliably be sought there

(H. L. Wullstein 1957 Int. Congress Washington). Beyond that point, it may adopt an atypical course and divide into two or three bundles; scarcely ever has it already divided up in the labyrinthine course. The inner cortex of the temporal squama is demonstrated using the cylindrical burr along the suspected site of the temporal line, from the anterior wall of the protympanic recess to the sinodural angle. At that point it passes from the lateral to the basal boundary of the middle cranial fossa. The cortex is followed deeply, using suitable cutting and diamond burrs, and the dura is exposed widely to allow the anterior crus of the anterior semicircular canal to be found close to the arcuate eminence. Two sides of the antelabyrinthine trigone (the dura and the labyrinthine ampule) are thus defined. Cutting out the third, the genu of the facial nerve, with the diamond burr, presents no difficulty.

Proceeding form this point to the tegmen tympani, the epitympanic space opens like a cleft above the head of the malleus and the incus. Preliminary definition of the desired depth is thus achieved.

The shaping of the anterior meatal wall starts from this point behind the anterior wall of the planum as far as the level of the epitympanic bony lid and from there to the future meatal wall. The anterior wall must curve slightly anteriorly. The future bony annulus lies deeper at that point than posteriorly in the plane of the future tympanic membrane, which sinks anteriorly into the tympanomeatal angle. The canal must be very wide to accommodate the full-thickness skin graft which is later placed on the bony walls.

Dissection of the middle ear can now begin. The head of the malleus and incus must be assessed through the easily extended subtegmental cleft to determine whether they are well formed or consist of only a misshaped mass. At the same time, palpation is used to determine whether and where one of the two ossicles is subject to bony fixation. The epitympanum and the second genu of the facial nerve can be evaluated endoscopically from an aditus-antrum inspection window if it is possible to create one. The endoscope is introduced along the line of the lateral semicircular canal in an arc along the antral wall and then running back to the canal, or very steeply on the posterior wall of the sinus tympani or very flatly over the oval niche and the pyramidal process. Knowledge of these courses (Nager 1983) facilitates drilling of the head of the malleus down to its neck from its adhesion with the atretic plate. Penetration of the instrument into the middle ear space is only allowed if the almost transparent bony plate over the mesotympanum has been cracked off earlier. Two to three bundles of the facial nerve can

possibly be recognized running freely through the middle ear, around or through the stapes to the stylomastoid foramen. The epitympanum is searched endoscopically for reddened and swollen membranes, since atypical folds can be present; mild unrecognized tubotympanic catarrh fairly commonly arises in atretic ears. Then the bony edges of the epitympanum and the future bony annulus are thinned sufficiently to allow the tympanic membrane repair to be glued to the epitympanic wall and to the handle of the malleus.

In favorable cases the customary lid can be developed to cover the epitympanum. In other cases a plate can be created from fragments of the epitympanic bone, embedded in plasticine, which close off an adequate epitympanum again. It is desirable to expose it if a concealed tubal ostium cannot otherwise be demonstrated. An open bony eustachian tube (even if it is very narrow) is a prerequisite for a middle ear with partially healthy mucosa.

The ossicles. If the long process of the incus is absent, the two ossicles usually form an ill-defined mass in the epitympanum, and the handle of the malleus is so defective that it no longer contacts the atretic plate. Construction of lever system in the narrow epitympanum is not to be considered. The epitympanic wall can be used in the presence of a high, robust stapes to allow a stapes build-up to be carried out and a Type III tympanoplasty with a deep tympanic cavity. The stapes is often atrophic, and a shallow Type III tympanoplasty can therefore lead to the formation of adhesions. If the window niches as well as the hypotympanum are well developed, cover of the oval window and niche to form a Type IV tympanoplasty should be considered after removal of the atrophic stapes. The simplest constructions under these circumstances are the most reliable. The stapedial artery, being very thick, can be retained and can penetrate the epitympanic space either through the stapes or freely, without contacting it. Damage causes brisk bleeding, and the vessel should therefore be coagulated early on.

Finally, *very extensive anomalies of the window niches* may be found. The subiculum of the promontory anterior to the round window niche can be absent, so that the round window is exposed and vulnerable. If it is closed, it should be opened up at the end of the operation using the diamond burr, and then be covered immediately. The oval window can be ossified as far as its edge, and only a small stapes head is visible. It is possible to drill out the oval window, including the stapes, so that it is open in its entire extent. All sides form a funnel of spongiosa with traumatized bony edges and therefore have a marked natural tendency to reossify, which is not prevented by cover with a split skin graft. Sound protection of the round window should therefore be created at the first operation; it is *undesirable* to remove the atretic plate over the hypotympanum *completely*; the lower aeration pathway thus remains open for a Type V tympanoplasty with fenestration.

The lateral semicircular canal is exposed for fenestration at a second sitting. Therefore, the small club-shaped cavity created to allow a view of the semicircular canal is covered with a thin, firm piece of full-thickness skin graft, which can easily be taken from the loose subcutis of the neck, for example. This can be done by making an oblique incision behind the sternocleidomastoid muscle (on the opposite side of the neck, because a pinnaplasty will be performed later on the operated side). The wound is closed, adhering to the principles of plastic surgery, and is scarcely visible.

The pedicled skin flaps are sutured from in front and below into the opening of the new meatus. The thin full-thickness covering of the depths of the wound is carefully adapted so that no cleft remains, and so that necrosis does not arise due to overlapping. The anterosuperior and posteroinferior accessory auricle are carefully fixed to serve as material for the pinnaplasty.

When the increased bleeding tendency of the free split skin graft is fully resolved ten to twelve weeks later, the cover is elevated beginning posteriorly, and a fenestration is carried out. It is advisable to model the dome first, and not to place the fenestration over the ampulla: adhesion of the graft to the ampulla causes mild attacks of dizziness even without any movement, but this is almost never observed when the fenestration lies more posteriorly (Fig. **65**).

All procedures developed so far for the pinnaplasty are unsatisfactory. They are not described in this monograph.

The most modest hearing result is a bilateral middle ear, with sound protection of the round window and fenestration of the lateral semicircular canal (Type V tympanoplasty). If the inner ear is normal, which is usually the case, there is a conductive loss of about 25 dB compared with about 60 dB before the operation. It is unnecessary to wear a hearing aid. Even in unilateral atresia with a normal ear and hearing on the opposite side, the operation is very valuable to improve communication.

If the anatomy of the middle ear is too narrow for effective creation of sound conduction, or the function of the ear or the facial nerve appears to be at risk, it is advisable to limit the procedure to thinning the meatal plate as far as possible to create a well-shaped external meatus, so that a *hearing aid* can be worn for the rest of the patient's life. Defects in the meatal wall in the epitympanic or mastoid region can easily be filled with plasticine.

The skin is sutured closely from in front into the newly created meatus to prevent stenosis. Thus, a replacement for the tragus is absent, a cosmetic and functional disadvantage. Its wind-deflecting action on the meatus is missing; even a light breeze causes a persistent sound of 30 dB (Feldmann 1986). The introduction of a suitably shaped autologous bone or cartilage with appropriate mobilization of the external skin and cover by free skin from the meatal side a few months later is only a minor plastic procedure.

Tympanoplasty for atresia and dysplasia of the middle ear may be limited by closure of the eustachian tube; this may be absolute because of inclusion in the anomaly or because of scar tissue, or functional because of severe narrowing in its bony course. It may be desirable to look for the eustachian tube carefully and to probe it, taking care not to create a false passage. If its function is lost, the only possible solution is a dry cavity lined by thin skin and a well-shaped meatus for the insertion of a hearing aid.

Facial Nerve

Surgery of the facial nerve cannot be covered in this monograph. This subject has already been referred to in individual chapters to allow paralysis to be seen in its original context. Tympanoplastic procedures are very often necessary for facial palsy.

In *chronic otitis media*, paralysis is due to *a very circumscribed* compression of the nerve. The cause is usually an *anterior paralabyrinthine cholesteatoma*, the inner ear and even the middle ear are otherwise undamaged. It may even arise from an *occult anteromedial cholesteatoma* causing strictly limited pressure in the narrow *antelabyrinthine trigone* over the geniculate ganglion. The diagnosis is made from plain films (Wullstein's view), but a CT scan gives clearer information. The paralysis can persist for years with slight variation, *without any other symptoms* (p. 119).

This type of compression paralysis also arises in *posteromedial cholesteatomas* which have penetrated so far into the labyrinthine block that they compress the nerve locally in the region of the vestibule. These paralabyrinthine cholesteatomas are hardly infected at all. Because there is an ever present danger of secondary infection and slow extension, these cholesteatomas must be eradicated by surgery.

Small neurinomas superior to the geniculate ganglion cause exactly the same symptoms and radiological findings as anterior paralabyrinthine cholesteatomas. Small facial nerve neurinomas are also found in the tympanic segment of the nerve. Compression paralysis does not occur, because they rapidly break through the thin layer of bone and interrupt sound transmission by erosion of the long process of the incus. The small medial epitympanic cholesteatomas behave in the same way. Differentiation of small neurinomas from cholesteatomas can only be made by local inspection.

If the facial nerve was not freed entirely from the matrix in the entrance to its labyrinthine course, it must remain accessible as far as the meatus to allow follow-up and drainage; i.e., the operation should be restricted to a shallow Type III tympanoplasty. (Compare "Operations for Para- and Retrolabyrinthine Cholesteatomas of the Middle Ear", p. 134.)

Compression paralysis in the mastoid due to osteitis is rare in comparison with idiopathic paralysis.

Often the *chorda tympani* is surrounded by matrix, and may be stretched during freeing. The resulting disorder of taste recovers more slowly than that due to division of the nerve. Resection of the chorda tympani is indicated in such cases.

Acute total inner ear osteitis with its rapidly progressive destruction of bone due to osteitis requires an early decompression of the nerve to prevent paralysis, or to restrict it to a short-lived paralysis.

Even the worst *pararetrolabyrinthine cholesteatoma* with complete isolation of the remnant of the inner ear over decades need not cause a facial paralysis. Occasionally the inner ear is sequestered, *due to a longstanding osteitis caused by a primary total or partial bone necrosis of the labyrinthine block* due to otitis media. Disintegration facilitates spontaneous rejection of the fragments if they have not been removed surgically.

Posttraumatic and postoperative paralysis due to entrapment by bone fragments, independent of site, require immediate exposure from the fundus of the internal auditory meatus to the fracture line in the mastoid canal. Osteoplastic exposure for access to the tympanic and labyrinthine segments of the nerve may be advisable to allow auditory function to be preserved and, if possible, the continuity of the ossicular chain to be reconstructed.

Severe anomalies in the course of the facial nerve are common in patients with congenital anomalies of the middle and internal ear (Miehlke 1982, second edition, Proctor 1982, 1990, Nager 1982). They extend from the labyrinthine region to the stylomastoid foramen. The nerve divides into two or three branches which run around the stapes, lateral to the malleus, free through the mesotympanum, above the lateral semicircular canal or even through the junction of the lateral semicircular canal with the subarcuate tract. Facial nerve fibers may be partially distributed with the chorda tympani (see operation for middle ear, "Congenital Anomalies," p. 167).

Dysplasias, Neoplasms and Craniosynostoses

Stapedial ankylosis due to otosclerosis will not be discussed here. There are many types of dysplasia of the skull base but as surgical cases they are infrequent, compared with otosclerosis. Few require surgery because of spatial constriction and conductive deafness. Only one of the dysplasias is an indication for a tympanoplasty, which is indeed life saving; this is sclerosteosis of the temporal bone, which also affects the skeleton elsewhere. It is a rare autosomal recessive progressive disease.

The lethal outcome in these cases is caused by the constriction of the sigmoid sinus and the jugular bulb, leading to venous congestion and increased intracranial pressure. Furthermore, a life-threatening constriction of the foramen magnum, narrowing the medulla oblongata, is an early feature of this disease. The remaining features include lesions of the cranial nerves, ranging from anosmia to compression of the nerves in the internal auditory meatus, but not affecting those in the medial part of the jugular foramen. The conductive deafness, the constriction of the external auditory meatus and the impaction of the ossicles in the narrowed epitympanum require surgery. The aditus and the antrum are also affected, both inner ear windows are narrowed, the stapes footplate is wedged, and later sclerosis of the labyrinthine block leads to sensorineural deafness and vestibular disorders. In addition to the severe deafness, the patient also becomes blind, due to narrowing of the optic foramen.

The management of one case was described by Nager et al. The venous congestion was eliminated by exposure of the entire course of the sinus in the ivory-hard temporal bone as far as the jugular foramen. The narrowed sinus thus regained its normal width. Next, the very narrowed antrum and epitympanum were sought, and the displaced and completely immobile malleus and incus resected. The stapedial crura were fractured, the oval window was narrowed and tilted, and the stapes footplate impacted. The middle ear was severely narrowed. A neurosurgeon widened the foramen magnum. After this decompression of the contents of the skull, the

Figs. **282—284 Osteoplastic epitympanotomy for Paget's disease.** In Fig. **282**, the constriction of the head of the malleus and the protympanic recess can be recognized after elevation of the bony lid. Fig. **283** shows the malleus and incus removed, followed by build-up of the stapes footplate using the sculpted autogenous head of the malleus to form a Type III tympanoplasty. Fig. **284** shows a plain anteroposterior radiograph of the skull, to demonstrate the extent of the bony disease

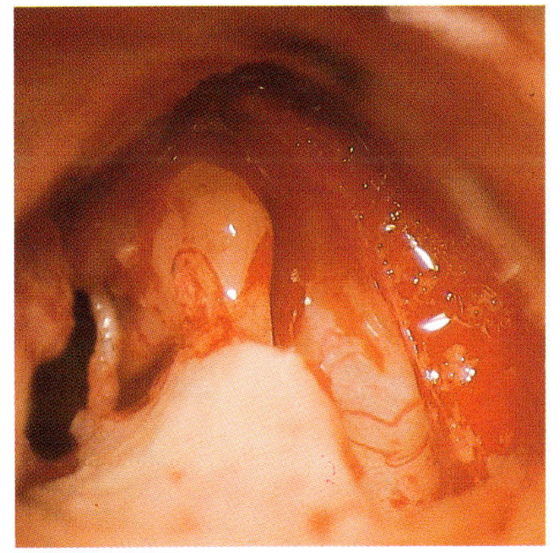

282

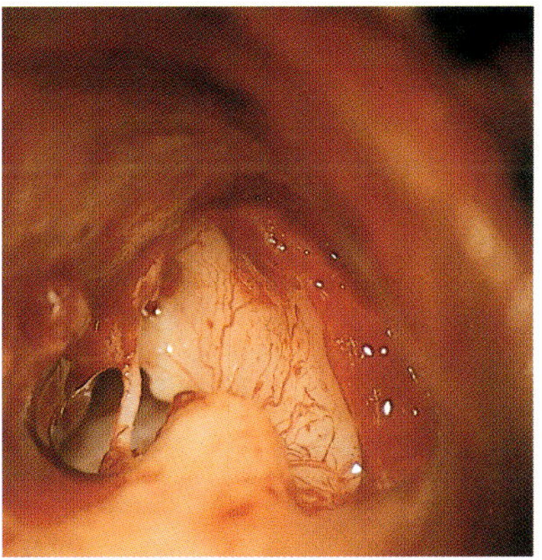

283

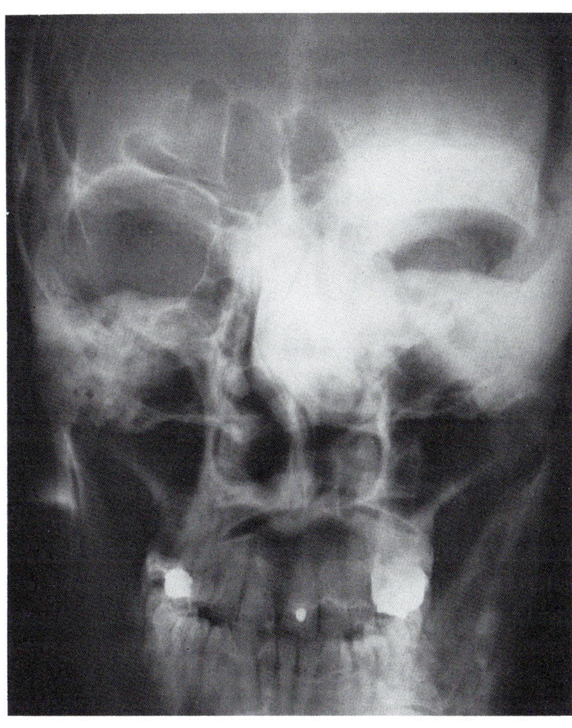

284

patient underwent an astonishing recovery and her sight improved.

Tympanoplasty provides only modest help in this type of extreme life-threatening disease. It is much more often considered for improvement of hearing in sclerosing lesions such as osteopetrosis, or for spongiotic lesions of the temporal bone such as osteodystrophia deformans in Paget's disease. These types of dysplasia can afflict the window of one niche and especially constrict the epitympanum. If the constriction reaches such an extent that the head of the malleus and the incus are completely fixed in the epitympanum, causing an appropriate degree of deafness, an osteoplastic epitympanotomy with resection of the head of the malleus and

incus is indicated, followed by stapedial build-up to form a tympanoplasty Type III (deep) (Figs. **282—284**).

Cutting and diamond burrs can be used to expand and reshape the niches of the middle ear, and the epitympanum. Removal of diseased bone can neither be totally successful nor halt the progress of the disease. Epithelialization of the diseased surface is distorted, so that it is advisable to cover them with fascia or plasticine. The sensorineural deafness may deteriorate, due to a new episode of dysplasia. This phenomenon has been well known since surgeons began to drill down extensive otosclerotic foci in the inner ear capsule during fenestration.

Benign neoplasm of the middle ear such as osteomas and semimalignant tumors are occasional indications for an operation to improve hearing. Paragangliomas arising from the tympanic glomus on the wall of the promontory produce a Schwartze's sign, destroy the incudostapedial joint and cause conductive deafness. Because they are diagnosed early, they can be easily removed. The surface of the bone of the promontory should be drilled down slightly to prevent a recurrence. This is followed by reconstruction of sound transmission.

Meningiomas should be regarded from a pathological point of view as hamartomas. They usually arise in the middle cranial fossa and, more rarely, in the posterior cranial fossa, and produce a wide range of symptoms. They penetrate the base of the skull, passing through the foramen lacerum and the jugular foramen along the trunks of the cranial nerves. The disease extends widely in the floor of the middle and posterior cranial fossas and penetrates the soft tissues of the neck, but there is only occasional limited involvement of the mastoid. Situations in which a tympanoplasty is still possible after thorough eradication are relatively unusual.

The craniosynostoses causing conductive deafness include Crouzon's and Apert's syndrome. The deafness is due both to constrictions of the bony meatus, impeding the conduction of sound, and to anomalies of the ossicles. These diseases are often associated with chronic otitis media. Tympanoplasty may therefore be indicated, but the number of corrective operations is extensive and, so far, little has been done for the deafness.

Healing and Hearing

Complete healing of the air-containing spaces of the temporal bone must always have priority over improvement of hearing (H. L. Wullstein 1952).

Healing

Subdivision of the Types of Tympanoplasty Before and After the Development of Osteoplastic Epitympanotomy

The results of 6,000 tympanoplasties reported in the monograph of H. L. Wullstein et al. (1968) are compared with those for osteoplastic epitympanotomy carried out between 1975 and 1985. In 1970, temporary resection and replacement of the lateral epitympanic wall to provide complete, unimpeded access to the original focus of disease was addressed. This phase of development ended in 1975, when evaluation began. Important improvements such as plasticine were only developed later.

In a population with good medical services, about 70% of patients undergoing tympanoplasty do so for some form of cholesteatoma (including the primary aquired, occult, i.e., early epitympanic, nonperforating type. In poorly developed countries, chronic otitis media is relatively much commoner, due to a high proportion of mucopolypoid and mucoperiostal forms.

Data on Osteoplastic Epitympanotomy

Two periods are compared in Table **2**: up to 1968 in the left-hand column, and from 1971 to 1985 in the right-hand column. In the first period, Type I included few cholesteatomas. Type III (shallow) and Type IV formed the largest groups.

In the second period the proportion of Type III (shallow) tympanoplasties is very small; this procedure is now only used to achieve an open tegmental gutter from the protympanum to the sinodural angle for monitoring of the paralabyrinthine danger zone. Type IV is no longer used, and Type V is used for congenital anomalies, but is very rare. Type I has become the most frequent type used because eradication of all cholesteatomas is the goal of osteoplastic epitympanotomy. Furthermore, this access provides better conditions for the repair of the ossicles, so that Type II tympanoplasty has also increased in frequency. The proportion of reconstruc-

tions of the ossicular chain (Types I and II) in the second period rose to 58% compared with 42% with a columellar system in the earlier period. The epitympanic wall was reimplanted in 97.5% of cases.

Data on Recurrent (Residual) Cholesteatoma

In order to test whether the above results satisfy clinical needs, the frequency of recurrent cholesteatoma is given for the two procedure (Table 3). The 3.5% recurrence rate of cholesteatoma is unsatisfactory. In the vast majority of cases, the recurrence lay medially in the protympanic recess at the ante-

Table **2** Percentage Distributions of Various Types

Tympanoplasty up to 1968 in %		Osteoplastic Epitympanotomy from 1971 to 1985 in %	
Type I	27.4	Type I	44.5
Type II	8.2	Type II	13.7
Type III (deep)	–	Type III (deep)	39.5
Type III (shallow)	30.9	Type III (shallow)	2.5
Type IV	23.2	Type IV	–
Type V (Ist stage)	4.2	Type V (Ist stage)	–
Type V (Ist and 2nd stage)	3.0	Type V (2nd stage)	–
Miscellaneous	3.1	Miscellaneous	–
	100%		100%

Table **3** Recurrent Cholesteatoma

	1976–1985 %	1971–1975 (the developmental phase) %
In all osteoplastic epitympanotomies	2.5	7.1
Exclusively in those carried out for cholesteatoma	3.5	9.6

labyrinthine trigone, due to remnants of the matrix concealed behind the head of the malleus during the operation. In these cases, Types I and II reconstructions were overused by the authors. A stricter assessment of pathological findings during the operation mandates Type III (deep) in cases of doubt, and Type III (shallow) if the paralabyrinthine area is at risk.

A residual cholesteatoma in a very narrow facial recess due to incomplete irradication of the matrix was an exception. Facial paralysis is a lesser danger than occult paralabyrinthine invasion of the vestibule by cholesteatoma. This mandates division of the stapedial tendon and drilling down the pyramidal process after sacrifice of the incus to achieve wide access to the tympanic sinus. The number of retracting cholesteatomas was negligeable.

In view of the 3.5% of residual cholesteatomas the proportion of Type I and Type II procedures should be reduced from 58.2% to 50%, so that the other 50% have a deep or shallow Type III tympanoplasty with an empty epitympanum. The hearing loss due to reduction of the middle ear component would be very slight and acceptable, compared with the danger of a concealed recurrence and the inconvenience of a second operation.

Local Healing of the Tympanoplasty — Disorders During Healing

A *one-stage* tympanoplasty, irrespective of the pathological process, is the prerequisite for the conservation of the entire *middle ear system* (H. L. Wullstein 1952).

After *osteoplastic epitympanotomy* the external ear and meatus are normal, the supra-auricular skin incision is hardly visible, the meatal skin is intact as far as the bony annulus, and the roof of the meatus has the same contours as before. In the interposition technique, the raw surface of the periosteum and fascia on the external surface of the tympanic membrane lies exposed. It is covered on all sides by the retained epidermis of the tympanic membrane, which rapidly provides optimal skin cover within a few days. The electrolyte milieu in the meatus must be maintained by saturated gelatin foam. Small strips are cut out of sterile compressed surgical cotton wool. They are the same length as the external meatus, and of such a size that three of them can be introduced without force. Then the meatus is filled with Ringer's solution, using a fine cannula, with a disinfectant added if the ear is severely infected. The cotton wool swells and exerts uniform pressure on all sides. The electrolyte solution is a

prerequisite for the survival of the *autogenic* fascial layer and for healing of a *xenogenic* membrane. The thin fascia contacting the surrounding edges forms the stroma for the newly formed capillaries.The cotton wool strips are left in place for 4 to 5 days, during which time they are repeatedly moistened to encourage epithelialization of the meatus. In this way a firmly adherant autogenous tissue layer of epidermis is achieved in the meatus. No other local aftercare is needed. Because no incisions are made into the meatal skin, the effects of surgery can no longer be recognized a few weeks later. A careful periosteal suture prevents sinking or protrusion of the auricle.

A slight widening of the normal contours of the meatus, extending as far as the tegmen tympani or even the tegmen antri, is unavoidable if the bony lid can no longer be replaced; for example, in an anteromedial cholesteatoma which has extended into the antelabyrinthine trigone so that the paralabyrinthine space can no longer be filled with plasticine after transtemporal-extradural dissection because of the danger of recurrence. In that case it is only possible to carry out a Type III (shallow) or possibly a Type IV reconstruction. If this procedure must be applied to the postlabyrinthine rhomboid, a narrow visible subtegmental groove covered with skin remains, running from the protympanic recess to the sinodural angle. Because the meatal skin and its accessory structures remain intact in these cases, the self-cleansing action of the meatus is preserved.

The control of chronic mucosal inflammation by *one-stage tympanoplasty* achieves regular healing of the middle ear and the eustachian tube, as can be recognized from the healthy tympanic membrane, the normal aeration, the hearing results, and the healthy epithelium, which is often found at further operations to improve hearing.

One underestimated means of overcoming infection at tympanoplasty is prolonged, vigorous suction-irrigation of all angles and niches during the entire operation. The effect can be increased by the addition of disinfectant for severe infection. It is advisable to roughen the bone surfaces, using a fine cutting drill at the point where it is intended to introduce a plasticine plug. The plasticine contains an antibiotic which acts directly over a long period on the bone wound. It is advisable to eradicate peripheral pneumatic cell groups such as those in the sinodural angle and to expose those in the approach to concealed sublabyrinthine cell groups between the posterior semicircular canal and the jugular bulb. The latter are seldom present in a poorly pneumatized bone and are then difficult of access.

If the classical radical mastoid cavity does not undergo spontaneous epithelialization, it becomes covered with a thick layer of granulation tissue that remains infected by mixed flora, and it therefore suppurates permanently. Local treatment by solutions is usually useless. For that reason radical operations were only carried out in earlier times for the most pressing indications. Because of these bad results the complete healing of the suppurating mucosa achieved by tympanoplasty was particularly well appreciated. The complete healing of the free tympanic membrane graft is the first prerequisite for healing of the mucosa of the internal walls.

Healing of the Epitympanic Flap

The pointed conical diamond burr used for the last stage of trephining of the bony lid has a diameter of 0.2−0.4 mm. The innermost part of the trephine cut behaves like a bone fissure. The orthotopic epitympanic bone lid remains viable after it has been reimplanted. In a few weeks perfect bony refixation has begun at the points of contact, as is shown by later revision operations. Absence of bony refixation is certainly due to an error on the part of the surgeon; this is true of revision procedures also. Reossification begins immediately if the groove for the bony incision is filled with plasticine. If a projecting bony edge on the tegmen was drilled off, producing a wide gap, or if the fulcrum at the genu of the facial nerve was taken down too far, bone dust (pâté) alone placed in this open groove of the epitympanum does not provide sufficient contact to hold the lid firmly in place, even if fibrin glue is used. In early cases a slight step could be recognized at the posterior tympanic spine, due to incorrect fitting of the lid and, in exceptional cases, the bony lid prolapsed too fair internally after it had healed, because the meatus was packed too tightly.

During the first attempts at osteoplastic epitympanotomy in 1971−1972, the release of the skinperiosteal sleeve in the meatus by an incision along the posteroinferior circumferance (a Stacke II flap) was thought to be necessary, and this incision was made tentatively on the anterosuperior wall. In these cases clefts remained over the anterior edge of the bony incision, and on two occasions the bony lid became infected and was unuseable as a result. One patient did not undergo the usual cleaning of the meatus immediately after the operation; this caused ulceration on the incision line in the posterosuperior meatal wall. The results were deep seated infection, and after a prolonged period the bony lid was rejected. A Type III (shallow) tympanoplasty was

created by adhesions of the new tympanic membrane with the facial canal, producing the best audiological results and a completely accessible, delicately healed subtegmental cavity extending as far as the sinodural angle. *There have been no more faults of this type in the fixation of the bony lid since the introduction of a supra-auricular approach without an incision in the meatal skin.*

Healing of the Tympanic Membrane Graft

Healing of the autogenous graft used as a replacement for the tympanic membrane rapidly became a reliable method in 1951−1952, with the underlay or overlay technique or, later, with the currently preferred interposition technique, which has become so much easier with access from above. If the membrane does not overlap the retained collagen fibers or the fibers of the bony annulus sufficiently, the margin can pull away, due to slight retraction during healing. This irritating event requires operative correction, usually by an underlay with fascia. This provides a good opportunity to inspect the middle ear.

Reperforation with suppuration following rapidly after the completion of healing was rare in the development phase of osteoplastic epitympanotomy (1971−1975) after careful dissection in the middle ear and tubal ostium. The cause lay in biologically incorrect solutions or unsatisfactory procedures.

It may be helpful to quote an example: in 1972, a Type I osteoplastic epitympanotomy was carried out to improve the hearing for an apparently dry central perforation in 1972. Tympanosclerosis and numerous mucosal cysts around the ossicles were found. The epitympanum was covered with an unsatisfactory, partially defective bony lid and fascia, and the remaining defect of the superior meatal wall was closed with a firm strip of *cutis-subcutis.* Six weeks later, a perforation developed in the cutis, which steadily enlarged, due to coagulation necrosis of the cutis, so that further operation was required several months later. The partial bony lid was found to have healed firmly to the bone; the entire ossicular chain was intact and very mobile; aeration was present as far as the antrum; there were lax adhesions and granulations in the epi- and hypotympanum. A Type I reconstruction was carried out. In the following years, *the patient complained of nasal obstruction due to seromucinous ethmoiditis* compromising the aeration of the eustachian tube and middle ear. Six years later, a further operation was carried out for suppuration arising from a bony lesion in the antrum. The bony lid had again adhered firmly, but the antrum was full of granulations extending around the ossicles into the epitympanum; the ossicular chain was fully mobile, the round window reflex positive; the mucosa was in good condition and the mesohypotympanum was well aerated. The bone defect was filled by plasticine covered by a pedicled periosteal flap from the intact surface of the mastoid process. A Type I repair was again carried out and healing proceeded smoothly. The functional result was poor, due to a conductive deafness of 30 dB with a *bilateral* progressive sensorineural deafness above 1,000 Hz of up to 70 dB, causing slight loss of discrimination in the operated ear. The *cause of the failure* lay in the use of a full-thickness skin graft with an unsatisfactory underlay in the narrow defect. Full-thickness grafts or transplants of this type were used in hundreds of fenestrations, and they healed over the cells on a broad surface, but they will not succeed in a narrow compressed position. Circumscribed coagulation necrosis led to a skin fistula and to a persisting, mild granulation which could only be healed by operation, again using a Type I. Satisfactory resolution of the middle ear component could no longer be achieved, due to the diffuse scar tissue.

Completely normal healing within 8—10 days is of decisive significance for achieving the best long-term results in any particular situation. Opening of the original area of disease in the epitympanum in all directions, with the most accurate and atraumatic dissection, is very important, even if this demands time and trouble. Otherwise, both the surgeon and the patient must waste even more time to achieve a satisfactory result.

Obviously, these new middle ears cannot be protected from later acute *infection ascending via the eustachian tube*, leading to *further perforation* of the tympanic membrane. Most of these perforations heal rapidly with *antibiotics* and *bed rest* instituted immediately, but large perforations may not heal.

The old methods in which the edge of the perforation was freshened with silver nitrate are not to be recommended because they do not produce a healthy capillary network in the pars tensa but only a thin scar, so that there is a risk that the perforation will enlarge. They are closed by excising the margin of the perforation from the meatus, so long as the tympanic membrane is still under tension on all sides; a fascial underlay is then introduced either from an endaural incision or under vision from a supra-auricular incision.

Re-inspections have repeatedly shown how the middle ear heals as soon as it is closed off and physiological aeration with mucociliary clearance is restored. Confirmation of this, using an angled endoscope to provide a view in the epitympanum, is standard procedure. The mucosa shrinks uniformly, but remains slightly thickened and flat and does not become transparent again. The outline of the wall of the promontory and the aeration pathways are re-established.

Plasticine added to the temporal squama or to the facial spur to build up the antral wall is found at reoperation to be firmly and uniformly adherent to bone and, after some time, can only be recognized by a slight difference in color. It does not retract, and is overgrown by thick transparent mucosa. If plasticine is used as a large disc to replace the entire bony lid, the greater part undergoes *alloplastic ossification* where it lies on the temporal bone over a wide surface. *Osteoid ground substance with atypical mineralization is converted in the long term into irregular fibrous bone with laminar bone over it.* The portion furthest from the surrounding bone does not ossify. More often it changes into a rigid plate, covered on its free surface with mucosa and skin; *this is alloplastic calcification and fibrous permeation to form a rigid cortex.*

Two-Stage or Three-Stage Tympanoplasty for Reconstruction of Sound Conduction

In exceptional cases problems arise which make a two-stage tympanoplasty advisable: at the first stage, an attempt is made to achieve healing by reconstruction of the tympanic cavity; in the second stage, sound conduction is reconstructed in a healthy middle ear cavity.

The reasons for such a procedure include:
1. risk to the inner ear;
2. a particularly severe mucosal inflammation with a perisinus or extradural abscess or wide extension of the mucosal defect;
3. narrow mesohypotympanic air space.

The bony lid may be cut and reimplanted a second or even a third time: it heals as smoothly and as rapidly as after the first operation. This ability facilitates the surgeon's decision to first reconstruct the three parts of the middle ear space to achieve healing, so that the functional reconstruction of sound transmission can be undertaken at a later stage.

Technical reasons for a two-stage operation include:
- overgrowth of the stapedial crura by cholesteatomatous matrix;
- fixation of the stapes by otosclerosis, osteitis or tympanosclerosis;
- defects of the stapes footplate;
- any type of residual cholesteatoma;
- correction or reconstruction of sound transmission in a middle ear healed by a previous procedure;

– release of sound transmission impeded by tympanosclerosis, osteophytes or scar tissue due to extensive mucosal defects;
– reconstitution of the round window niche or the tympanic ostium of the tube;
– vigorous bleeding.

The inner ear is at risk at every attempt to free *the crura of the stapes* from adherent matrix, and a residual cholesteatoma cannot be prevented, even with very great attention to detail. In this case the middle ear is healed by a first-stage tympanoplasty, and a stapedectomy is carried out at a second stage. If firm healing of the window is necessary so that a high columella can be achieved for a Type III (deep) repair, a third stage may be required.

If both crura of the stapes are defective, the *long process of the incus* is also often absent. One possibility for the suspension of a stapedial replacement is then not available. The footplate is often so weakened by osteitis that it is not capable of withstanding the pressure of a high columella without the danger of perforation at a one-stage operation, especially if the pressure is increased by scar tissue contraction during healing of the myringoplasty. A thin plate of cartilage used to cover it should not unite with the bony edges of the window. Tissue contact of a high, thin columella cut with a suitable arch for the tympanic membrane graft can be provided at the two-stage operation. It is embedded between the two layers of fascia by transfixing its very slender shaft by overlapping thin fascia to achieve adherence to the internal surface of the tympanic membrane graft.

It is possible for *otosclerosis* to coexist with *chronic otitis media*. They may not be distinguished initially, because both produce a conductive deafness.

Fixation of the stapes footplate by osteitis is quite common. Stapes mobilization for otosclerosis has been regarded as unsatisfactory for a long time, and this is also true of firm fixation by osteitis. If the long process of the incus is present to allow suspension of the replacement stapes, it was our practice to carry out stapedectomy with tympanoplasty in one stage, provided that the ear was virtually free of inflammation. This procedure does not cause inner ear damage, but cannot be routinely recommended. Stapedectomy as a second-stage operation once the middle ear cavity has been healed for several months causes no great difficulty; it hardly disturbs the patient, and carries a much lower risk of inner ear damage.

In *fixation of the malleus and/or incus by tympanosclerosis*, but with a very mobile stapes, the incu-

dostapedial joint should be released first in all cases. This interruption of the ossicular chain prevents massive movements being transmitted to the stapes when the malleus and incus are released. *Indirect movement during epitympanic manipulation is the most serious cause of iatrogenic trauma of the cochlea. It is therefore most frequent in Type I operations.*

A second operation is necessary for the correction of unsatisfactory sound transmission. The operative procedure can only be decided upon at that time.

The mucosal disease can exceptionally be so severe, the ossicles so embedded and the window so obstructed that there is little hope of restoring normal function to the middle ear in one operation. The first stage ensures that no new adhesions arise, that the mucosa resolves and that the eustachian tube reopens. The second stage corrects the sound transmission either by Type I, Type II or Type III (deep) tympanoplasty.

If the stapes is so tilted by massive granulations on the facial side of the niche or adhesions on the promontorial side that it cannot safely be permanently straightened up in the annular ligament to restore function, it must be removed at a second stage and immediately reintroduced in the correct position.

Severe extradural and perisinus infections may require antibiotics and short-term drainage of the mastoid process. The details of the anatomy are only established and the correction of sound transmission undertaken in the second stage.

Injury of the middle cranial fossa dura is very unlikely if sufficient care is taken during dissection of the tegmen after drilling the temporal squama down to the inner cortex. Occasional bleeding from the underlying pachymeningeal veins can require compression for a short time. The authors are aware of one death in a foreign clinic from injury of the dura, leading to meningitis due to anaerobes which were not isolated and for which antibiotic treatment was not considered.

A foreign surgeon referred a patient with *injury to the facial nerve* during creation of the bony lid. A reoperation demonstrated the mistake against which warnings are always being made; the posterior groove at the edge of the bony lid, which should serve as a fulcrum during fracture, did *not run vertical* to the course of the facial nerve over the incudal fossa, but ran obliquely to the antrum, and therefore inevitably met the facial nerve at the second genu. Careful observation of this rule is an absolutely reliable protection against injury to the facial nerve. Facial paralysis at the end of the procedure demands immediate reoperation. *It is certain that damage to the facial nerve in the presence of a very narrow aditus and antrum, a low-lying dura and a high facial genu, or a Koerner's septum, can more easily be prevented by using osteoplastic epitympanotomy than by a transmastoid search for the antrum and the aditus, in which the semicircular canal is also at risk.*

Osteoplastic epitympanotomy permits injuries of the facial nerve to be exposed rapidly from the labyrinthine to the mastoid segment via a tympanic approach. Thereafter, the epitympanic wall and the sound conduction can be reconstructed; previously, they had to be sacrificed in any lesion of the facial nerve.

Recurrent Cholesteatoma

Recurrent cholesteatoma may be subdivided as follows:
- residual, including the dangerous invasive recurrent type;
- recurrent;
- annulus cholesteatoma;
- graft cholesteatoma;
- inverted cholesteatoma;
- recurrence of traumatic cholesteatoma;
- cholesteatoma due to tympanostomy tubes.

All recurrent cholesteatomas are iatrogenic. Most are now due to the use of the closed technique; previously, occasional recurrence followed radical mastoidectomy. Residual cholesteatomas after osteoplastic epitympanotomy are even more disappointing, as this operation was created to prevent recurrent cholesteatoma. After a period of trial of the access from the facial-chordal angle to the tegmen tympani for eradication of middle ear cholesteatoma, H. L. Wullstein (1952–1955) restricted the use of the closed technique to polypoid and muco-periosteal middle ear inflammation. The retention of the epitympanum in the presence of cholesteatoma remained the great problem. Other surgeons have also gradually resumed radical mastoidectomy for cholesteatoma (Charachon, Smyth, Steinbach, and the members of the panel at the International E.N.T. Congress in 1985 in Miami).

Residual cholesteatoma is almost always found in the protympanic and supratubal recess, the sinus tympani, the facial recess and as an invasive form in the labyrinthine wall. Many surgeons remove the incus in the closed technique to prevent this type of recurrence. Although the access to the epitympanum is extended, the necessary view is not achieved and a Type I tympanoplasty cannot be carried out. The head of the malleus is left behind, but this has no value in bridging the defect from the neck of the malleus to the head of the stapes. Pearls of noninvasive cholesteatoma are occasionally discovered incidentally on the epitympanic mucosa at a second-look operation. They have little tendency to grow without renewed irritation and can be removed easily. Few detailed descriptions are available in the literature about the findings and results of large epitympanic residual cholesteatomas, and especially of invasive cholesteatomas.

The risk of development of a paralabyrinthine cholesteatoma is less posterior to the labyrinth than anterior to it, because anterior cholesteatomas are in any case more frequent than posterior ones and because the antrum is always opened widely at mastoidectomy, both in the open and closed techniques.

Residual cholesteatoma can grow into the posterior point of danger in the open technique. In this operative procedure there is now a tendency to reduce the size of the mastoid cavity, possibly to the level of the meatus, using a pedicled periosteal or aponeurotic flap; for example, the Palva flap, which lies on lyophilized dura, bone dust, etc. These materials have entirely different resorption and reorganization times. The pedicled skin-aponeurosis flap described by H. L. Wullstein (1968) is also being used more. All these soft tissues fill the sinodural angle and thus cover the postlabyrinthine rhomboid and the tractus niche. Residual cholesteatomas in the mastoid, extending to the posterior paralabyrinthine cells or the spongiosa, are thus hidden from view, despite the open technique.

Obliteration of the mastoid cavity up to the level of the facial spine using plasticine leaves the antrum and sinodural angle open as a wide, subtegmental groove. If a Type III (shallow) tympanoplasty was necessary, this subtegmental groove covered with a split-thickness skin graft remains open from the protympanum to the sinus for inspection.

The surgeon carrying out osteoplastic epitympanotomy must decide the limits which justify complete reconstruction of the middle ear spaces for cholesteatoma. A surgeon who uses only the open technique avoids this decision. Those who wish to retain the anatomical and functional advantages of the closed technique have made the decision easier by making a second operation obligatory.

The first task of ostoplastic epitympanotomy is to determine the type and extent of the reconstruction. The surgeon must know when the risk of recurrence of the cholesteatoma *in the protympanic recess or in the sinodural angle* becomes so great that reintroduction of the bone lid is not permissible; the patient must be satisfied with a Type III (shallow) tympanoplasty and an open subtegmental groove to allow long-term monitoring of the antelabyrinthine trigone and the postlabyrinthine rhomboid.

In the closed technique it is impossible to assess the medial wall or the inner surface of the lateral wall of the epitympanum using the microscope for *invasion by a cholesteatoma*. In contrast, the bony lid is very accurately inspected on its medial side under high magnification and is drilled down with the diamond burr as far as necessary, either over the entire surface or only partially. Because these cholesteatomas are invasive, they are likely to recur. In this case the lid can be replaced by a plasticine wall, possibly mixed with bone dust from the temporal squama, which is always free of cholesteatoma.

The matrix of a cholesteatoma is not so easily concealed in a widely opened *sinus tympani* as in a narrow, curved sinus hidden under a steep, overhanging mastoid segment of the facial nerve. Inaccessibility when using the closed technique makes finding and complete eradication through the usually narrow facial-chordal angle more uncertain than from the middle ear. Residual cholesteatomas after osteoplastic epitympanotomy are best prevented by polishing with the diamond burr after removal of the pyramidal process, and maximal opening of the sinus, even as far as the facial nerve from the tympanic surface, using undercuts. They are not excluded in the sinus tympani and the facial recess by a Type III (shallow).

Reimplantation of a bony lid containing invasive remnants of cholesteatoma is a great error. They are easy to avoid, in the light of knowledge of the danger of the various concealed forms of residual cholesteatomas.

The conditions for *retraction cholesteatoma* in the epitympanum are seldom present after osteoplastic epitympanotomy. After removal of the bony lid, dissection of the compartments around the ossicles is so thorough that no inflammatory soft tissue which might lead to renewed retractions remains. The membrane used for closure of a large tympanic membrane defect must be of sufficient strength. The depth of indrawing of the new atrophic membrane can be seen with an angled endoscope, allowing deposition of debris containing keratin at this point to be assessed.

Because the wall of the sinus tympani and the mastoid process remains intact, the function of the lower aeration pathway leading to the aditus is retained. Prolapse of an atrophic membrane through the sinus and then into the mastoid is not possible.

A planned second look through the facial-chordal angle has no place here. In transmastoid operations for cholesteatomas, large recurrences at the second operation for restitution of function mandate the creation of a large mastoid activity with an extensive wound surface.

Symptoms of a *residual cholesteatoma in the epitympanum* include a slowly progressive deafness, vestibular disturbance, and a peripheral facial palsy which varies, but slowly progresses if the cholesteatoma penetrates the antelabyrinthine trigone. The symptoms of a posterior cholesteatoma are a dural headache and occasional tinnitus, but epitympanic secretion is rare. When the cholesteatoma has become relatively large, the posterosuperior meatal wall may sag, due to erosion of the surgically thinned epitympanic wall. Before the introduction of antibiotics, it was often the classical symptom of early penetration of acute otitis media into the meatus from the antrum. Residual cholesteatoma in the mesotympanum (for example, in the sinus tympani), is usually visible through the tympanic membrane.

A case will now be described as an example of an incorrect indication for osteoplastic epitympanotomy. The permissible limits were far overstepped by the surgeon (H. L. Wullstein) during the early period in February 1972.

The patient was a woman with primary acquired cholesteatoma on both sides. *Osteoplastic epitympanotomy was carried out on the left side using a broad bony lid. Extensive cholesteatoma was found filling the entire epitympanum, antrum and mastoid, as well as the sinus tympani.* There were defects of both incudal processes, and the remnant of the incus and the head of the malleus were fixed to the medial wall by bone. *Cholesteatoma lay between osteophytes in the epitympanum, with deep niches and roots between the lateral semicircular canal and the second facial genu.*

All bony walls were drilled down so that no mucosa remained. The bony lid was replaced to form a Type III (deep) tympanoplasty. Six months later the lid began to retract, and twelve months later a progressive sensorineural deafness set in. The patient was followed up in subsequent years in a nearby clinic. She refused a revision operation for severe progression of deafness. A year later she complained of vomiting, dizziness and deafness. A revision operation showed erosion of the anterior semicircular canal by cholesteatoma extending under the dura of the middle cranial fossa and in a paralabyrinthine direction along the facial nerve toward the petrous apex as well as toward the lateral semicircular canal and the oval window niche, but there was no osteitis. The mastoid cavity was left open.

The operation on the left ear can be criticized because the cholesteatoma with severe mucoperiosteal inflammation and osteophytes on the wall of the inner ear with early paralabyrinthine extension and exposed dura did not justify the creation of a closed epitympanum. A Type III (shallow) tympanoplasty with an exposed medial epitympanic wall and antrum should have been performed.

At the first admission, an osteoplastic epitympanotomy was carried out on the right ear because of *cholesteatoma*, and again later on the right side when the left was revised. The primary operation on the right side showed an epitympanic defect. There was an extensive posterolateral cholesteatoma over the entire width of the epitympanum between the bony wall and the ossicles. The long process of the incus was destroyed. The head of the malleus and the stapes were incorporated in massively infiltrated folds. The cholesteatoma was dissected out after exposure of the upper aeration pathway. Silicone sheet was introduced under the lid to prevent adhesions: at that time, there was great uncertainty about healing of a freestanding bony lid and fear of scar tissue retraction. In addition a tantalum wire suture was used to fix the lid to the tympanic spine.

Healing was uneventful. Three and a half years later, the graft and the meatal wall were unremarkable. The patient had a conductive deafness of 10 dB from 500—6,000 Hz with normal bone conduction. At the time of the revision operation on the left side, the right side was also revised. The bony lid was now fixed firmly; the wire suture had come undone and was therefore removed, as was the silicone sheet. A residual cholesteatoma in the facial recess was exposed and removed. The reconstructed incus and stapes were still retained in their position. The bony lid was replaced and covered with meatal skin.

The small residual cholesteatoma found in the facial recess on the right side was an incidental finding. The tantalum wire and the silicone sheet formed a focus of tissue irritation.

The development and prevention of an annulus cholesteatoma, graft cholesteatoma and inversion cholesteatoma of the tensa epidermis have already been discussed. They are visible on clinical examination and should be removed through the meatus, provided they are small. Cholesteatoma due to *inversion* of tympanic membrane epithelium after interposition of fascia can form a pocket that only needs to be opened up. The *annulus cholesteatomas*, particularly those due to an incorrectly placed, full-thickness skin graft leading to a transplant cholesteatoma, may remain concealed while the matrix grows over the inner walls. A skillful myringoplasty is necessary.

The same points apply to *recurrent traumatic cholesteatomas* as to recurrent tensa lesions. Recurrences arising from remnants of matrix in the pneumatic system can remain concealed for a long time and require extensive mastoid surgery. Cholesteatoma due to inversion of the thin, nonpapillary epidermis of the pars tensa through a *tympanostomy tube* requires myringoplasty for the same reason, particularly if the perforation in the pars tensa has closed spontaneously.

Recurrence of Otitis Media with Effusion

The insertion of a *tympanostomy tube* for severe conductive deafness initially gives the impression of being a very successful form of treatment. If it needs to be repeated several times, it become an iatrogenic disaster. The effects on hearing of repeated tympanotomy militate against successful results in the long term, even if long-term antibiotics are administered; it has been shown that the correct antibiotic enters various forms of effusion. The secretion, infected or noninfected, need not drain into the mesotympanum, but is retained in the adherent compartments of the epitympanum. Later it becomes thickened and leads to fibrosis and tympanosclerosis, which block the interossicular air spaces, causing severe conductive deafness which is almost impossible to eradicate by surgery because of the absence of mucosa capable of regeneration.

In order to avoid this very undesirable outcome of otitis media with effusion, several surgeons have elected to carry out mastoidectomy and atticoantrotomy, and remove relatively late-stage cholesterol granulomas from this site; however, thorough, permanent success was not achieved. The explanation is to be sought in the fact that the inspissated secretion behind the massively infiltrated folds is not eradicated through this single opening. Minimal treatment requires simultaneous elevation of Shrapnell's membrane and the superior quadrants of the tympanic membrane to allow the epitympanum to be aspirated and irrigated with continuous irrigation from the antrum.

An experienced surgeon would prefer to carry out osteoplastic epitympanotomy for these patients, exposing and opening the often firmly closed compartments, and thoroughly eradicating all cholesterol granulomas, adhesions of the folds and infiltrations. Only then is normal aeration restored, allowing the mucosa to recover. Treatment of the anterior middle ear sector (mesohypotympanum) as far as the tympanic diaphragm is inadequate. This procedure is indicated because of the danger of later massive adhesive processes in the epitympanum.

The repeated trauma of long-term tympanostomy tubes causes a severe disturbance of the fine structure of the pars tensa. The results are: firstly, circumscribed atrophic areas consisting only of external and internal epithelium without a collagenous fiber layer and possibly with a ring of scar tissue; and secondly, myringitis with fibrosis and myringosclerosis. A purely serous noninfected effusion should be treated by management of the ethmoids and the eustachian tube, supplemented by single or repeated puncture and aspiration of the secretions through the tympanic membrane. However, recurrent mucous effusions, especially during the development of the lymphatic system and in the second growth phase of the temporal bone (Figs. **6, 7**) resolve rapidly, with reliable long-term results and minimal trauma to the middle ear by the use of osteoplastic epitympanotomy.

Iatrogenic infections during tympanoplasty. The introduction of tympanostomy tubes exposes the ear to bacteria. Antibiotics are effective against seromucinous effusions if they are correctly chosen and the treatment is short. However, it is difficult to obtain secretions for culture and sensitivity tests. The resistance of the organisms increases with long-term use. An effusion in the compartments sterilized by antibiotics is less likely to liquify and drain, the longer it persists (see above).

Allogenic Grafts and Virus Infection

Allogenic ossicles have great merit for the replacement of the ossicular chain, and mucosa can grow over them smoothly and well. After implantation of a prepared ossicle host, granulation tissue begins to sprout two weeks later along the vessels of the graft, and vascularization follows this pathway (Eitschberger 1980). The risk of transmission of the HIV-III virus has created an entirely new and difficult situation, because it is incorporated into the DNA molecule. It is rendered inactive by warming to 57°. Human biological fibrin glue is maintained at a temperature of 60° for 30 hours to inactivate the virus. But further research is required to determine the efficacy of allograft sterilization against HIV and Creutzfeld-Jakob disease (Glasscock 1988). The preparation of the plasticine during the operation is thus made even more reliable. Tests have not yet confirmed whether inactivation of the virus by cialit reaches as far as the center of the ossicles. The change to xenogenic ossicles of young animals, such as lambs or calves, has abolished the danger due to human pathogenic viruses. However, some remnants of antigenicity remain, and a mural hyalinosis with constriction of the lumen occurs rather than vascularization. It is therefore important at the beginning of every operation to take as much autogenous bone dust from the temporal squama as possible so that a replacement bony lid, whose periphery has become too small for whatever reason, can be augmented by plasticine mixed with this bone dust.

Chronic Seromucinous Ethmoiditis

The healing and prevention of ethmoiditis is one of the provisions for smooth healing within the otobase. The ethmoid bone, with the anterior end of the middle turbinate and the ostia of the pneumatized spaces of the viscerocranium lying posterior to it, is the portal of access for the most frequent of all human infections.

Investigation of the middle ear is incomplete *without endoscopy of the middle and inferior nasal meatus* supplemented by radiology of the paranasal sinuses in the frontal and axial planes. For this reason, it would be wrong to restrict the specialty to the practice of otology only. A meticulous, thorough endoscopic, endonasal operation on the entire ethmoid sinus, opening of the sphenoid and of Haller's cells lying inferior to the floor of the orbit, using the various angled endoscopes either in one stage together with tympanoplasty, or as a two-stage procedure, must be part of the repertoire of the otorhinolaryngologist.

S. R. Wullstein has investigated the anterior, middle and posterior ethmoid sinuses (Figs. **233–234**), finding *seromucinous inflammation* extending immediately anterior to the ostium of the tympanic tube in the cells of the ethmoid sinus, similar to that found in the compartments of the epitympanum and sealed off by adhesions. Healing of this chronic inflammation is a prerequisite for the healing of the pharyngeal ostium of the eustachian tube and thus the restitution of the function of the tube and of the middle ear. The mucosa of these cavities with their natural drainage pathways usually heals after the creation of a wide, healthy ethmoid with a free view into its recesses and into the wide drainage ducts of the frontal sinus, the maxillary sinus and the sphenoid sinus, followed by aspiration and inhalations through the anatomical ostium. Operations for infection of the maxillary and frontal sinus are now only exceptionally carried out.

In children with the quite common infection of the maxillary sinuses, there is a high probability of a subacute inflammation of the ethmoids. The treatment is similar to that for persistent seromucinous otitis media with effusion (see p. 137 ff.).

Hearing

Improvement in hearing takes second place to reliable healing, so that it may be necessary to destroy a functioning sound conduction apparatus and to use a replacement which is inferior. Therefore, the operative results with regard to hearing cannot be compared with those expected in otosclerosis. Because of the numerous anatomical and pathological factors, the severity of the infection, the tendency to severe scarring, and the properties of the reconstructed sound conduction apparatus, it is astonishing that useful hearing is so often achieved.

Serious pathology *with almost normal sound conduction before the operation demands destruction of the ossicular chain, so that the hearing often becomes worse after successful healing.* This adversely affects the statistics twice; firstly by increasing the mean preoperative values and secondly, by lowering the mean postoperative values.

In a few cases with previously good inner ear function, the operation causes severe damage to the inner ear (see below). Because the data ought to represent an average result, such extremes are not reported, but are treated separately as iatrogenic damage.

The results quoted below (Figs. **286–290**) since the introduction of osteoplastic epitympanotomy are compared with those for 6,000 tympanoplasties which were calculated by Schmitt for the author's monograph, *Operationen zur Verbesserung des Gehöres* (Fig. **285**).

Mean Hearing Values After Tympanoplasty

Because cochlear damage in chronic otitis media is very variable, only mean changes in conductive deafness are given in Figs. **286–290**, and the *preoperative bone conduction* is adjusted to the base line.

It is remarkable that the postoperative air conduction curve is better than 27 dB in all the types which depend on sound pressure transformation [Types I, II and III (deep)]. Thus, hearing in these types is achieved via sound pressure transformation.

Statistical Comparison

The curves of the mean values from 0.25 kHz to 6 kHz in each of the types are very similar in the earlier and in the more recent measurements of air and bone conduction before and after operation. The change in hearing for speech is given as the speech sound level.

The improvement in hearing is greater after osteoplastic epitympanotomy: the air conduction improved by 10–15 or even 20 dB over the entire range. In Type III (shallow) and Type IV, it amounts from 25 dB to 30 dB.

The air conduction audiogram remains constant for many years, except for those patients who must be considered for revision surgery.

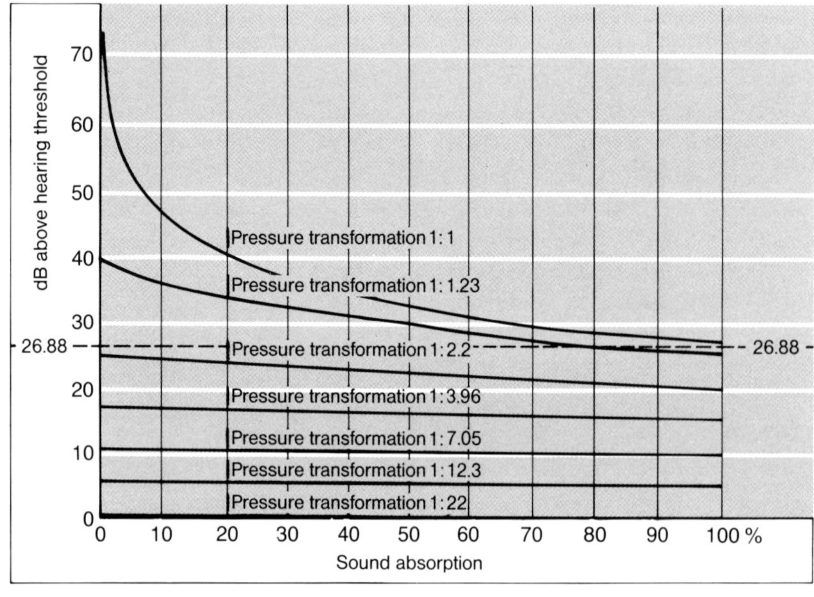

Fig. **285** **Dependence of the hearing threshold on the sound pressure transformation.** The abscissa shows the sound absorption. The ordinate shows the hearing loss in dB above normal threshold (Schmitt 1968)

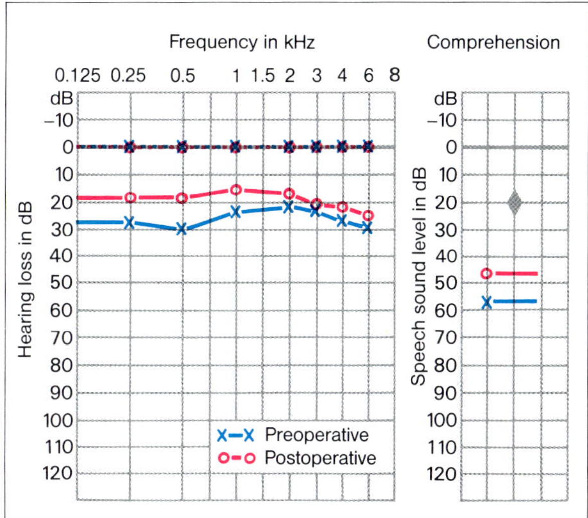

Fig. **286a**   **Results of tympanoplasty Type I, up to 1968**

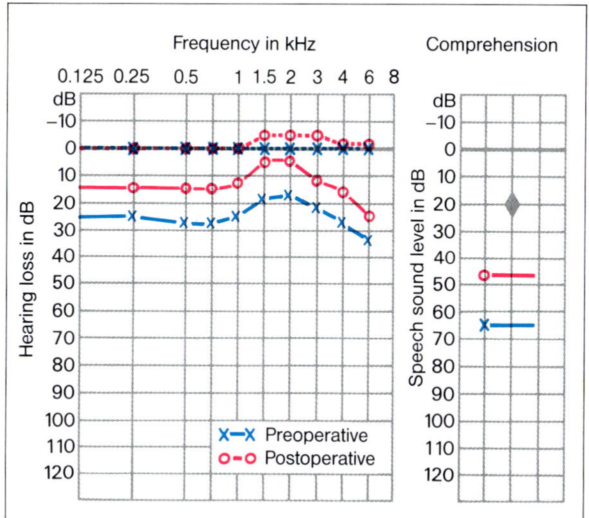

Fig. **286b**   **Results of osteoplastic epitympanotomy Type I (1975−1985)**

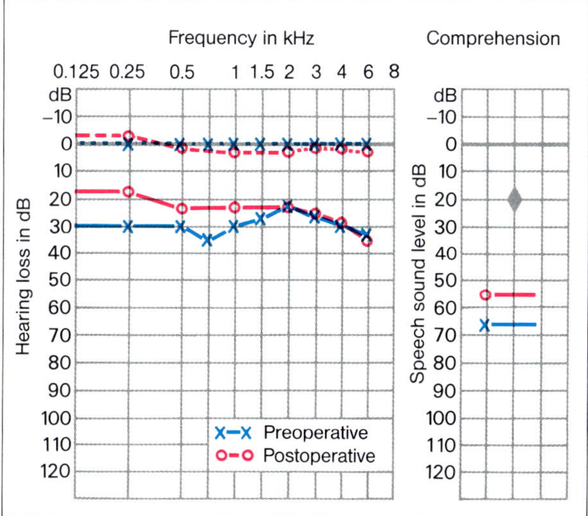

Fig. **287a**   **Results of tympanoplasty Type II, up to 1968**

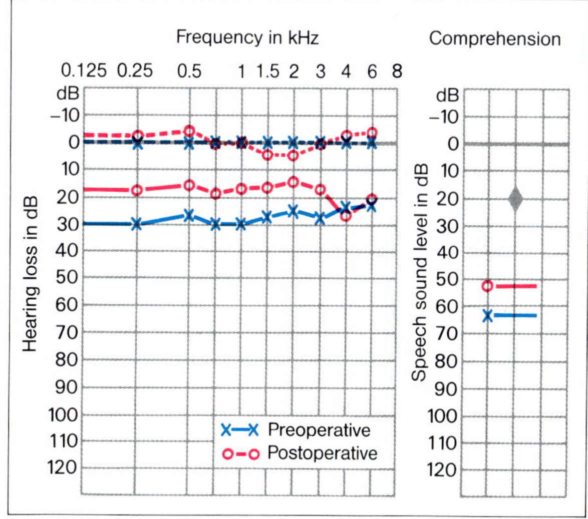

Fig. **287b**   **Results of osteoplastic epitympanotomy Type II (1975−1985)**

Fig. **288**   **Results of osteoplastic epitympanotomy Type III (deep) (1975−1985).** * 50% comprehension = 20 dB in normal hearing. 100% = 30 dB

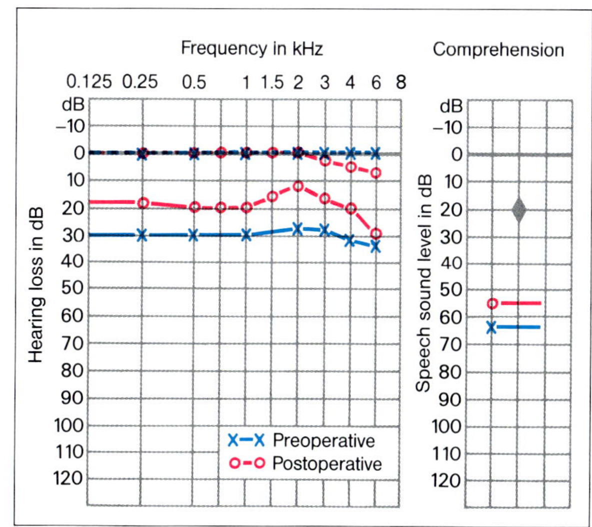

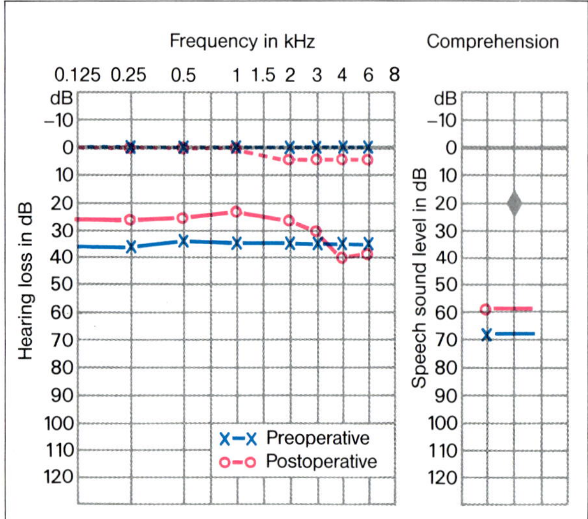

Fig. **289** **Results of tympanoplasty Type III (shallow), up to 1968**

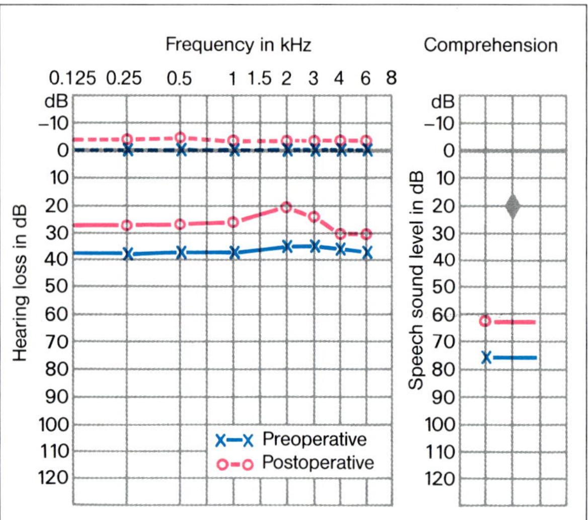

Fig. **290** **Results of tympanoplasty Type IV, up to 1968**

In anatomical functional and audiological terms. Type III (deep) is more similar to the original Type III, which is today called Type III (shallow). The air content of the middle ear space is considerably larger and better attuned for the various frequencies. The active tympanic membrane surface is also larger and reaches beyond the facial canal. The lever system of the middle ear is absent.

Assessment of Hearing Capability

The mean values do not allow recognition of wide variation in the values for the sound conduction component before the operation. A large stable pars tensa which is minimally diseased offers the best prospect for good hearing, even with defects of ossicular transmission, as Zöllner 1957 recognized quite early.

The demands on the capability for sound pressure reception on the tissue of a new tympanic membrane and the sound transmission via the ossicles as a result of tympanoplasty can be deduced from the fact that a change of 6 dB at 1000 Hz indicates a twofold change in the sound pressure, and a change of 20 dB indicates a tenfold alteration. An improvement in a conductive hearing loss from 25 dB to 15 dB indicates an increase of sound pressure transformation from 1:2.2 to 1:4; a rise from 10 dB to 5 dB indicates an increase of sound transformation from 1:7 to 1:12. Raising a conductive hearing loss from 5 dB to 0 dB (i.e., to a normal threshold value) would require a further increase of pressure transformation from 1:12 to 1:22. This is an impossible demand on an operation which must simultaneously eradicate inflammation and prevent adhesions while it heals and reconstructs, using free transplanted tissue. The similarity of the curves in large numbers of cases over the range from 0.25 to 6 kHz is astonishing.

Fate and Function of the Middle Ear Muscles after the Operation

In a Type I tympanoplasty, the middle ear muscles remain in their normal anatomical relationships as long as one of the tendons has not been divided because of tympanosclerosis. In a Type II, the muscles are usually intact, and any myositis is of such a slight degree that it heals. In a Type III (deep or shallow), the tensor tympani muscle never functions, and myositis of this structure can be very severe. In order to aid the healing of the tubal ostium, it may be advisable to drill its canal with the diamond burr and possibly resect it. The pyramidal process and the stapes tendon are often destroyed.

The surgeon can always see the tendons of both muscles, but the muscles themselves can only be exposed by dissection. Chronic inflammation and scarring of the two muscles are frequent. Severe disease can only be assessed after exposure.

The stapedius muscle reflex is elicited by a stimulus; for example, the sound of very loud suction anterior to the round window niche. If the reflex is absent, the muscle must be scarred if bone conduction had been shown to be normal before the operation; the stapedius tendon must then be divided.

The average hearing results only worsen very slightly on passing from Type I to Type III (shallow). However, there is no information about the function of the muscles in comparison with the information available about the tympanic membrane and the vibratory ability of the ossicular chain. In Type III (shallow), the head of the stapes adheres to the displaced membrane and is thus limited in movement, as it is in Type III (deep), with stapes build-up due to the bipartite reconstruction of the columella.

The sensitive interplay of the middle ear muscles in response to the marked variation in character of sound of different speakers cannot be measured by pure tone threshold audiometry, nor with brief and uniform suprathreshold word tests.

The continuous control of the middle ear structures by the muscles makes the unwieldy middle ear system receptive for successive sounds. This control cannot be recorded with standard audiology, nor can the very sensitive control of ossicular damping, which is achieved by the ossicles in the epitympanum with the help of the epitympanic air cushions. These functions facilitate the understanding of speech if they are well preserved, but it is only possible to compare them if the opposite ear is well preserved. For this reason music remains an enjoyment for the deaf for a long time, even if the highest frequencies are lost, because the analysis of music causes less difficulty than the analysis of the rapidly changing, complicated sound patterns of speech.

Postoperative High-Tone Loss

A steep loss for air conduction at about 3 kHz with well-maintained bone conduction indicates a resonance loss in the middle ear system. A steep loss of air and bone conduction together indicates iatrogenic cochlear trauma.

Problems of Unilateral Chronic Otitis Media Associated with Deafness in the Opposite Ear

Because of the possibility of cochlear damage, surgery should be as atraumatic as possible in preparing the hearing ear for the wearing of a hearing aid. A concealed cholesteatoma should be eradicated and chronic suppuration healed. The posterior meatal wall remains intact, the epitympanic wall is removed and the mastoid is cleared and obliterated. The mucosa of the mesohypotympanum heals, protected by a Type III or IV tympanoplasty. The labyrinthine-paralabyrinthine area above the facial nerve is covered as usual with a split-thickness skin graft, but reconstructive procedures in the middle ear are not undertaken.

0.6% of our patients suffered *iatrogenic postoperative inner ear damage* during osteoplastic epitympanotomy, which made the operated ear almost unusable despite a good anatomical and pathological result. The highest risk is in severe tympanosclerosis with a well-preserved ossicular chain. If the malleus and incus alone are fixed, the connection to the stapes must be divided before all manipulations in the epitympanum. In extensive mucosal defects due to tympanosclerosis in the epitympanum, the functional aftercare is facilitated by dispensing with Type I and II tympanoplasty. A fixed incus or head of malleus that can only be mobilized with great difficulty is resected. A good result is achieved more quickly by a Type III (deep) and the result is hardly worse than that of a difficult Type I. In severe adhesions the results of Type I become much worse.

The greatest risk to function lies in persistent attempts at mobilizing a massively fixed stapes. Although the authors have carried out one-stage mobilization or stapedectomy for ankylosis without causing cochlear damage, they would prefer to carry out the operation in two stages if there is the slightest risk. A repeat epitympanotomy is an easy, reliable procedure for exposing the oval window niche. Again the surgeon must decide how far he ought to go in a one-stage procedure and when he ought to choose a two-stage procedure for the sake of function.

Demands on Sound Transmission Mechanism of the New Middle Ear

The above results based on threshold values show that demands made on the middle ear sound transmission of the operated ear are usually fulfilled. The patients are normally satisfied, provided that the inner ear function is good. The expected results are astonishingly good over a wide frequency range. Such results were initially achieved with labyrinthine fenestration, which has its own handicaps, including the loss of sound pressure transformation in the middle ear. Later, similar results were achieved with stapedectomy, and then under completely dissimilar conditions, with tympanoplasty. In the early period of surgery, to improve hearing when no useful electronic hearing aids were available, patients with massive otosclerotic deafness were happy with any improvement of comprehension, and those with chronic otitis media were no less happy. If they regained social and economical hearing (Lempert 1941) (above 30 dB with satisfactory inner ear function), their demands were regarded as having been fulfilled.

Goode (1977) tested not only the resonance of the external ear and the meatus but also the changed conditions after operation. The following data are important in operations aimed at improving hearing; they are based on measurements made on Knowles Electronic Mannikin for Acoustic Research, on the temporal bone and on patients, and on sources quoted by Goode: the free standing edge of the auricle contributes little to resonance but, in conjunction with the conchal fossa, it achieves an increase of sound pressure of about 10 dB at 4 kHz, and at 3 kHz also, if the conchal fossa is deep. Surgical flattening causes the opposite. The removal of cartilage from this point is therefore ill advised.

The theoretical peak of the resonance of the external meatus can be calculated from two factors: the length of the canal and the impedance at the tympanic membrane. The best sound pressure gain is achieved with impact of the sound at an angle of 45° to the sagittal midline. The resonance of the normal meatus causes an increase of up to 20 dB at 3−5 kHz in the air conduction threshold; the higher the impedance, the higher and narrower the resonance peak. The shape of the *natural* meatus has no decisive influence on this. Once again the very wide variations in the growth of the base of the skull have no effect on the astonishingly uniform hearing capacity. Variations are either too little, or they are compensated by developments of the sound conduction apparatus at other points. A constriction of the meatus to 3 mm or less causes a loss of air conduction threshold of up to 15 dB at 2−4 kHz.

If the meatus and the antrum are joined by surgery, the resonance peak can fall by 20 dB and anti-resonance may even occur. In the lined operative cavity, the fall is less and not uniform. In many cases the open mastoid cavity even acts as a resonator with a wide band width. H. L. Wullstein has previously stated that *in Type IV tympanoplasty covered with a split skin graft* a conduction loss is often no longer present over the entire frequency range. The result achieved by sound protection therefore resembles that achieved by sound pressure transformation, and is thus better than theoretically expected. Later, Goday-Rodriguez and Schuknecht 1977 confirmed this observation.

It would be preferable if the ideal operative result could be achieved deliberately and not only accidentally. Therefore H. L. Wullstein asked von Bèkèsy in 1957 whether the paramenters of the shape of the antral cavity could be calculated to allow the wide resonance reinforcement to be led into the depth of the oval window niche. Sadly, von Bèkèsy had to answer in the negative.

The individual external meatus is tailored to its middle ear and constructed to ensure the best hearing. Any necessary extensive surgical change can lead to either improvement or to deterioration. It is therefore most advisable not to change the shape of the auricle and external meatus; indeed, the acoustic properties of the skin, the subcutaneous layers and the periosteum should remain completely unaltered. In a Type III (shallow) tympanoplasty, the necessity for an open subtegmental gutter outweight the insignificant hearing loss caused by the change in shape.

The value of the new hearing levels after an anatomically and functionally successful tympanoplasty depends on the function of the inner ear. In otosclerosis, surgery is only justifiable if the inner ear hearing for speech is satisfactory, whereas in chronic otitis media, a tympanoplasty is unavoidable, even in the presence of severe sensorineural deafness. This component can even improve after the operation, because of the prolonged toxic inflammation of the windows. Furthermore, it can never be known beforehand how long the patient will live and whether a premature presbycusis will develop. A tympanoplasty should therefore be so designed that a hearing aid can be worn later. This requires a normal external meatus completely lined by healthy epithelium in which the capacity to transport wax and debris is retained to allow the patient to wear a hearing aid continuously. The planning of the operation must therefore consider how the patient will be able to understand speech, even in old age, with the help of a hearing aid.

The assessment of function of the new middle ear by impedance measurement is limited by the fact that it is restricted to a frequency of 220 Hz and, possibly, also 660 Hz. It provides only one value, which is a composite of the functional disturbance of various parts of the middle ear system. The result is unequivocal if the clinician is certain that only one factor is responsible for the abnormality. This is true in a young child in the years of rapid development of the lymphatic and immunological systems. However, it is no longer true in later years; firstly, because a tympanic membrane perforation is usually present in chronic otitis media, and secondly, because the various pathological factors in a closed middle ear have equally affected the impedance. As a result of protection by immunization and timely treatment by antibiotics, the number of recurrent acute purulent middle ear inflammations has markedly decreased. However, the number of upper respiratory infections has not fallen, so that otitis media with effusion (serous and seromucinous otitis media) is very important at this age. Its careful control is of great significance because of the results of marked deafness; firstly, the development of speech, and therefore of education, can be at risk in early childhood, and secondly, severe adhesions can arise from the persisting epitympanic sequelae. Despite the limitation, measurement of impedance is a leading parameter for defining the pathological status of the middle ear, as is the stapedius reflex.

Measurement of the impedance is still successful if only a partial segment of the tympanic membrane remains capable of movement, a fact which the investigator, however, cannot simultaneously observe. Holography permits a view of the entire range of the tympanic membrane.

Otoscopic investigations with the holographic interferometer have become possible in the last few years, both in probands and also in patients, using the flexible endoscope (Bally 1979). These investigations showed that the vibration pattern as deduced by von Bèkèsy is erroneous. The vibration patterns demonstrate several centers which break up into sectional vibrations at frequencies of only 2 kHz in the healthy tympanic membrane (Tonndorf and Khanna 1972). Vibration centers can also be recognized in the pars flaccida. The purpose of the investigations includes:

1. the differential diagnosis of sound transmission disorders in the unopened hearing organ, for example, after removal of the incus in congenital anomalies of the ossicular chain;
2. follow-up after operations to improve hearing;
3. basic investigations of the transmission function of the middle ear.

The results of point 2 are especially important for the surgeon at the present time, and they include the postoperative investigations of the aptitude and long-term adaptation of *materials used for the reconstruction of the middle ear, the membrane and the columella.*

The pars tensa should be so constructed that it always ensures firm union to the manubrium during slow adaptation of tension of the graft. The purpose is to create unimpeded aeration pathways to the antrum by careful dissection of the open epitympanum; if necessary, even by strengthening of the membrane using two layers of glued temporal periosteum in which the rapid capillary attachment to the host tissue occurs for each layer. In contrast, a replacement for the pars flaccida with its papillary epidermis should not heal with this type of tension.

This kind of information about the tissue used as a replacement tympanic membrane, in comparison with the pars tensa and its collagenous fiber system,

would be valuable. At present, only empirical experience forms a basis for deciding the most suitable tissue for the tympanic membrane and for the transmission of sound.

If a persistent conductive deafness is paired with a sensorineural deafness, a hearing aid (particularly an in-the-ear apparatus with relatively weak capacity) may be necessary for heavy occupational use. Obstruction of the conchal fossa by the hearing aid removes the amplifying effect of the fossa, which ideally should be retained.

Unfortunately, very severe inner ear damage with disorders of frequency resolution are common in chronic middle ear inflammation. Comprehension is then only possible with a very high performance aid in which hearing is achieved via *the supra-auricular fold and the temporal bone with the microphone on the end of the fold and the receiver behind the superior otobasion.* This was introduced by H. L. Wullstein and employed by industry under the definition *frontal hearing.* The sound impinges from 45° in front, and not from all sides, as in the nondirectional microphones which lie either posteroinferior (causing marked disturbance due to noise) or free in front of the auricle on the temporal bone. Once the microphone was placed at the end of the supra-auricular fold, it became possible to use a microphone with cardioid-shaped characteristics. Furthermore, a microphone worn free on the temple is exposed to the slightest wind noise, which is otherwise broken up on hearing via the meatus through the tragus and the concha. The problem of the conduction to the microphone through the contours of the helix with the placement on the auricle at the superior otobasion is solved by hearing along the supraauricular fold.

In order to improve bilateral hearing loss by bilateral digital hearing aids tuned to each other, a simultaneous bilateral continuous audiogram performed by the patient is helpful. It is an extremely subjective method for measurement and adjustment of hearing sensitivity. A special measuring apparatus, the Audioanalysator, was developed by Schlitt (1985), Wullstein and Wullstein (1985). The otaudion described by Schwarz in 1925 was the first electronic audiometer acting as a continually functioning apparatus. For ease of manufacture, industry has limited measurement to unchangeable tone increments, whereas von Bèkèsy used continuous recording for this purpose. Frequency and time analysis, particularly in noise from all sides, demand an appropriate hearing aid worn in the meatus, even in slight degrees of deafness. But in high degrees of deafness in an occupation which demands the comprehension of speech, the air space of the meatus must be preserved for coupling to the tympanic membrane. For all these reasons it is the duty of the surgeon to leave all parts of the external ear undisturbed.

Patients undergoing tympanoplasty seldom demand "purity" of sound and the restoration of harmonics in binaural hearing for music. The reason is that these patients have long forgotton this capability, due to the difficulty of comprehension or to the fact that because of illness-related familial and occupational problems, this refined hearing no longer appears to be important to them. Only seldom do they express a wish to play in a quartet, for example. More rarely, unilateral improvement to provide almost normal hearing in one ear with an abnormal opposite ear can be a catastrophe, as in the left ear of an orchestral violinist. In a violinist the left ear lies close to the body of the violin so that the sound from all sides of the player is drowned by his own instrument. In this case the right ear should be operated on first, if at all possible. For this reason, as well as because of the possible necessary sound protection due to the absence of the middle ear muscles, questions about the occupational requirements and the patient's interests are a necessary part of the history and planning of the operation.

Summary

Untreated inflammatory complications of the air spaces of the petrous bone *have always been inevitably fatal, and this remains true to this day.* Even after the introduction of antrotomy and radical mastoidectomy, the mortality rate was still high.

In the textbook of otology published by Marx (the successor of von Tröltsch and Manasse) in 1947, acute and chronic inflammations of the middle ear take up almost half of the 850 pages. This was after the discovery of sulphonamides but before the use of penicillin and the introduction of microsurgery. *Complications* took up more than *20% of the text, labyrinthitis* 50 pages, *extradural* and *subdural abscesses* 20, *cerebral abscess* 30, *sinus thrombosis* 30, and *otogenic meningitis* 60 pages. On the other hand, benign tumors were dealt with in 10 pages and malignant tumors in 5 pages. Otogenic meningitis was regarded as being uniformly fatal, but after generous exposure and treatment by sulphonamides, it became potentially curable. More than 50% of these dural inflammations were of labyrinthine origin. Only 25% to 30% of *all forms of labyrinthitis* were lethal, because the acute form was only occasionally fatal, and serous membranous labyrinthitis was included in the total. There was no *clinical differential diagnosis.*

The first and most important duty of otology was therefore to save life, very often that of an adolescent. The first planned step for prevention of complications was *antrotomy* described by Schwarzte in 1873. It was a blessing which, for the first time, brought hope of relief from the threat posed by every middle ear inflammation, provided that the operation was carried out in good time. The later marked reduction in frequency of *acute otitis media* was firstly, the result of infantile immunization, and secondly, the introduction of antibiotics for the treatment of the unavoidable infections of the mucosa of the upper airway.

Chronic otitis media then became less common, but even today, no antibiotic therapy is capable of healing it, but serves only to tide the patient over the dangerous phase until an operation eradicates it.

When surgery was the only solution for chronic otitis media, radical procedures as described by Zaufal (1890) and Stacke (1893) were used. They were destructive operations with disappointing, unsatisfactory results. For this reason the operation was carried out as late as possible.

Extension of the infection to the posterior cranial fossa or to the middle cranial fossa was easily recognized, if it had not been suppressed by antibiotics. The development of the lethal phase of osteitis of the tiny inner ear capsule progressed subclinically for many months or years. It was unknown whether the infection spread directly to the two cranial fossae or from the frequent arachnoid abscess in the subarachnoid space of the internal meatus. The question was whether the adhesions would prove resistant or whether the infection would break through in a few hours, leading to basal meningitis and death in a few days.

The treatment of cholesteatoma, particularly primary acquired cholesteatoma, will remain a surgical task for the forseeable future.

Tympanoplasty eradicates the danger and, at the same time, restores function and heals. It is thus now easy to recommend a prophylactic procedure for all types of otitis media. The decisive fall in the intracranial complications of chronic otitis media is solely due to the use of tympanoplasty.

In countries with well-organized medical services, such complications have become rare, and their clinical features relatively unknown to modern generations of doctors. However, large numbers of articles on this subject can be found in the literature originating from less developed countries. Recently, the chief of a clinic in a large city in a developing country told the author that 30 otogenic brain abscesses in a year was the rule.

In 1936, H. L. Wullstein investigated the pathological processes in the epitympanum, the labyrinthine block and the surface of the petrous pyramid, in an attempt to explain whether the destructive processes could be recognized early, using the technology available at that time. The subject stimulated him to follow up each patient at risk for several months. The results of this longitudinal study of membranous labyrinthitis and the entirely different course of osteitis of the labyrinth appeared in 1948 in the monograph *Labyrinthitis und Paralabyrinthitis im Röntgenbilde*. A small number of radiographs from this collection have been reproduced for this monograph because they are truly unique. The authors have purposefully confined themselves to these few samples of CT and MRI.

With this scientific foundation, the author regarded it as justified to seal off inflammatory processes from the inner ear windows in one stage. From this arose tympanoplasty, which was then further developed to osteoplastic epitympanotomy by the junior author.

Otosurgery of the pneumatized base of the skull and the viscerocranium remains the central point of operative surgery. The results which are achieved with osteoplastic epitympanotomy are excellent. The first requirement is thorough study of pathological anatomy and histology of this very crowded region, which is rich in variations, and its closely related structures.

Within the period of a few years, more than 2,000 operating microscopes came into use in otological surgery. Other disciplines then adopted the microscope: first, ophthalmology; then, many years later, neurosurgery (which was fundamentally changed), followed by vascular and nerve surgery, traumatology (with the possibility of reimplantation of divided limbs), hand surgery, organ transplantation and, finally, plastic surgery (pedicled or free-muscle grafts). The otological surgeon has prepared the pathway for them all.

An entirely new era of surgery, that of microsurgery, was inaugurated by otological surgery because of the high demands in the relatively inaccessible petrous bone.

Finally, tympanoplasty is a prototype for reconstructive surgery, with the multitude of requirements it has to fulfil simultaneously. It involves the use of various tissues as grafts, both for the construction of air spaces and the establishment of sound transmission, as well as for the reconstruction of body surfaces — all in a delicate, usually infected, organ surrounded by other organs in which infection is life-threatening.

References

Aimi, K. The clinical significance of epitympanic mucosal folds. Arch Otolaryngol 1971; 94: 499–508.

Aimi, K. The tympanic isthmus: its anatomy and clinical significance. Laryngoscope 1978; 88: 1067–81.

Aimi, K. The role of the tympanic ring in congenital cholesteatoma pathogenesis. Laryngoscope 1983; 93: 1140–6.

Akle, C. et al. Expression of HLA antigens, β_2-microglobulin and enzymes by human amniotic epithelial cells. Nature 1982; 295: 325.

Anson, BJ., Bast, TH. The fetal and early postnatal development of the tympanic ring and related structure in man. Ann Otol 1955; 64: 802–24.

Anson, BJ., Donaldson, AJ. Surgical anatomy of the temporal bone and ear. Philadelphia: Saunders, 1973.

Armstrong, BW. A new treatment for chronic secretory otitis media. Arch Otolaryngol 1954; 59: 653–4.

Arnold, W. Reaktionsformen der Mittelohrschleimhaut. Arch Otolaryngol 1977; 216: 369–473.

Austin, DF. Reporting results in tympanoplasty. Am J Otol 1985; 6: 85–8.

Bally, G. von Holographische Schwingungsanalyse des Trommelfelles. Laryngol Rhinol, Otol 1978; 57: 444–50.

Bally, G. von, Baumeister S. Otologische Untersuchungen mittels holographischer Interferometrie. Arch Otolaryngol 1979; 223: 181–3.

Bandtlow, O. Experimentelle Untersuchungen zur plastischen Wiederherstellung des Trommelfelles. Heidelberg: Hüthig, 1967.

Baumann, RR. Die Schädelentwicklung bei den Vertebraten. HNO 1978; 26: 1–8.

Bebear, JP., Stoll, D., Bagot d'Arc M. Primary tumors of the facial nerve: a ten-case study. In: Portman M., ed. The facial nerve. New York: Masson, 1984: 322–325.

Becker, W., Buckingham, RA, Holinger, PH, Steiner, W., Jaumann MP. Atlas of ear, nose and throat diseases, including bronchcesophagology. 2nd ed. Stuttgart: Thieme, 1984.

Becker, W., Naumann HH., Pfaltz CR. Hals-Nasen-Ohren-Heilkunde. 3rd ed. Stuttgart: Thieme, 1986.

Beickert, P. Einige Schwierigkeiten und Komplikationen nach Schalleitungsplastiken. Arch Ohren-Nasen-Kehlkopfheilkd. 1957; 58: 109–16.

Beighton, P., Hamersma H. Sclerosteosis in South Africa. S Afr Med J 1979; 55: 783–8.

Békésy, G. von. Über die Schwingungen der Schneckentrennwand beim Präparat und Ohrenmodell. Akust. Zeitung 1942; 7: 173.

Békésy, G. von. Personal communication, 1957.

Békésy, G. von Experiments in hearing. New York: McGraw-Hill, 1960.

Berendes, J., Link R., Zöllner F. Hals-Nasen-Ohren-Heilkunde in Praxis und Klinik, vol. 5. Stuttgart: Thieme, 1979.

Berendes, J., Link, R., Zöllner, F. Hals-Nasen-Ohren-Heilkunde in Praxis und Klinik, vol. 6. Stuttgart: Thieme, 1980.

Berthold, E. Über Myringoplastik. Wien Med Bl 1978; 1: 1627.

Bess, FH., Harington DA, Bluestone CD. Use of acoustic impedance measurement in screening for middle ear disease in children. Ann Otol Rhinol Laryngol 1978; 87: 288–92.

Bluestone, CD., Beery QC. Concepts on the pathogenesis of middle ear effusions. Ann Otol Rhinol Laryngol 1976; 25 (suppl): 182.

Bluestone, CD., Doyle, WJ. Eustachian tube function: physiology and role in otitis media. Ann Otol Rhinol Laryngol 1985; Part III, Suppl. 120.

Bluestone, CD., Beery, QC., Paradise, JL. Audiometry and tympanometry in relation to middle ear effusions in children. Laryngoscope 1973; 83: 594–604.

Bluestone, CD., Caselbrant, ML., Cantekin, EI. Functional obstruction of the eustachian tube in the pathogenesis of aural cholesteatoma in children. In SADÉ, J. ed.: Tel. Aviv: Proceedings Second International Conference on Cholesteatoma and Mastoid Surgery, 1981: 211–224.

Bocca, E. Risultati della timpanoplastica ed età dei pazienti. Arch Ital Otol 1958; 69: 1–7.

Bocca, E., Cis C., Zernotti, E. L'impiego di lembi liberi di periostio nella timpanoplastica. Arch Ital Otol 1959; 40 (suppl): 205–11.

Bollobás, B. Ahalloszerv mikrochirurgiai anatomiaja. Budapest: Medicina Könyvkiado, 1972.

Bollobás, B., Hajdu, B. Ätiologische Faktoren bei Aditus-Verschluß (occlusio aditus). Arch Ohren-Nasen-Kehlkopfheilkd. 1971; 198: 350–9.

Bosma, JB. Development of the basicranium. Washington, DC: National Institutes of Health, 1976. (Dept. of Health, Education, and Welfare, publication no. 76989).

Bostroem, E. Über die pialen Epidermoide. Dermoide und Lipome und duralen Dermoide. Zentralbl. Pathol. 1897; 8: 1.

Brackmann, DE., Sheehy, JL. Tympanoplasty: torps and porps. Laryngoscope 1979; 89: 108–14.

Brown, JS. Statistical ten-year follow-up of 1142 consecutive cholesteatomas: a comparison of the closed and open techniques. Laryngoscope 1982; 92: 390–6.

Buckingham, RA. Cholesteatoma and chronic otitis media following tympanic drainage. Laryngoscope 1982; 91: 1450–6.

Buckingham, RA., Ferrer, JL. Reversibility of chronic adhesive otitis media with polyethylene tube, middle ear air vent: Kodachrome time-lapse study. Laryngoscope 1966; 76: 993–1014.

Buckingham, RA., Ferrer, JL. Middle ear cholesteatoma: etiology, relation to chronic adhesive otitis media, and treatment: an otophotographic study. Trans Am Acad Ophthalmol Otolaryngol 1969; 73: 873–85.

Cantekin, EI., Bluestone, CD., Parkin LP. Eustachian tube ventilatory function in children. Ann Otol Rhinol Laryngol 1976; 25: 171–7.

Cawthorne, T. Congenital cholesteatoma. Arch Otolaryngol 1963; 78: 248–52.

Chang, TM. Personal communication, 1963.

Charachon, R., Roux O., Eyraud S. Le cholestéatome de l'oreille moyenne: choix des techniques et résultats chez l'adulte et chez l'enfant. Ann Otolaryngol 1980; 97: 1–2, 65–78.

Charachon, R., Eyraud, S., Guenoun, A., Egal, F. Le traitement chirurgical du cholestéatome de l'enfant. Rev Laryngol Otol Rhinol 1984; 105: 465–74.

Chatelier, HP., Lemoine, J. Le diaphragme interatticotympanique du nouveau-né. Ann Otolaryngol 1946; 13: 534–6.

Chilla, R., Schröder, M. Rezidivrate und Hörvermögen nach operativer Behandlung von Mittelohrcholesteatomen mit und ohne Erhalt der hinteren Gehörgangswand. HNO 1980; 28: 1–9.

Clemis, JD. Allergic factors in management of middle ear effusions. Ann Otol Rhinol Laryngol 1976); 25 (suppl): 259–62.

Crysdale, WS. Conservative treatment of serous otitis media. Otolaryngol Clin North Am 1984; 17: 653–57.

Curtis, AW., Clemis, JD. Tympanic effusions: clinical aspects. Extracta Otorhinolaryngol 1980; 2: 79–103.

Dahm, P. Über die postnatale Entwicklung der Form und Größe des menschlichen os temporale [dissertation]. University of Würzburg, West Germany, 1970.

Dahmann, H. Zur Physiologie des Hörens. Experimentelle Untersuchungen über die Mechanik der Gehörknöchelchenkette sowie über deren Verhalten auf Ton- und Lichtdruck, Teil 1. Z Hals-Nasen-Ohrenheilkd. 1929; 24: 462.

Dahmann, H. Zur Physiologie des Hörens. Experimentelle Untersuchungen über die Mechanik der Gehörknöchelchenkette sowie über deren Verhalten auf Ton- und Lichtdruck, Teile 2–4. Z Hals-Nasen-Ohrenheilkd. 1930; 27: 329.

Debruyne, F. Laterale Sinusthrombose in den achtziger Jahren. J. Laryngol 1985; 99: 91–3.

Deguine, C., Desaulty, A. La réparation du conduit osseux dans la chirurgie du cholestéatome. Rev. Laryngol. 1984; 105: 461–3.

Derlacki, EL. Congenital cholesteatoma of the middle ear and mastoid: a third report. Arch. Otolaryngol. 1973; 97: 177.

Derlacki, EL. Congenital cholesteatoma of the middle ear and mastoid: a fourth report. In: Shambaugh GE Jr., Shea JJ, eds. Proceedings of the Fifth Shambaugh International Workshop on Middle Ear Microsurgery and Fluctuant Hearing Loss, February 29-March 5, 1976 Northwestern University Medical School, Chicago. Huntsville, AL: Strode, 1977: 156–161.

Derlacki, EL. Congenital cholesteatoma today. Am. J. Otol. 1985; 6: 19–21.

Derlacki, EL., Clemis, JD. Congenital cholesteatoma of the middle ear and mastoid. Ann. Otol. 1965; 74: 706.

Derlacki, EL., Clemis, JD., Harrison, WH. Congenital cholesteatoma of the middle ear and mastoid: a second report, presenting seven additional cases. Laryngoscope 1968; 78: 1050.

Diamant, M. Anatomic and etiological factors in chronic middle ear effusion. In: Proceedings. Sixth International Conference on Otolaryngology. Washington, DC: 1957: 185–186.

Djupesland, G., Zwislocki, JJ. Sound pressure distribution in the outer ear. Acta Otolaryngol 1973; 75: 305–2.

Doyle, WJ. Animal models of eustachian tube function. In: Extraordinary International Symposium on Recent Advances in Otitis Media with Effusion, Kyoto, January 12–15, 1985

Drettner, B., Ekvall, L. Tympanomaxillary shunt. Acta otolaryngol 75 1973; 75 (4): 277–8.

Eitschberger, E. Gefäßentwicklung in Ossikulatransplantaten und -implantaten. Laryngol Rhinol Otol 1980; 59: 238–43.

Eitschberger, E., Gammert, C., Heine WD. Über das histologische Verhalten von Knorpel (Amboßgelenkpfanne) im Mittelohrraum nach unterschiedlicher Konservierung. HNO 1977; 25: 419–23.

Elis, W., Zeimer, H., Hacke, W., Buchner, H. Die ektopische A. carotis interna in der Paukenhöhle. Intraoperative Komplikationen und ihre Behandlung. Laryngol. Rhinol. Otol. 1985; 64: 202–5.

Elner, A., Ingelstedt, S., Ivarsson, A. The normal function of the eustachian tube. Acta Otolaryngol 1971; 72: 320–8.

Ely, ET. Haut-Transplantation bei chronischer Eiterung des Mittelohres. Z. Ohrenheilkd. 1881; 10: 145.

Escher, F. Das Schädelbasistrauma in oto-rhinologischer Sicht. Ein Überblick über 3 Jahrzehnte. HNO 1973; 21: 129–44.

Escher, F. Die Therapie des Mittelohrcholesteatoms. HNO 1979; 27: 145–8.

Falk, B. Eustachian tube closing failure: studies on sniff-induced negative middle ear pressure [dissertation]. Linköping University, 1984.

Falk, B., Magnuson, B., Drainage of the middle ear by sniffing: a cause of high negative pressure and developing middle ear infection. Otolaryngol Head Neck Surg 1984; 92: 312–8.

Falk, B., Magnuson, B., Test-retest variability of eustachian tube responses in children with persistent middle ear effusion. Arch. Otolaryngol 1984; 240: 145–52.

Farrior, JB. Atlas of tympanology in 3-D, vol 3: Cholesteatoma in 3–D. Portland, OR: American Academy of Ophthalmology and Otolaryngology, 1972.

Farrior, JB. Recurrent and residual cholesteatoma, Am J. Otol. (1985) 13–18.

Feldmann, H. Eine Stichsäge für die Mikrochirurgie. Neue Möglichkeiten zu osteoplstischen Eingriffen am Ohr und den Nebenhöhlen. Arch. Ohren-Nasen-Kehlkopfheilkd. 1977; 216: 507–8.

Feldmann, H. Osteoplastische Meato-Attiko-Antrotomie. Laryngol Rhinol Otol 1977; 56: 785.

Feldmann, H., Steinmann, G. Die Bedeutung des äußeren Ohres für das Hören im Wind. Arch. Ohren-Nasen-Kehlkopfheilkd. 1968; 190: 69.

Fisch, U. Tympanoplasty and stapedectomy. Stuttgart: Thieme, 1981.

Fisch, U. Intracranial complications of cholesteatoma, In: Sadé, J., ed. Cholesteatoma and mastoid surgery. Amsterdam; Kugler, 1982: 369–79.

Fisch, U., Fragan, P., Valavanis, A. Der Zugang zur lateralen Schädelbasis durch die Fossa infratemporalis. Extracta Otorhinolaryngol 1985; 7: 151–200.

Fleischer, G. Evolutionary principles of the mammalian middle ear. Adv. Anat. Embryol. Cell. Biol. 1978; 55-5.

Fleury, P. Techniken der Ohrchirurgie. Stuttgart: Schattauer, 1976.

Frei, O. Natürliche Konstruktionen. Stuttgart: Deutsche Verlagsanstalt, 1982.

Frei, O., et al. Pneus in nature and technics. Stuttgart: Kammer 1976.

Friedmann, I. Pathology of the ear. Oxford: Blackwell, 1974.

Fritze, W., Kreitlow, H., Winter, D. Zur Form der Trommelfellschwingung. Arch. Otolaryngol. 1979; 223: 184–185.

Gaceck, RR. Evaluation and management of primary petrous apex cholesteatoma. Otolaryngol Head Neck Surg 1980; 88: 519–23.

Glasscock, ME., Jackson, CG., Knox, GW. Can acquired immuno-deficiency syndrome and Creutzfeldt-Jakob disease be transmitted via otologic homgrafts? Arch Otolaryngol Head Neck Surg 1988; 114: 1252–1255.

Goday-Rodriguez, VM., Schulknecht, HF. Experiences with type IV tympanomastoidectomy. Laryngoscope 1977; 87: 522–8.

Goode, RL., Glasscock, ME. The tympanofrontal shunt: a procedure for treatment of chronic eustachian tube insufficiency. Laryngoscope 1975; 85: 100–12.

Goode, RL., Friedrichs, R., Stephen, F. Effect on hearing

threshholds of surgical modifications of the exteral ear. Trans Am. Otol. Soc. 1977; 65: 45−55.

Goodhill, V. Circumferential tympanomastoid access in the sinus tympani area. Ann. Otol. 1973; 82: 547−53.

Griesemer, C., Pfaltz, DR., Werdenberg, D. Perikard − erste Erfahrungen mit einem neuen Ersatzmaterial für die Tympanoplastik. ORL J. Otorhinolaryngol Relat Spec 1985; 8: 201−6.

Griessmann, Schwarz, Zur exakten Gehörmessung mit Vorführung eines Otaudion. Z. Hals-Nasen-Ohrenheilkd. 1927; 9: 885−6.

Grote, JJ., ed. Biomaterials in otology: proceedings of the First International Symposium, April 21−23, 1983, Leiden, the Netherlands. The Hague: Nijhoff, 1984.

Grünberg, H. Mikrokarzinom und Resorption der gesunden und kranken Mittelohrschleimhaut [postdoctoral thesis]. University of Würzburg, West Germany, 1985.

Guerrier, Y., Andrea, M., Paco, J. Les repaires anatomiques du cholestéatome dans la caisse du tympan. Ann Otolaryngol. 1980; 97: 15−28.

Gussen, R. Pacinian corpuscles in the middle ear. J. Laryngol 1970; 84: 71−6.

Gussen, R. The human incudomalleal joint. Arthritis Rheum 1971; 14: 465−74.

Hammar, JA. Studien über die Entwicklung des Vorderdarms und einiger angrenzenden Organe. Arch. Mikroskop. Anat. 1902; 59: 471−628.

Hansen, CC. Vascular anatomy of the human temporal bone, 1: anastomoses between the membranous labyrinth and its bony capsule. Arch Ohren-Nasen-Kehlkopfheilkd. 1971; 200: 83−98.

Hansen, CC. Vascular anatomy of the human temporal bone, 2: anastomoses inside the labyrinthine capsule. Arch. Ohren-Nasen-Kehlkopfheilkd. 1971; 200: 99−114.

Hansen, CC. Vascular anatomy of the human temporal bone, 3: the vascularization of the vestibulocochlear nerve. Arch. Ohren-Nasen-Kehlkopfheilkd. 1971; 200: 115−24.

Hansen, HG. Sklerosteose. In: Opitz, J. Schmid, F., eds. Handbuch der Kinderheilkunde, vol. 6. Berlin: Springer, 1967: 351−5.

Heermann, H. Trommelfellplastik mit Fasciengewebe vom Musculus temporalis nach Begradigung der voderen Gehörgangswand. HNO 1960; 9: 136.

Heermann, J. Auricular cartilage palisade tympano-epitympano-antrum and mastoid-plasties. Clin. Otolaryngol. 1978; 3: 443.

Helms, J. Specific treatment in ear trauma: abstracts of papers presented at the 13th Greek−Yugoslav Congress of Oto-Neuro-Ophthalmo-Neurosurgery, Corfu, September 23−26, 1982. Thessaloniki.

Holmgren, G. Die chirugische Behandlung der Otosklerose. Nord Tidsskr Otorhinolaryngol 1917; 2: 217.

Holmquist, J. Middle ear ventilation [dissertation]. University of Göteborg, Sweden, 1969.

Honjo, J., Kumazawa, T., Hondo, K., Shimojo, S. Electromyographic study of patients with dysfunction of the eustachian tube. Arch. Otolaryngol 1979; 222: 47−51.

Hoshino, T., Suzuki, JI. Anterior attic wall anatomy. Arch. Otolaryngol. 1978; 104: 588−90.

House, HP. An apparent primary cholesteatoma: case report. Laryngoscope 1953; 63: 712−13.

House, W., Histelberge, WE. The transcochlear approach to the skull base. Arch. Otolaryngol. 1976; 102: 334−42.

House, WF., Belal, A. Jr. Translabyrinthine surgery, anatomy, and pathology. Am J. Otol. 1980; 1: 189−98.

House, WF., Glasscock, ME., Miles, J. Eustachian tuboplasty. Laryngoscope 1969; 79: 1765−82.

Ingelstedt, S., Örtegren, U. Qualitative testing of the eustachian tube function. Acta Otolaryngol 1963; 182 (suppl.): 7.

Jansen, C. Über Radikaloperation und Tympanoplastik. Sitz. Ber. Ärztek. Ob v. 18. 2. 1958.

Jansen, C. Combined approach tympanoplasty in cholesteatoma surgery: a report on 1904 adults and 472 children. In: SADÉ, J., ed. Proceedings J. Second Conference on Cholesteatoma. Tel Aviv: 1981: 455−459.

Jansen, CW. Intact canal wall for cholesteatoma. Am J. Otol. 1985; 6: 3−4.

Jerger, J. Clinical experience with impedance audiometry. Arch. Otolaryngol. 1970; 92: 311−24.

Jerger, J. Handbook of clinical impedance audiometry. Acton, MA: American Electromedics Corporation, 1975.

Kastenbauer, ER., Hochstrasser, K. Der Einfluß des Konservierungsmittels Cialit auf die Proteinlöslichkeit und die Antigenität von allogenen und xenogenen Gehörknöchelchen- und Trommelfelltransplantaten. Arch. Ohren-Nasen-Kehlkopfheilkd. 1973; 203: 173−205.

Kelemen, G. Diseases of the ear. In: Benirschke, K., Garner, FM., Jones, TC. Pathology of laboratory animals. Berlin: Springer, 1978.

Kirikae, I. The structure and function of the middle ear. Tokyo: University of Tokyo Press, 1960

Kumazawa, T. Autonomic nerve regulation in eustachian tube function. In: Proceedings Extraordinary International Symposium on Recent Advances in Otitis Media with Effusion, Kyoto, January 12−15, 1985. 5−7

Kumazawa, T., Honjo, I., Honda, K. Aerodynamic evaluation of eustachian tube function. Arch. Otolaryngol. 1974; 208: 147−56.

Kup, W. Die 3-Schichtenplastik des Trommelfells unter Verwendung eines Hilfstransplantates aus lyophilisierter Dura. Arch. Ohren-Nasen-Kehlkopfheilkd. 1967; 188: 593−603.

Lang, J., Klinische Anatomie des Kopfes. Berlin: Springer, 1981.

Lang, WH., Muchel, F. Zeiss microscopes for microsurgery. Berlin: Springer, 1981.

Lapidot, A., Brandow, EC. A method for preserving the posterior canal wall and bridge in the surgery of cholesteatoma. Acta Otolaryngol 1966; 62: 88−92.

Lapiod, A., Terrée, D., Rezvani, F., et al. Eustachian tube bypass: experimental evidence for total Eustachian tube substitution. ORL J. Otorhinolaryngol Relat Spec 1977; 86: 498−505.

Lehnhardt, E. Pathophysiologie der Schalleitung, einschließlich Ohrtrompete. In: Berendes, J., Link, R., Zöllner, F., eds. Hals-Nasen-Ohren-Heilkunde in Praxis und Klinik, vol. 6. Stuttgart: Thieme, 1980; 27: 1−27.

Lehnhardt, E. Praxis der Audiometrie. 6th ed. Stuttgart: Thieme, 1987.

Lempert, J. Improvement of hearing in cases of otosclerosis: new one-stage surgical technique. Arch. Otolaryngol. 1938; 28: 42.

Lempert, J. Enaural fenestration of the horizontal semicircular canal for otosclerosis: indications, technique, observations as to early and late postoperative results. Laryngoscope 1941; 51: 330.

Lempert, J. Lempert fenestra nov-ovalis with mobile stopple. Arch. Otolaryngol. 1945; 41: 1.

Lim, DJ. Pathogenesis and pathology of chronic otitis media with effusion. In: Proceedings Extraordinary International Symposium on Recent Advances in Otitis Media with Effusion, Kyoto, January 12−15, 1985. 8−10

Lim, DJ., Bluestone, CD., Klein, JO., Nelson, JD. Recent advances in otitis media with effusion. Philadelphia: Becker, 1984.

Lim, DJ., Bluestone, CD., Klein, JO., Nelson, JD. Proceedings of the fourth international Symposium recent advances in otitis media. Philadelphia: BC. Decker Inc., 1987.

Lim, DJ., et al. Acquired cholesteatoma: light- and electron-microscopic observations. Ann. Otol. 1972; 81: 2.

Lim, DJ., Jackson, D., Bennet, J. Human middle ear corpuscles: a light- and electron-microscopic study. Laryngoscope 1975; 85: 1725.

Lo, WWM., Solti-Bohmann, LG., Brackmann, DE., Gruskin, P. Cholesterin-Granulom der Spitze des Os petrosum: CT-Diagnostik. Radiology 1984; 153: 705—11.

McCabe, BF., Sadé, J., Abramson, M. eds. Cholesteatoma: First International Conference. Birmingham, AL: Aesculapius, 1977.

McDonald, C., Ryan, RE. Congenital cholesteatoma of the ear. Ann. Otol. Rhinol. Laryngol 1984; 93: 637—40.

Magnuson, B. Tubal closing failure in retraction-type cholesteatoma and adhesive middle ear lesions. Acta Otolaryngol 1978; 86: 408—17.

Mann, W., Jonas, I., Müncker, G. Growth influence on tubal function. Acta Otolaryngol 1979; 87: 451—7.

Marquet, J. Technique inédite de myringoplastie par homogreffe de tympan. Acta Otorhinolaryngol. Belg. 1967; 21: 127—32.

Marquet, J. The incudomalleal joint. J. Laryngol. 1981; 95: 543—65.

Marx, H. Kurzes Handbuch der Ohrenheilkunde. Jena: Fischer, 1947.

Melsen, B. The postnatal development of the cranial base studied histologically in human autopsy material. Acta Odontol Scand 1974; 62 (suppl.): 126.

Messerklinger, W. Endoskopie des unteren Nasenganges. Monatsschr. Ohrenheilkd. 1972; 106: 569—72.

Messerklinger, W. Endoscopy of the nose. Munich: Urban and Schwarzenberg, 1978.

Messerklinger, W. Zur Endoskopietechnik des mittleren Nasenganges. Arch. Otorhinolaryngol. 1978; 221: 297—305.

Miehlke, A. Surgery of the facial nerve. 2nd ed. Munich: Urban and Schwarzenberg, 1973.

Miehlke, A., Arold, R., Chilla, R., Evers, K., Haubrich, J., Schätzle, W. Arbeitsbuch HNO. Munich: Urban and Schwarzenberg, 1980.

Montgomery, NW. Cystic lesions of the petrous apex: transsphenoid approach. Ann. Otol. Rhinol. Laryngol 1977; 86: 429.

Montgomery, NW, Turner, PA. Benign lesions of the petrous apex. In: Silverstein, H., Norrel, H., eds. Neurological surgery of the ear, vol. 2. Birgmingham, AL. Aesculapius, 1979

Moritz, W. Plastische Eingriffe am Mittelohr zur Wiederherstellung der Innenohrschalleitung. Z. Laryngol. Rhinol. 1952; 31: 338.

Moser, L., Kley, W., Seiler, CF. Die Lärmbelastung des Ohres während der Ohroperation. HNO 1982; 30: 232—3.

Mündnich, K., Über das Hamartom im Bereich der Paukenhöhle. Monatsschr. Ohrenheilkd. 1939; 73: 239—44.

Mündnich, K., Terrahe, K. Mißbildungen des Ohres. In: Berendes, J., Linke, R., Zöllner, F., eds. Hals-Nasen-Ohrenheilkunde in Praxis und Klinik, vol 5 (1). Stuttgart: Thieme, 1979: 18.1.—18.4.5.

Münker, G., Arnold, W. eds. Physiology and pathophysiology of eustachian tube and middle ear: international symposium, Freiburg im Breisgau, 1977. Stuttgart: Thieme, 1980.

Münker, G., Arnold, W. Das Funktionssystem Mittelohr-Ohrtrompete. Symposium über Physiologie und Pathophysiologie, 28.9.—1.10.1977, Freiburg. Biberach an der Riß, West Germany: Thomae, 1980.

Nager, GT. Epidermoids (congenital cholesteatomas) involving the temporal bone. In: SADÉ, J. Cholesteatoma and mastoid surgery: proceedings of the Second International Conference, Tel Aviv, 22—27 March 1981. Amsterdam: Kugler, 1982: 41—59.

Nager, GT., Holliday, MJ. Fibröse Dysplasie des Fesenbeines. Ann. Otol. Rhinol. Laryngol 1984; 93: 630—3.

Nager, GT., Stein, SA., Dorst, JP, et al. Sclerosteosis involving the temporal bone: clinical and radiologic aspects. Am J. Otolaryngol. 1983; 4: 1—17.

Naumann, HH. Kopf- und Hals-Chirurgie, vol. 3. Stuttgart: Thieme, 1976.

Ortiz, P., Gonzáles, E., Pedregal, MA, et al. Current survery of brain abscesses as complications of ENT infections. Acta Otorrhinolaringol Esp 1984; 35: 393—406.

Padovan, I. Stapedo-vestibularna i endolabirintarna mikrokirurgija. Vojnosanit Pregl 1961; 9: 751—60.

Padovan, I. Otorhinolaringologija, 1: kirurgija uha. Zagreb: Skolska Knjiga, 1982.

Palva, T., Palva, A., Kärjä, J. Musculoperiosteal flap in cavity obliteration. Arch. Otolaryngol. 1972; 95: 172.

Palva, T., Karma, P., Palva, A. Cholesteatoma surgery: canal wall down and mastoid obliteration. In: McCabe, BF., Sadé, J., Abramson, M. eds. Cholesteatoma: first international conference. Birmingham, AL: Aesculapius, 1976: 373—7.

Palva, T., Karma, P., Kärjä, J. Cholesteatoma. Arch. Otolaryngol, 1977; 103: 74—7.

Palva, T., Virtanen, H., Mäkinen, J. Akute und latente Mastoiditis bei Kindern. J. Laryngol 1985; 99: 127—36.

Palva, T. The pathogenesis and treatment of cholesteatoma. Acta Otolaryngol (Stockh) 1990; 109: 323—330.

Pankow, G. Untersuchungen über die Schädelbasisknickung beim Menschen. Z. Menschliche Vererbungs-Konstitutions-Lehre 1949—50; 19: 69—139.

Paulsen, K. Einführung in die rekonstruktive Mikrochirurgie des Mittel- und Innenohres. Stuttgart: Schattauer Verlag 1974.

Perkins, R. Human homograft otologic tissue transplantation: buffered formaldehyde preparations. Trans Am Acad Ophthalmol Otolaryngol 1970; 74: 278.

Pernkopf, E. Topographische Anatomie, vol. 4 (2). Munich: Urban and Schwarzenberg, 1960.

Pfeifer, G. Über Meßmethoden und Maßverhältnisse des Gesichts und des Gesichtsschädels. In: Schuchart, K., ed. Fortschritte der Kiefer- und Gesichts-Chirurgie, vol. 3. Stuttgart: Thieme, 1957.

Pfeifer, G. Die relativen Maßverhältnisse des wachsenden Gesichtes im Hinblick auf die zeitliche Indikation zu operativen Eingriffen. In: Schuchart, K., ed. Fortschritte der Kiefer- und Gesichts-Chirurgie, vol. 4. Stuttgart: Thieme, 1958.

Piyakov, VP., Shlychkov, IP. Frequency and treatment of labyrinthitis in patients with acute or chronic middle ear effusion [in Russian]. Z. Usn. Nos Gorlov Bolezn (Moscow) 1985; 1: 56—8.

Plester, D., Zöllner, F. Behandlung der chronischen Mittelohrentzündungen. In: Berendes, J., Link, R., Zöllner, F. eds. Hals-Nasen-Ohren-Heilkunde in Praxis und Klinik, vol. 6. Stuttgart: Thieme, 1980; 28: 1—28.

Politzer, A. Lehrbuch für Ohrenheilkunde, vol. 1. Stuttgart: Enke, 1878.

Politzer, A. Über primäre Erkrankung der knöchernen Labyrinthkapsel. Z. Ohrenheilkd. 1893; 25: 309.

Portmann, M. "Open" or "closed" technique in surgery of the middle ear. Ann. Otol. Rhinol. Laryngol 1968; 77: 927.

Portmann, M. Les voies d'accès dans la chirurgie tympnoplastique. Rev Laryngol 1970; 91: 61—79.

Portmann, M. Offene oder geschlossene Technik für die Tympanoplastik. HNO 1973; 21: 169—71.

Portmann, M. Traité de technique chirurgicale O.R.L. et cervicofaciale, vol. 1. Paris. Masson, 1975.

Portmann, M. ed. Proceedings of the Fifth International Symposium on the Facial Nerve, Bordeaux, September 3—6, 1984. New York: Masson, 1985.

Portmann, M., Poncet, E., Roulleau, P., Lacher, G. Les homogreffes tympano-ossiculares. Paris: Amette, 1978.

Proctor, B. The development of the middle ear spaces and their surgical significance. J. Laryngol 1964; 87: 631-48.

Proctor, B. Surgical anatomy of the posterior tympanum. Ann Otol. Rhinol. Laryngol 1969; 78: 1026−40.

Proctor, B. Attic-aditus block and the tympanic diaphragma. Ann. Otol. Rhinol. Laryngol 1971; 80: 371−5.

Proctor, B., Nager, GT. The facial canal: normal anatomy, variations, and anomalies. Trans. Am. Otol. Soc. 1982; 70: 49−77.

Proctor, B. Surgical anatomy of the ear and temporal bone. Stuttgart: Thieme, 1989.

Reck, R. Erste tierexperimentelle und klinische Erfahrungen mit bioaktiver Glaskeramik in der rekonstruktiven Mittelohrchirurgie. Arch. Otorhinolaryngol 1979; 223: 369−73.

Rettig, H. Biomaterialien und Nahtmaterial. Berlin: 1984, Springer.

Richardson, GS. Aditus block. Ann. Otol. Rhinol. Laryngol. 1963; 72: 223−36.

Rius, M. La aticotmia osteoplastica transmeatal en la cirurgia del colesteatoma, y algunas consideraciones sobre nuevos aportes en timpanoplastia. Ann. Otorinolaringol. Urug. 1965; 35: 1−10.

Roulleau, P., François, M., Receveur, M., Candeau, P.: Ann Otolaryngol 1984; 101: 53−61.

Rüedi, L. Mittelohrentwicklung vom 5. Embryonalmonat bis zum 10. Lebensjahr. Acta Otolaryngol 1937; 22 (suppl.).

Rüedi, L. Mittelohrraumentwicklung und Mittelohrentzündung. Z. Hals-Nasen-Ohrenheilkd. 1939; 45: 175.

Rüedi, L. Pathogenesis and treatment of cholesteatoma in chronic suppuration of the temporal bone. Ann. Otol. Rhinol. Laryngol. 1957; 66: 283.

Rüedi, L. Cholesteatoma formation in the middle ear in animal experiments. Acta Otolaryngol 1959; 50: 233−42.

Rüedi, L. Acquired cholesteatoma. Arch. Otolaryngol. 1963; 79: 252−61.

Rüedi, L. Pathogenesis and surgical treatment of the middle ear cholesteatoma. Acta Otolaryngol 361 1978; 361 (suppl): 1−45.

Sadé, J. Middle ear mucosa. Arch. Otolaryngol. 1966; 84: 137−43.

Sadé, J. Secretory otitis media and its sequelae. Edinburgh: Churchill-Livingstone, 1979.

Sadé, J. Cholesteatoma and mastoid surgery. Amsterdam: Kugler 1982.

Sadé, J., Berco, E. Atelectasis and secretory otitis media. Ann. Otol. Rhinol. Laryngol. 1976; 25 (suppl.): 66−72.

Sadé, J., Halevy, A., Hadas, E. Clearance of middle ear effusions and middle ear pressures. Ann. Otol. Rhinol. Laryngol. 1976; 25 (suppl.): 58−62.

Sadé, J. Acute and secretory otitis media. Amsterdam: Kugler & Ghedini Publications, 1986.

Sadé, J. The eustachian tube. Amsterdam: Kugler & Ghedini Publications, 1987.

Saito, R., Igarashi, M., Alford, BR, et al. Anatomical measurement of the sinus tympani. Arch. Otolaryngol. 1971; 94: 418−25.

Schmidt, HM., Dahm,. P. Die postnatale Entwicklung des menschlichen Os temporale, 1: Einleitung, Material und Methode, Pars squamosa et petromastoida; 2. Pars mastoidea, Pars tympanica und Facies lateralis ossis temporalis; 3: Wachstumszunahme der Schläfenbeinabschnitte. Gegenbaurs Morphol Jahrb. 1977; 123: 484−513, 589−620, 689−98.

Schmitt, H. Über die Bedeutung der Schalldrucktransformation und der Schallprotektion für die Hörschwelle. Acta Otolaryngol 1958; 49: 71.

Schnee, IM., Paterson, NJ. Tympanoplasty: a modification in technique. Arch. Otolaryngol. 1963; 77: 87−91.

Schuknecht, HF., Gao, YZ. Arachnoidal cyst in the internal auditory canal. Trans Am. Otol. Soc. 1983; 71: 17−23.

Schuknecht, HF. Congenital aural atresia. Laryngoscope 1989; 99: 908−917.

Schwartze, HH., Eysell, CG. Über die künstliche Entfaltung des Warzenfortsatzes. Arch. Ohrenheilkd. 1873; 7: 157−62.

Schwarz, M. Das Cholesteatom im Gehörgang und im Mittelohr. Stuttgart: Thieme, 1966. (Abhandlungen aus dem Gebiet der Hals-Nasen-Ohren-Heilkunde, 8.)

Senturia BH., Bluestone, CD., Lim, DJ, Saunders, WH. Recent advances in otitis media with effusion: proceedings of the Second International Symposium, May 9−11, 1979. Columbus, OH: Annals, 1980.

Sercer, A. L'angulation de la base cranienne et le problème d'otospongiose. Bull. Acad. Natl. Med. 1959; 143: 727−31.

Sercer, A. Etiopathogénie de l'otosclérose, Prog. ORL 1961; 8: 188.

Sercer, A. Otorhinolaryngologija, vol. 1. Zagreb: 1966.

Sercer, A., Krmpotic, J. La transformation de la base cranienne au cours de la vie: contribution à l'étude de l'otospongiose. Rev. Laryngol 1960; 81: 324−81.

Sexton, Cited after Chatellier, HP., Lemoine, J., Le diaphragme interattico − tympanique du nauveau − né. Ann. Oto-Laryng. (Paris) 13 (1946) 534−566, GE, Jr. ed. Shambaugh First International Workshop on Middle Ear Microsurgery, March 1959. Chicago.

Shambaugh, GE. Jr., Glasscock, ME. III. Surgery of the ear. 3rd. ed. Philadelphia: Saunders, 1980.

Shambaugh, GE., Jr. Shea, JJ., eds. Proceedings of the Fifth Shambaugh International Workshop on Middle Ear Microsurgery and Fluctuant Hearing Loss, February 29-March 5, 1976, Northwestern University Medical School, Chicago, Huntsville, AL: Strode, 1977.

Shambaugh, GE. Jr., Shea, JJ., eds. Proceedings of the Sixth Shambaugh International Workshop an Otomicrosurgery and Third Shea Fluctuant Hearing Loss Symposium, March 2−7, 1980, Northwestern University Medical School, Chicago. Hunstville; AL: Strode, 1981.

Shambaugh, GE., J., Shea, JJ., eds. Seventh Shambaugh-Shea International Workshop on Otology, March 1−4, 1984. Am J. Otol. 1985; Vol. 6.

Shea, JJ., Jr., Homsy, CA. The use of Proplast in otologic surgery. Laryngoscope 1974; 84: 1835−45.

Sheehy, JL. Testing eustachian tube function. Ann. Otol. Rhinol. Laryngol. 1981; 90: 562−4.

Sheehy, JL. TORPs and PORPs: Ursachen von Mißerfolgen bei 446 Operationen. Otolaryngol. Head Neck Surg 1984; 92: 583−7.

Sheehy, JL. Obliterative procedures in cholesteatoma surgery. Am J. Otol. 1985; 6: 9−12.

Sheehy, JL., Anderson, RE. A review of 472 cases. Ann. Otol. Rhinol. Laryngol 1980; 89: 331−3.

Sheehy, JL., Crabtree, JA. Tympanoplasty: staging the operation. Laryngoscope 1973; 83: 1594−1621.

Sheehy, JL., Linthicum, FH., Greenfield, EC. Chronic serous mastoiditis, idiopathic hemotympanum, and cholesterol granuloma of the mastoid. Laryngoscope 1969; 79: 1189−1217.

Sheehy, JL., Robinson, JV. Cholesteatom surgery at the Otologic Medical Group: residual and recurrent disease − a report on 307 revision operations. Am J. Otol. 1982; 3: 209−15.

Sheehy, JL. Cholesteatoma surgery: Canal wall down procedures. Ann Otol Rhinol Laryngol 1988; 97: 30−35.

Shimada, T., Lim, DJ. Distribution of ciliated cells in the human middle ear: SEM, TEM and light-microscopic observation. Ann. Otol. 1972; 81: 203.

Siebenmann, F., Cited after Hammar, J.

Siirala, K. Otitis media adhesiva. Arch. Otolaryngol. 1964; 80: 287.

Smith, MFW., Proffitt, SD., Shinn, JB. Autologic tissue bank. Trans Am Acad Ophthalmol Otolaryngol 1972; 76: 134−41.

Smyth, GDL. Postoperative cholesteatoma in combined approach tympanoplasty: fifteen-year report on tympanoplasty, part 1. J. Laryngol 1976; 90: 597−611.

Smyth, GDL. Tympanic reconstruction: fifteen-year report on tympanoplasty, part 2. J. Laryngol 1976; 90: 713.

Smyth, GDL. Chronic ear disease. Edinburgh: Churchill Livingstone, 1980 (Monographs in clinical otorhinolaryngology, 2.)

Smyth, GDL. Canal wall for cholesteatoma: up or down? Am J. Otol. 1985; 6: 1−2.

Smyth, GDL. Cholesteatoma surgery: the influence of the canal wall. Laryngoscope 1985; 95: 92−6.

Smyth, GDL., Hassard, TH. What do we find at the revision of mastoid surgery? In: Sade, J., ed. Cholesteatoma and mastoid surgery. Amsterdam: Kugler, 1982: 439−42.

Smyth, GDL. Surgical treatment of cholesteatoma: The role of staging in closed operations. Ann Otol Rhinol Laryngol 1988; 97: 667−669.

Stacke, L. Stackes Operationsmethode. Arch. Ohrenheilkd. 1893; 35: 145.

Starck, D. Embryologie. 3rd. ed. Stuttgart: Thieme, 1975.

Steinbach, E. Das Mittelohrcholesteatom. Pathogenese und Therapie. In: Ganz, H., Schätzle, W. HNO Praxis Heute, vol. 5. Berlin: Springer 1985: 1−20.

Sterkers, JM., Batisse, R., Gandom, J., Cannoni, M., Vaneecloo, FM. Les voies d'abord du rocher. Paris: Arnette, 1984.

Swartz, JD. Imaging of the temporal bone. Stuttgart: Thieme, 1986.

Tangemann, W. Ersatz des Trommelfeldes durch Hauttransplantationen. Z. Ohrenheilkd. 13 1883; 13: 174.

Tonndorf, J., Khanna, SM. The tympanic membrane as a part of the middle ear transformer. Acta Otolaryngol. 1971; 71: 177−80.

Tonndorf, J., Khanna, SM. Tympanic membrane vibrations in human cadaver ears studied by time-averaged holography. J. Acoust. Soc. Am. 1972; 52: 1221.

Tos, M. Epidemiology and natural history of secretory otitis. Am. J. Otol. 1984; 5: 459−62.

Tos, M., Poulsen, G. Secretory otitis media: late results of treatment with grommets. Arch. Otolaryngol. 1976; 102: 672−5.

Tos, M., Thomsen, J. Cholesteatoma and mastoid surgery 3. Amsterdam: Kugler & Ghedini Publications, 1989.

Tröltsch, A. von. Beiträge zur Anatomie des menschlichen Trommelfells. Z. Wiss. Zool. IX 1858.

Tröltsch, A. von. Lehrbuch der Ohrenheilkunde. 7th ed. Leipzig. Vogel, 1881.

Venker, J. Die Technik der Fensteroperation. Ned. Tijdschr. Geneeskd. 1949; 93: 307.

Waddington, CH. The evolution of an evolutionist. New York: Cornell University Press, 1975

Wang, R., Zubick, HH., Vernick, DM., Strome, M. Bilateral congenital middle ear cholesteatoma. Laryngoscope 1984; 94: 1461−3.

Wayoff, M., Charachon, R., Roulleau, P., Lacher, G., Deguine, C. Le traitement chirurgical du cholestéatome de l'oreille moyenne. Paris: Arnette, 1982

Weiss, P., Cellular dynamics. In: Oncley J., et al., eds. Biophysical science: a study program. New York: Wiley, 1959: 11−20.

Wiener, FM., Ross, DA. The pressure distribution in the auditory canal in a progressive sound field. J. Acoust Soc. Am. 1946; 18: 401.

Wigand, ME. Tympano-méatoplastie endaurale pour les atrésies congénitales sévères de l'oreille. Rev Laryngol 1978; 99: 15−28.

Wilson, JG. Cited after Gussen R 1970.

Wullstein, HL. Die Klinik der Labyrinthitis und Paralabyrinthitis aufgrund des Röntgenbefundes. Stuttgart: Thieme, 1948.

Wullstein, HL. Die extratympanale endocranielle Fensterung bei chronischer Otitis media und Labyrinth-Innendruck-Störung im Vergleich zur typischen Fensterung am seitlichen Bogengange. Z. Laryngol Rhinol 1951; 30: 203−16.

Wullstein, HL. Operationen am Mittelohr mit Hilfe des freien Spaltlappentransplantates. Arch. Ohren-Nasen-Kehlkopfheilkd. 1952; 161: 422−35.

Wullstein, HL. Audiology of hearing improvement operations. Acta Otolaryngol 1955a; 45: 440−54.

Wullstein, HL. Die Tympanoplastik als gehörverbessernde Operation bei Otitis media chronica und ihre Resultate. In: Proceedings of the Fifth International Congress of Otorhinolaryngology, Amsterdam 1953, Assen, Netherlands: Koninklijke van Gorcum, 1955b: 104−118.

Wullstein, HL. Die Methode der Dekompression des Nervus facialis vom Austritt aus dem Labyrinth bis zu dem Foramen stylomastoideus ohne Beeinträchtigung des Mittelohres. Z. Hals-Nasen-Ohrenheilkd. 1958; 172: 582−7.

Wullstein, HL. Techniques of tympanoplasty, 4 and 5. Arch. Otolaryngol 1960; 71: 451−3.

Wullstein, HL. Operationen zur Verbesserung des Gehöres. Stuttgart: Thieme, 1968

Wullstein, HL. Tympanoplastik heute. Laryngol Rhinol 1975; 54: 202−8.

Wullstein, HL. Das paralabyrinthäre Cholesteatom und die Tympanoplastik, HNO 1977; 25: 389−92.

Wullstein, HL. Die Osteomyelitis der viszerokranialen Otobasis. Laryngol Rhinol 1978a; 57: 1032−4.

Wullstein, HL. Tympanoplasty: the fundamentals of the concept. Clin. Otolaryngol 1978b; 3: 431−5.

Wullstein, HL. Von der Weichteillabyrinthitis und der Osteitis des knöchernen Innenohres zur osteoplastischen Epitympanotomie. HNO 1981; 29: 143-9, 255−62, 315−20.

Wullstein, HL. Antrotomie, Mastoidektomie, Radikaloperationshöhlen, Tympanoplastikhöhlen, Tympanum und Gehörgang [lecture at the 52nd Annual Meeting of the German ENT Association, Wiesbaden, West Germany, 31 May-4 June 1981]. Z. Hals-Nasen-Ohrenheilkd 1982; 128: 759.

Wullstein, HL. Die operativen Aufgaben in der Basis cranii für die HNO-Heilkunde. HNO 1984; 32: 225−29, 313−19, 401−12.

Wullstein, HL, Wullstein, SR. Die Verletzungen der Rhino- und Otobasis unter dem Gesichtspunkt des pneumatischen Systems im Schädel. Chirurg 1970; 41: 490−4.

Wullstein, HL., Wullstein SR. The altered metabolism of the full-thickness skin graft. Laryngoscope 1972a; 82: 1990−9.

Wullstein, HL., Wullstein, SR. Problem epitimpanalnog zarista bolesti za reparativnu kirurgiju uha. In: Proc. IX Kongress der Otorhinolaryngologen Jugoslawiens, Sarajevo, Mai 1972. Zbornik Radova, 1972b: 231−40.

Wullstein, HL., Wullstein, SR. L'épitympanotomie osteoplastique. ORL J Otorhinolaryngol Relat Spec 1973a; 22: 639−45.

Wullstein, HL., Wullstein, SR. The problem of the hidden primary cholesteatoma in tympanoplasty. Arch Otolaryngol 97 1973b: 194−7.

Wullstein, HL., Wullstein, SR. Chirurgie der Tumoren des Mittelohres. In: Naumann, HH., ed. Kopf. und Hals-Chirurgie, vol 3. Stuttgart: Thieme, 1976: 407−56.

Wullstein, HL., Wullstein, SR. Cholesteatoma; etiology, nosology and tympanoplasty. ORL J. Otorhinolaryngol. Relat. Spec. 1980; 42: 313−72.

Wullstein, HL., Wullstein, SR. Surgery of tumors of the middle ear and the otobase. In: Naumann, HH., ed. Head and Neck Surgery, vol. 3. Stuttgart: Thieme, 1982: 415−64.

Wullstein, HL., Zöllner, F. Panel on myringoplasty methods. Arch. Otolaryngol. 1963; 78: 296−304.

Wullstein, HL., Wullstein, SR., Köster, K., Heide, H. Human biologic tissue adhesive and ceramics in surgical reconstruction. In: Bernstein, L., ed. Plastic and reconstructive surgery of the head and neck, vol. 2: Rehabilitative surgery. New York: Grune and Stratton, 1981: 354−6.

Wullstein, HL., Wullstein, SR., Schlitt, H. Audioanalysator: Eine Brücke zwischen Audiometrie und Psychoakoustik. Laryngol Rhinol 1985; 64: 249−51.

Wullstein, SR. Die osteoplastische Epitympanotomie und ihre Resultate. Arch. Ohren-Nasen-Kehlkopfheilkd. 1972; 202: 655−8.

Wullstein, SR. Die osteoplastische Epitympanotomie und die Pathologie des Mittelohrs, 1: Das operative Vorgehen. Laryngol Rhinol 1973; 52: 34−44.

Wullstein, SR. Die Cholesteatomtheorien gewertet mit Hilfe mikrochirurgischer Befunde. Berichte Phys Med Ges Würzburg 1974a; 82: 191−203.

Wullstein, SR. Feinstrukturen der Paukenhöhle als bestimmender Faktor für die Entwicklung und den Ablauf der entzündlichen Mittelohrerkrankungen [postdoctoral thesis]. University of Würzburg, 1974b.

Wullstein, SR. Osteoplastic epitympanotomy. Ann. Otol. Rhinol. Laryngol 1974c; 83: 663.

Wullstein, SR. Die osteoplastische Epitympanotomie und die Pathologie des Mittelohres, 2: Die Feinstrukturen des Epitympanums und ihre Bedeutung für die Pathologie der retrotympanalen Räume. Laryngol Rhinol 1975a; 54: 32−9.

Wullstein, SR. Le radiogramme de l'oreille moyenne avant et après la chirurgie fonctionelle et ostéoplastique. In: Trujillo, M., ed. Progresos en Radiologica ORL. Madrid: Marban, 1975b: 585−587.

Wullstein, SR. Histopathological alterations of the mucosal folds in chronic otitis media. Acta Otolaryngol 1976; 81: 197−9.

Wullstein, SR. Die Folgen des Hochstandes des Bulbus venae jugularis für den unteren Durchlüftungsweg der Paukenhöhle. HNO 1977a; 25: 393−7.

Wullstein, SR. The surgical principles in cholesteatoma surgery. In: Shambaugh GE., Jr., Shea, JJ., eds. Proceedings of the Fifth Shambaugh International Workshop on Middle Ear Microsurgery and Fluctuant Hearing Loss, February 29−March 5, 1976, Northwestern University Medical School, Chicago. Huntsville, AL: Strode, 1977b: 169−172.

Wullstein, SR. Therapy for cholesteatoma in children. In: Shambaugh, GE. Jr., Shea, JJ., eds. Proceedings of the Fifth Shambaugh International Workshop on Middle Ear Microsurgery and Fluctuant Hearing Loss, February 29−March 5, 1976, Northwestern University Medical School, Chicago. Huntsville, AL: Strode, 1977c: 173−176.

Wullstein, SR. Cholesteatoma in children: is the disease different in childhood? Clin Otolaryngol 1978; 3: 353−62.

Wullstein, SR. Die Septumplastik bzw. submuköse Septumresektion ohne postoperative Nasentamponade. Schonung der Schleimhäute der oberen Luftwege durch die Anwendung des humanbiologischen Gewebeklebers, HNO 1979; 27: 322−4.

Wullstein, SR. The interrelationship and interdependency of the first and second bottleneck regarding the ventilation and drainage of the middle ear. In: Münker, G., Arnold, W. eds. Physiology and pathophysiology of eustachian tube and middle ear: international symposium Freiburg (Breisgau), 1977. Stuttgart: Thieme, 1980: 145−55.

Wullstein, SR. Keramik und Humankleber beim Aufbau der Tympanoplastik und Implantate in der plastischen und Wiederherstellungschirurgie [offprint for the 17th Annual Meeting of the Deutsche Gesellschaft für Plastische und Wiederherstellungschirurgie]. Berlin: Springer, 1981a.

Wullstein, SR. Epitympanic air cushions. In: Shambaugh, GE., Jr., Shea, JJ., eds. Proceedings of the Sixth Shambaugh International Workshop on Otomicrosurgery and Third Shea Fluctuant Hearing Loss Symposium, March 2−7, 1980, Northwestern University Medical School, Chicago. Huntsville, AL: Strode, 1981b: 396−402.

Wullstein, SR. Die postnatale Entwicklung − Formgebung und Formveränderung des Hirn-, Kau-, und Atmungsschädels und Pathomorphologie des Mittelohres. Zentralbl. Hals-Nasen-Ohrenheilkd. 1982; 128: 759.

Wullstein, SR. Ceramics in tympanoplasty. Am J. Otol. 1985a; 6: 31−3.

Wullstein, SR. Immunologic and allergic aspects regarding the interrelationship of the middle ear and ethmoid effusions: a clinical and morphological study. In: Proc. Extraordinary International Symposium on Recent Advances in Otitis Media with Effusion, Kyoto, January 12−15, 1985. 89−90.

Wullstein, SR. Osteoplastic epitympanotomy: tympanoplasty types I, II, III − a review of 15 years of experience. Am J. Otol. 1985c; 6: 5−8.

Wullstein, SR., Schindler, K., Döll, W. Further observations on application of plasticine in ear surgery. In: Grote JJ. ed. Proceedings of the First International Symposium on Biomaterials in Otology, April 21−21, 1983, Leiden, the Netherlands. The Hague: Nijhoff, 1984: 250−261.

Zange, J. Pathologische Anatomie und Physiologie der mittelohrentspringenden Labyrinthentzündungen. Wiesbaden: 1919: Bergmann.

Zaufal, F. Technik der Trepanation des Processus mastoideus nach Küsterschen Grundsätzen. Arch. Ohrenheilkd. 1890; 30: 291.

Zechner, G. Zur Entstehung des erworbenen Mittelohrcholesteatoms. Laryngol Rhinol. Otol. 1985; 64: 67−72.

Zehm, S. Personal communication, 1984.

Zini, C., Bacciu, S., Sanna, M., Jemmi, G. Cinq années d'expériencedes hétérogreffes tympaniques moulées. In: Compus Rendus des Séanus 76e Congrès Français ORL. Paris: Arnette, 1979: 83−8.

Zini, C., Sanna, M., Bacciu, S. Hétérogreffes tympaniques en tympanoplastie fermée: techniques et résultats. In: Compus Rendus des Séames 73e Congrès Français ORL. Paris: Arnette, 1976: 249−56.

Zini, C., Sheehy, JL., Sanna, M. Microsurgery of cholesteatoma of the middle ear. Milan: Ghedini, 1983.

Zöllner, F. Anatomie, Physiologie, Pathologie und Klinik der Ohrtrompete und ihrer diagnostisch-therapeutischen Beziehungen zu allen Nachbarschaftserkrankungen. Berlin: Springer, 1942.

Zöllner, F. Plastische Eingriffe an den Labyrinthfenstern. Arch. Ohren-Nasen-Kehlkopfheilkd. 1952; 161: 419−20.

Zölner, F. Hörverbessernde Operationen bei entzündlich bedingten Mittelohrveränderungen. Arch. Ohren-Nasen-Kehlkopfheilkd. 1957; 171: 1−62.

Zöllner, F. Tympanosclerosis. Arch. Otolaryngol. 1963; 78: 538−44.